Anatomy of the Temporal Bone with Surgical Implications

Anatomy of the Temporal Bone with Surgical Implications

HAROLD F. SCHUKNECHT, M.D.

Walter Augustus LeCompte Professor of Otology
Harvard Medical School
Emeritus Chief of Otolaryngology
Massachusetts Eye and Ear Infirmary
Boston, Massachusetts

A. JULIANNA GULYA, M.D.

Assistant Professor, Department of Surgery
Division of Otolaryngology
George Washington University School of Medicine
Washington, District of Columbia

LEA & FEBIGER · 1986 · PHILADELPHIA

LEA & FEBIGER
600 Washington Square
Philadelphia, Pennsylvania 19106–4198
U.S.A.
(215)922–1330

Library of Congress Cataloging-in-Publication Data

Schuknecht, Harold F. (Harold Frederick), 1917–
   Anatomy of the temporal bone with surgical implications.

   Bibliography: p.
   Includes index.
   1. Ear—Anatomy.   2. Temporal bone—Anatomy.   3. Anatomy,
Surgical and topographical.   I. Gulya, Aina J.   II.
Title.   [DNLM: 1. Temporal Bone—anatomy & histology.   2.
Temporal Bone—surgery.   WV 201 S385a]
QM507.S38   1986   611'.85   85–23834
ISBN 0–8121–1011–0

PRINTED IN THE UNITED STATES OF AMERICA
Print No.   3   2   1

Preface

The principal source of material for this book is the human temporal bone collection housed at the Massachusetts Eye and Ear Infirmary. The collection consists of 1,500 temporal bones from 850 subjects, most of whom had otologic disorders. The specimens were prepared for light microscopic study by fixation, decalcification, embedding in celloidin, and serial sectioning at a thickness of 20 μ, with every tenth section stained and mounted on glass slides. The primary purpose for collecting these temporal bones was to study the pathologic basis of ear disease. The extent to which this objective was realized is evidenced in a book entitled *Pathology of the Ear* (Schuknecht, 1974). The temporal bone collection also provides numerous examples of normal anatomy and its variations which provides the basis for this book on anatomy and its surgical implications. It is meant to be a practical compendium written by clinicians for clinicians. As such, it contains a minimum of cellular and ultrastructural detail, which would have little relevance to the practicing otologist. It is meant to complement the excellent books *Surgical and Microscopic Anatomy of the Temporal Bone* (Wolff, Bellucci, & Eggston, 1971) and *Surgical Anatomy of the Temporal Bone* (Anson & Donaldson, 1981).

The sequence of presentation of the material begins with Chapter 1 showing low-power photomicrographs of serial sections in horizontal and vertical planes. Chapters 2 through 7 present selected views in the following sequence: pinna and external canal, middle ear, pneumatization, inner ear, neuroanatomy and vascular anatomy.

Photomicrographs present a two-dimensional display of anatomy in a single plane which leads to an appreciation, although somewhat imperfect, of the size and spatial relationships of these structures. Realizing that we live in a three-dimensional world and that the temporal bone is a three-dimensional structure, part of Chapter 1 and all of Chapter 8 have been devoted to stereoscopic anatomy. The photographs were made with a Donaldson camera (designed by Dr. David Donaldson, ophthalmologist at the Massachusetts Eye and Ear Infirmary and Harvard Medical School). These color stereoscopic transparencies are mounted into View-Master reels (Sawyer's Inc., Portland, Oregon) and can be viewed with the View-Master three-dimensional viewer that can be purchased at department and toy stores. To assist in orientation of anatomic structures, the book contains labeled photographs matching each of the stereo views.

Chapter 1 features two reels (14 views) of partially sectioned temporal bones in celloidin blocks that expose to view the intimate anatomy of the middle and inner ears. Chapter 8 provides a set of four reels (28 views) showing a method of progressive dissection of the fresh temporal bone, as well as one (seven views) of pathologic anatomy, and two (14 views) of otologic surgery.

Congenital anomalies of the ear are often the result of faulty or arrested development and present in recurring patterns of dysplasia which are best understood by a knowledge of the normal embryologic process. With this in mind we present in Chapter 9 a series of photomicrographs from three embryos of progressive gestational ages.

The appendices present a glossary of terms and a history of anatomic discoveries of the ear. We had originally hoped that the history section could be brought up-to-date. However, the recent contributors to ear morphology have been so numerous and the assessment of relative importance to new knowledge so difficult to judge that we are limiting the presentation to those who are deceased, leaving to subsequent generations the task of pinpointing the principal contributors of our time.

Finally, we are making available a set of 163 selected color, 35-mm paper-mounted transparencies, each of which matches a photomicrograph in the book. This teaching set should be useful in augmenting lectures in both the basic and clinical sciences.

We are grateful to the histologic technicians, especially Diane DeLeo Jones, Barbara Burgess, Richard Cortese and Clarinda Northrop DuBois, who have provided such technically excellent temporal bone sections. We appreciate the superb quality of the photomicrographs prepared by Arthur Bowden. To Carol Ota and Linda Joyce we are especially grateful for preparation and editing of the manuscript as well as mounting and labeling of photomicrographs. Others who contributed significantly to editing and preparation were Eileen Nims, Cheryl Hurley, Anne Schuknecht, and Tomomi Kimura; we thank them. Finally, we are indebted to the publishing house of Lea & Febiger, and especially to R. Kenneth Bussy, for their willingness to publish a book with so many illustrations as well as View-Master reels and slide sets.

Otology is both a medical and surgical specialty. The anatomy is complex with many important structures sequestered deeply in bone. A sophisticated knowledge of anatomy is necessary if invasive therapeutic procedures are to be performed safely. We believe this book will serve that end.

Boston, Massachusetts   HAROLD F. SCHUKNECHT

Washington, District of Columbia   A. JULIANNA GULYA

Acknowledgments

This book represents the accumulated experience and observations of the authors (and their clinical and research associates) in a single volume. As a result, numerous illustrations were previously published in several journals and books.

The authors are grateful to these publishers for permission to use illustrations that have appeared previously as indicated below (the corresponding figure number in this book is set in boldface).

ALAN R. LISS FOR THE MARCH OF DIMES BIRTH DEFECTS FOUNDATION
Morphogenesis and Malformation of the Ear, Gorlin, 1980
Figure 1, page 48   **Figure 5.39**

AMERICAN JOURNAL OF OTOLOGY (Thieme Stratton)
5:262, 1984—Figure in "Letter to the Editor"   **Figure 7.34**

ANNALS OF OTOLOGY, RHINOLOGY, LARYNGOLOGY (Annals Publishing Company)

72:689, 1963—Figure 1	**Figure 5.39**
78:794, 1969—Figure 2	**Figure 3.78**
79:109, 1970—Figure 4	**Figure 5.24**
Supplement 11, 83:13, 1974—Figure 8	**Figure 3.110**
83:49–53, 1974—Figure 1	**Figure 3.60**
Figure 2	**Figure 3.65**
Figure 3	**Figure 3.68**
Figure 5	**Figure 3.69**
Figure 6	**Figure 3.70**
Figure 7	**Figure 3.72**
Figure 8	**Figure 3.73**
88:317, 1979—Figure 2	**Figure 5.45**
Supplement 78, 90:7, 1981—Figure 6	**Figure 7.36**
Figure 7A	**Figure 7.37**

ARCHIVES OF OTOLARYNGOLOGY (American Medical Association)

86:499, 1967—Figure 2	**Figure 4.20**
Figure 3	**Figure 7.2**
91:599, 601, 1970—Figure 1	**Figure 6.19**
Figure 3	**Figure 6.20**
110:479, 1984—Figure 6	**Figure 5.23**
111:120, 1985—Figure 3	**Figure 5.41**

AURIS NASUS LARYNX

Figure from Sando et al., in press	**Figure 3.109**

HARVARD UNIVERSITY PRESS

Pathology of the Ear, Schuknecht, 1974

Figure 2.5, page 24	**Figure 3.62**
Figure 2.6, page 24	**Figure 3.63**
Figure 2.7, page 26	**Figure 3.77**
Figure 2.8, page 26	**Figure 3.74**
Figure 2.9, page 26	**Figure 3.76**
Figure 2.10, page 28	**Figure 3.1**
Figure 2.11, page 28	**Figure 6.23**
Figure 2.12, page 29	**Figure 3.84**
Figure 2.13, page 29	**Figure 3.92**
Figures 2.14–2.16, pages 31–32	**Figures 7.26–7.28**
Figure 2.19, page 34	**Figure 7.25**
Figure 2.20, page 35	**Figure 6.31**
Figure 2.21, page 36	**Figure 6.22**
Figure 2.25, page 41	**Figure 6.18**
Figure 2.26, page 41	**Figure 5.3**
Figure 2.59, page 59	**Figure 5.24**
Figure 2.60, page 60	**Figure 5.19**
Figure 2.62, page 61	**Figure 7.11**
Figure 2.63, page 62	**Figure 7.32**
Figure 2.64, page 62	**Figure 7.33**
Figure 2.65, page 63	**Figure 7.38**
Figure 2.89, page 79	**Figure 4.1**
Figure 2.90, page 80	**Figure 3.53**
Figure 2.91, page 80	**Figure 4.3**
Figure 2.92, page 81	**Figure 4.5**
Figure 2.93, page 82	**Figure 4.15**
Figure 2.95, page 83	**Figure 4.20**
Figure 2.96, page 84	**Figure 4.26**
Figure 2.97, page 84	**Figure 4.29**

Figure 2.98, page 84   Figure 4.30
Figures 2.99–2.118, pages 85–92   Figures 1.1–1.20
Figure 3.47, page 145   Figure 5.39
Figure 4.18, page 185   Figure 3.58
Figure 4.23, page 187   Figure 7.30
Figure 4.25, page 188   Figure 3.40
Figure 4.26, page 189   Figure 3.42
Figure 4.29, page 190   Figure 3.57
Figure 4.30, page 192   Figure 7.19
Figure 5.8, page 219   Figure 3.5
Figure 5.40, page 234   Figure 3.4
Figure 7.15, page 301   Figure 3.59
Figures 8.12–8.14, page 328   Figures 7.3–7.5
Figure 10.68, page 385   Figure 2.10
Figure 10.70, page 385   Figure 2.12
Figure 11.11, page 422   Figures 3.115 & 3.116
Table 2.1, page 79   Table, page 111
Teaching slide set

JOURNAL OF LARYNGOLOGY AND OTOLOGY
87:281, 1973—Figure 1   Figure 3.80
89:987–995, 1975—Figure 1   Figure 5.18
                 Figure 7   Figure 5.26
                 Figure 10   Figures 9.1–9.4
                 Figure 11   Figure 5.25

LARYNGOSCOPE
69:629, 1959—Figure 9B   Figure 2.9
79:641, 1969—Figure 1   Figure 9.5
85:1730, 1975—Figure 4   Figure 3.113
86:1166, 1976—Figure 1   Figure 2.5

LITTLE, BROWN AND COMPANY
Stapedectomy, Schuknecht, 1971
Figure 86, page 76   Figure 3.25
Figure 91, page 78   Figure 3.48

OTOLARYNGOLOGY CLINICS OF NORTH AMERICA (W.B. Saunders Company)
1:298, 1968—Figure 26B   Figure 5.28

Contents

Anatomy of the Temporal Bone with Surgical Implications

1. Serial Photographs of Sections of the Temporal Bone

The temporal bone is made up of the squamous, mastoid, petrous, and tympanic parts. It articulates with the occipital, parietal, sphenoid, and zygomatic bones. It contributes to the lateral wall and base of the skull and forms part of the middle and posterior cranial fossae. For study of the osteology of the temporal bone the reader is referred to the superb illustrations of Anson and Donaldson (1981).

The squama is a vertical plate of bone which forms the lateral wall of the middle cranial fossa. It articulates with the sphenoid bone anteriorly and the parietal bone superiorly. The anteriorly projecting zygomatic process articulates with the zygoma of the maxillary bone. The lateral surface of the squama provides an anchor for the temporalis muscle while the masseter muscle attaches to the zygomatic process. On its lateral surface is the sulcus for the middle temporal artery and on the medial surface the sulcus for the middle meningeal artery.

The mastoid part of the temporal bone is made up of the inferior protrusions of the squamous and petrous bones. The sternocleidomastoid, posterior auricular, and occipital muscles attach to the lateral aspect of the mastoid, while the posterior belly of the digastric muscle attaches to a groove medial to the mastoid process. The mastoid branch of the occipital artery and mastoid emissary vein pierce its lateral surface. The mastoid fossa is a cribriform area immediately posterior to the suprameatal spine of Henle. The latter projection is located at the posterosuperior margin of the external auditory canal. Medially the mastoid is indented by a deep furrow for the sigmoid portion of the lateral venous sinus.

The petrous part of the temporal bone is pyramidally shaped and contains the inner ear structures. It extends from the mastoid part posteriorly to the angle between the occipital and sphenoid bones anteriorly. Its anterosuperior surface contributes to the floor of the middle cranial fossa and is marked by the arcuate eminence denoting the location of the superior semicircular canal, the tympanic tegmen overlying the tympanic cavity, and the trigeminal impression for the Vth cranial nerve. Anterior to the arcuate eminence is the facial hiatus, an opening which leads to the geniculate ganglion and genu of the facial nerve and from which emerges the greater superficial petrosal nerve. The posterior surface of the petrous pyramid lies in a vertical plane and forms the anterolateral wall of the posterior cranial fossa. It is bounded above by the sulcus for the superior petrosal sinus and below by the sulcus of the inferior petrosal sinus. The meatus of the inter-

3

nal auditory canal is located on the posterior surface at the midpoint between the base and apex of the petrous pyramid. Other structures on the posterior surface of the petrous bone are the subarcuate fossa leading into the petromastoid canal and the cranial orifice of the vestibular aqueduct. Located at the apex of the petrous pyramid are the internal carotid artery, the hiatus for the lesser superficial petrosal nerve, and the semicanal for the tensor tympani muscle. The inferior aspect of the petrous pyramid is irregular and provides attachment for several deep neck muscles. A ridge of bone separates the jugular bulb from the more anteriorly located canal for the internal carotid artery. The inferior aperture of the inferior tympanic canaliculus (containing Jacobson's nerve and the tympanic branch of the ascending pharyngeal artery) is located medially in this ridge as is the cranial orifice of the cochlear aqueduct. The styloid process arises just lateral to the posterior aspect of the jugular fossa. The stylomastoid foramen for the facial nerve lies posterior to the styloid process.

The tympanic bone forms the inferior, anterior, and part of the posterior wall of the bony external auditory canal. Its juncture with the mastoid forms the tympanomastoid suture while its anterior interface with the petrous bone results in the petrotympanic fissure. Superiorly the tympanosquamous fissure represents the union of the tympanic bone with the squama. Its inferior projection forms the sheath (vaginal process) of the styloid. At the medial end of the tympanic bone is a narrow groove, the tympanic sulcus, which is deficient superiorly and which harbors the tympanic annulus.

Horizontal Two-Dimensional Serial Photographs

The following photomicrographs (Figs. 1.1 to 1.20) depict horizontal sections of the right ear of a 5-year-old male. The temporal bone was mounted on the cutting block in the standard method with the plane of sectioning passing through the axis of the modiolus of the cochlea. Each section was cut at a thickness of 20 μ, and sectioning proceeded from superior to inferior. Every 20th section was photographed for this series.

This temporal bone, like most of the others in the collection, was removed with the bone plug cutter which is a circular oscillating saw blade 1-1/2 inches (38 mm) in diameter. After the brain has been removed at the time of autopsy, the saw is centered on the arcuate eminence and advanced in an inferior direction until it has passed through the skull base. This plug of bone contains the bony part of the external auditory canal, the middle ear, the bony labyrinth, the internal auditory canal, the petrous apex, part of the eustachian tube and most of the mastoid. After the decalcification and embedding process has been completed, the block is trimmed to a size that allows each section to be accommodated on a 1- × 3-inch (25- × 76-mm) glass slide. This routine procedure of horizontal sectioning at 20 μ thickness generates about 500 sections; normally every tenth is stained and mounted for study, resulting in a set of about 50 slides.

The posterior cranial fossa is located medially and posteriorly, while the middle cranial fossa is situated anteriorly. The external auditory canal and mandibular fossa are located laterally and the internal auditory canal lies medially.

In preparation for the material that follows, the student of ear anatomy would do well to pass sequentially back and forth through these serial sections until he/she is thoroughly familiar with the anatomic relationships.

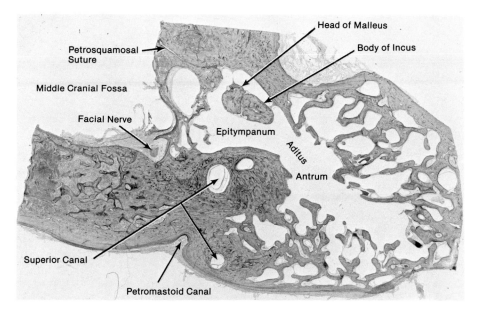

Labels for Fig. 1.1:
- Petrosquamosal Suture
- Middle Cranial Fossa
- Facial Nerve
- Superior Canal
- Petromastoid Canal
- Head of Malleus
- Body of Incus
- Epitympanum
- Aditus
- Antrum

FIG. 1.1: The petrosquamosal suture marks the apposition of the petrous pyramid and the squama. The head of the malleus, the most superior component of the ossicular system, is visible in the epitympanum anterolateral to the body of the incus. The facial nerve is evident at the facial hiatus in the floor of the middle cranial fossa. The lateral (ampullated) and the medial (nonampullated) limbs of the superior canal are seen in cross section. The cranial aperture of the petromastoid canal which carries the subarcuate artery and its venae comites is seen. This artery is a branch of the labyrinthine artery (or less frequently a branch of the anterior inferior cerebellar artery) and distributes to the mastoid air cells. The aditus ad antrum leads posteriorly from the epitympanum to the mastoid antrum.

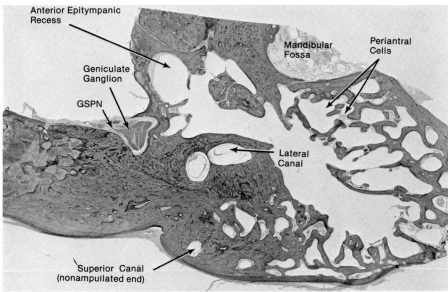

Labels for Fig. 1.2:
- Anterior Epitympanic Recess
- Geniculate Ganglion
- GSPN
- Superior Canal (nonampullated end)
- Mandibular Fossa
- Periantral Cells
- Lateral Canal

FIG. 1.2: The greater superficial petrosal nerve (GSPN) emerges from the geniculate ganglion and passes anteriorly into the intracranial cavity via the facial hiatus en route to the foramen lacerum. The anterior epitympanic recess, mastoid antrum, and periantral cells are well demonstrated. Laterally lies the mandibular fossa.

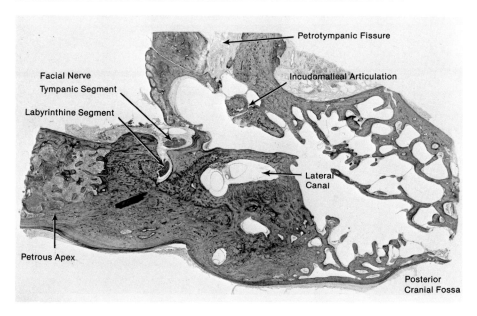

Labels for Fig. 1.3:
- Facial Nerve Tympanic Segment
- Labyrinthine Segment
- Petrous Apex
- Petrotympanic Fissure
- Incudomalleal Articulation
- Lateral Canal
- Posterior Cranial Fossa

FIG. 1.3: There is an exceptionally wide petrotympanic (Glaserian) fissure. The facial nerve is seen in its labyrinthine and tympanic segments.

FIG. 1.4: The incus extends toward the aditus as the crus breve or short process. The facial nerve is seen entering its labyrinthine segment as it leaves the internal auditory canal (IAC). The lateral canal bulges prominently into the mastoid antrum. The petrosquamosal (Koerner's) septum divides the mastoid into squamous and petrous parts.

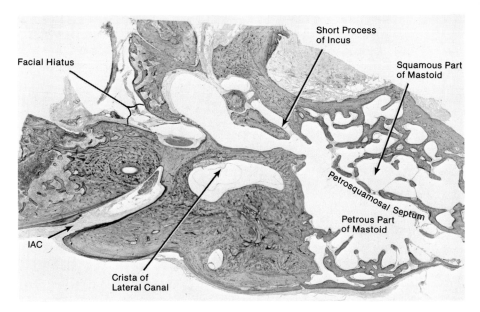

FIG. 1.5: The external auditory canal (EAC) has come into view. Tethering the short process of the incus to the walls of the incudal recess is the fan-shaped posterior incudal ligament. Within the internal auditory canal are the facial nerve and the superior division of the vestibular nerve. The superior-most aspect of the basal turn of the cochlea is apparent. The ampullated end of the lateral semicircular duct joins the utricle. As the superior canal recedes from view, the posterior semicircular canal emerges.

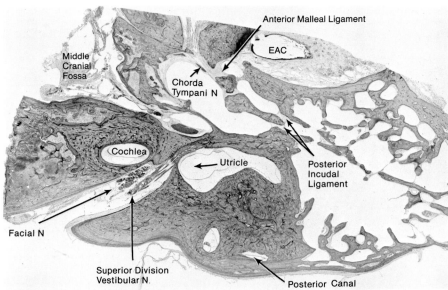

FIG. 1.6: The anterior malleal ligament envelopes the anterior process of the malleus (processus Folianus, also known as processus gracilis). Fibers of the tensor tympani muscle are visible in its semicanal and the cochleariform (spoon-shaped) process is beginning to assume its characteristic form. The facial nerve courses in its bony canal on the medial wall of the middle ear, accompanied in this case by a large vein. The posterior canal continues its emergence. The macula of the utricle lies in its elliptical recess.

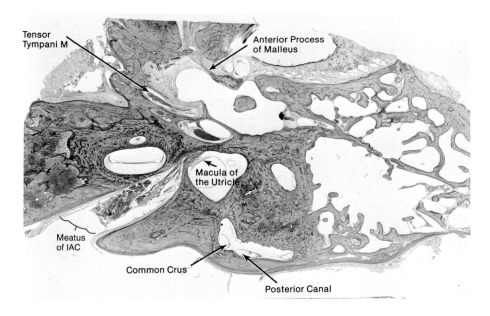

6 Anatomy of the Temporal Bone with Surgical Implications

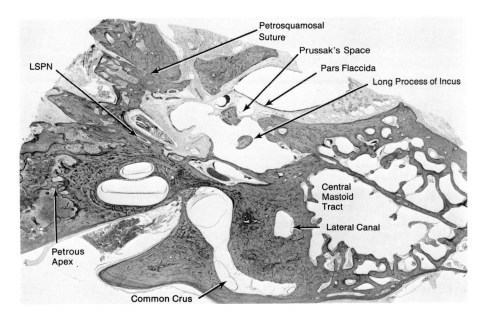

Labels for Fig. 1.7 image:
- Petrosquamosal Suture
- Prussak's Space
- Pars Flaccida
- Long Process of Incus
- LSPN
- Central Mastoid Tract
- Lateral Canal
- Petrous Apex
- Common Crus

FIG. 1.7: The pars flaccida of the tympanic membrane (Shrapnell's membrane) forms the lateral wall of Prussak's recess. The body of the incus narrows to its long process. The chorda tympani nerve is seen passing medial to the neck of the malleus. The cochleariform process is now distinct as are the bundles of the tensor tympani muscle. The common crus, formed by the junction of the nonampullated limbs of the superior and posterior canals, approaches the utricle. The lesser superficial petrosal nerve (LSPN) is located in the superior tympanic canaliculus medial to the tensor tympani muscle. The middle turn of the cochlea is exposed.

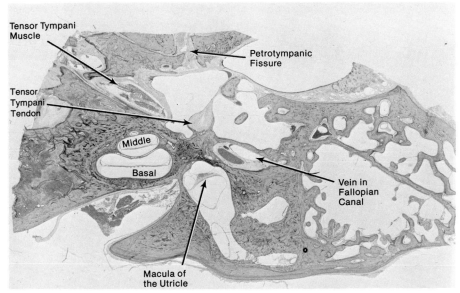

Labels for Fig. 1.8 image:
- Tensor Tympani Muscle
- Petrotympanic Fissure
- Tensor Tympani Tendon
- Middle
- Basal
- Vein in Fallopian Canal
- Macula of the Utricle

FIG. 1.8: The tensor tympani tendon bridges the middle ear on its way to the malleus. The macula of the utricle faces posteromedially.

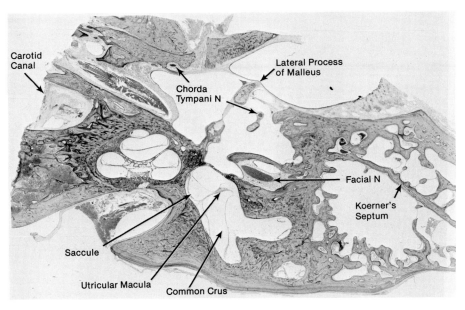

Labels for Fig. 1.9 image:
- Carotid Canal
- Lateral Process of Malleus
- Chorda Tympani N
- Vein in Fallopian Canal
- Facial N
- Koerner's Septum
- Saccule
- Utricular Macula
- Common Crus

FIG. 1.9: The lateral process of the malleus is evident. The chorda tympani nerve is seen lateral to the long process of the incus. This nerve is also seen more anteriorly in its iter chordae anterius. More often than not, the tympanic segment of the facial canal is dehiscent, as shown here. The common crus communicates with the utricle. The bony lateral canal joins the vestibule. All three turns of the cochlea are visible. The carotid canal is seen anteriorly.

FIG. 1.10: The manubrium, long process of the incus, and footplate are apparent. Lateral to the facial nerve is the facial recess. Within the internal auditory canal, one can distinguish the cochlear nerve as it passes to the cribrose area of the cochlea. Posterior to it is the inferior division of the vestibular nerve. The saccule is visible in its spherical recess. The endolymphatic duct courses posterolaterally, paralleling the common crus.

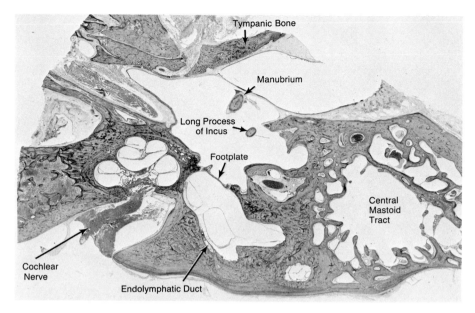

FIG. 1.11: The manubrium continues its descent separated from the pars tensa by a mucosal fold. The stapes is now evident in its characteristic stirrup form. The facial nerve descends in its mastoid segment. The protympanum extends anteriorly from the mesotympanum. The apical turn of the cochlea is visible as well as the helicotrema which marks the wide communication of the scala tympani and scala vestibuli. The nonampullated end of the membranous lateral semicircular duct enters the utricle.

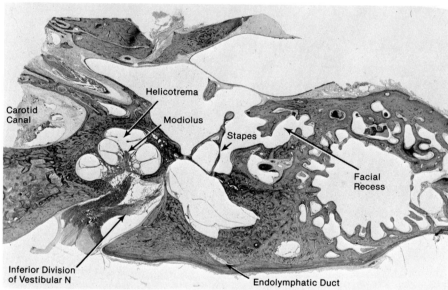

FIG. 1.12: Note the normal thinness of the skin lining the anterior wall of the bony external auditory canal. The fibrous annulus of the tympanic membrane is seated within its bony sulcus. The manubrium narrows as it extends downward. The incudostapedial articulation is seen. The bone which overlies the facial nerve protrudes toward the oval window niche, forming the pyramidal eminence which houses the stapedius tendon. The tendon attaches to the head of the stapes. The saccule is seen at the anteromedial aspect of the perilymphatic cistern of the vestibule. The glial-Schwann sheath junctions of the cochlear and vestibular nerve trunks are seen in the internal auditory canal.

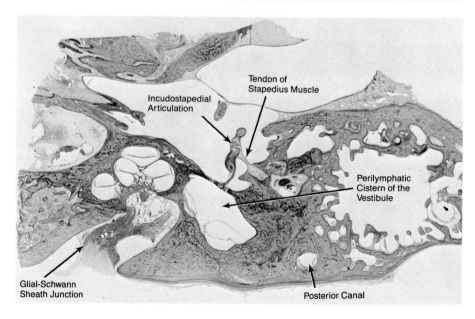

8 Anatomy of the Temporal Bone with Surgical Implications

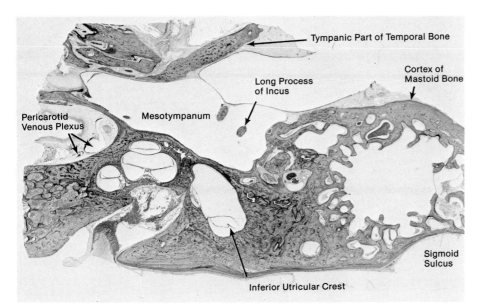

FIG. 1.13: The manubrium and inferior tip of the long process of the incus are seen. The facial nerve continues its descent in its fallopian canal. The posterior semicircular canal remains visible. The utricle narrows as the nonampullated end of the lateral duct enters at the utricular crest. The saccular nerve traverses the cribrose area to the saccular macula. The carotid artery is surrounded by a connective tissue sheath in which the pericarotid venous plexus and pericarotid sympathetic nerve plexus are embedded. The sigmoid sulcus is visible posteriorly.

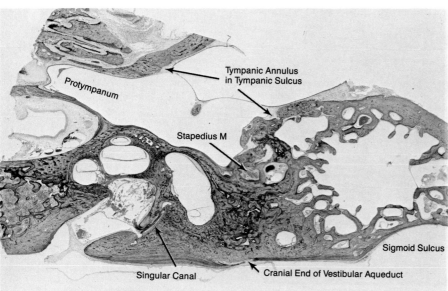

FIG. 1.14: The tympanic membrane is circumferentially fixed by the tympanic annulus to the walls of the tympanic sulcus. The singular canal carries the posterior ampullary nerve, a branch of the inferior division of the vestibular nerve, to the ampulla of the posterior canal. The vestibular aqueduct containing the endolymphatic (otic) duct approaches the dura. Shielding its exit is a thin scale of bone, the operculum.

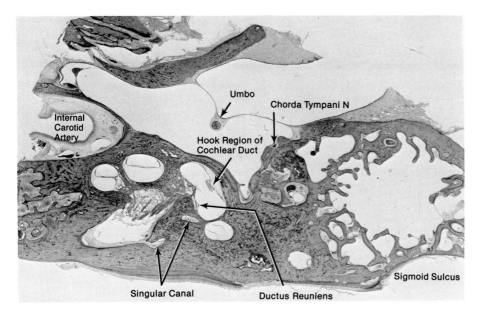

FIG. 1.15: The umbo marks the approximate center of the tympanic membrane and corresponds to the end of the manubrium which at this level is completely enveloped by the pars propria of the tympanic membrane. The basal turn of the cochlea turns into the vestibule. The ductus reuniens links the cochlear duct and saccule. The singular canal is seen traveling toward the ampullated end of the posterior canal.

FIG. 1.16: The internal auditory canal gradually recedes from view as does the middle turn of the cochlea. The bony wall of the basal turn forms the promontory on the medial wall of the middle ear.

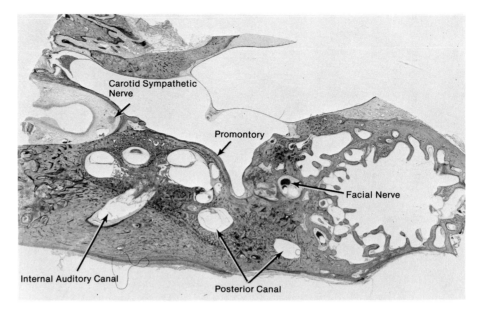

FIG. 1.17: The facial nerve continues its descent in the mastoid segment of the fallopian canal. Only the basal turn of the cochlea remains visible. The scala tympani of the basal turn lies adjacent to the round window membrane. The endolymphatic sac lies between two layers of dura in its foveate fossa, paralleling the posterior wall of the temporal bone.

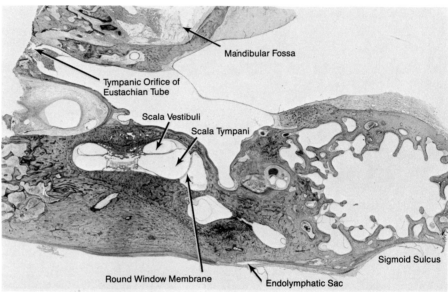

FIG. 1.18: The round window niche lies inferior to the promontory. The tympanic ostium of the cochlear aqueduct is situated at the posteromedial aspect of the basal turn of the cochlea. The subiculum is a ridge of bone that defines the inferior limit of the sinus tympani. The lumen of the bony posterior semicircular canal is seen with the ampullated and nonampullated ends of the membranous duct. Anteriorly lies the petrous apex containing, in this case, highly cellular marrow.

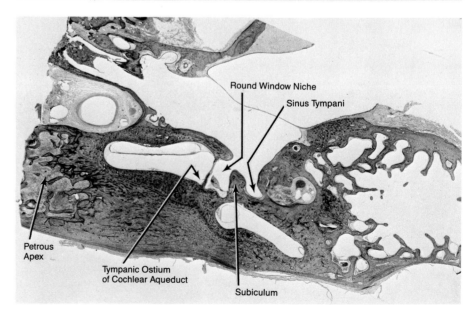

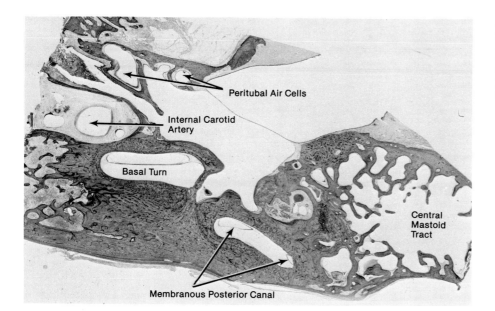

FIG. 1.19: The pericarotid venous plexus is visible on both the anterior and posterior aspects of the internal carotid artery. The peritubal air cells comprise the lateral components of pneumatization of the petrous apex region.

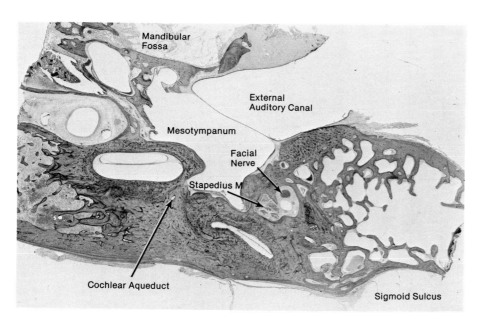

FIG. 1.20: The anatomic juxtaposition of the stapedius muscle and the facial nerve is evident. The bony posterior semicircular canal recedes from view. The cochlear aqueduct proceeds postero-inferiorly towards the subarachnoid space.

FIG. 1.21: The external auditory canal (EAC) is seen in cross section. The chorda tympani nerve heads anteriorly and laterally toward the tympanic cavity. The bony posterior canal is opened and its enclosed duct is seen. The break in the tegmen of the mastoid is an artifact of preparation.

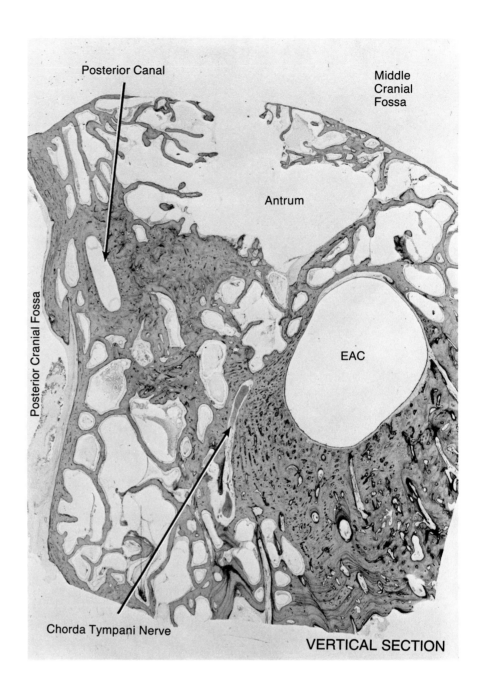

Vertical Two-Dimensional Serial Photographs

The following series of photomicrographs (Figs. 1.21 to 1.37) show the right temporal bone of a 32-year-old female as it appears in vertical cross section, cut perpendicular to the long axis of the petrous bone. Vertical sections are smaller than horizontal sections but there are more of them. The trimmed specimen cut at 20 μ generates about 800 sections and every tenth is stained and mounted on glass slides. In this case two vertical sections can be mounted on each 1- × 3-inch slide, resulting in a final series of about 40 such slides. Vertical sections are particularly useful for the study of pathologic conditions located in the most superior and inferior parts of the temporal bone.

The sections are arranged sequentially from posterolateral to anteromedial; approximately every fiftieth section has been selected for this series. The tegmen lies superiorly separating the mastoid and middle ear from the temporal lobe. The posterior cranial fossa is located posteriorly. The carotid canal and jugular vein are seen inferiorly, the external auditory canal laterally, and the middle ear space medially. The inner ear structures begin with the canals, then the vestibule, and finally the cochlea.

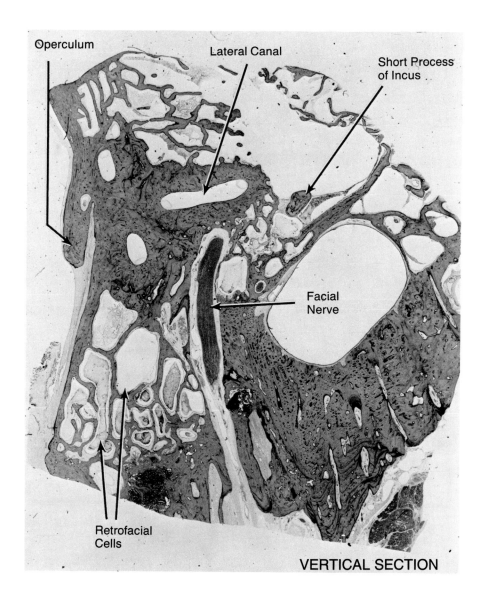

FIG. 1.22: The facial nerve descends in its mastoid segment and the chorda tympani nerve approaches the iter chordae posterius. The short process of the incus is tethered in the incudal fossa by the posterior incudal ligament. The lateral canal is now evident; an extension through its long axis bisects the posterior canal. Cells of the supralabyrinthine area are visible posterosuperiorly. Posteriorly, the endolymphatic sac is capped by the operculum. The retrofacial group of mastoid air cells is seen.

Operculum

Lateral Canal

Short Process of Incus

Facial Nerve

Retrofacial Cells

VERTICAL SECTION

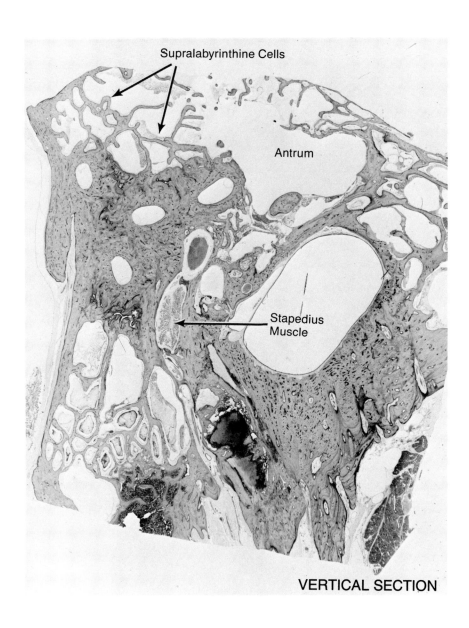

FIG. 1.23: Progressing anteromedially the tympanic membrane, tympanic sulcus, and fibrous annulus come into view. The stapedius muscle is inferior and posterior to the facial nerve.

Supralabyrinthine Cells

Antrum

Stapedius
Muscle

VERTICAL SECTION

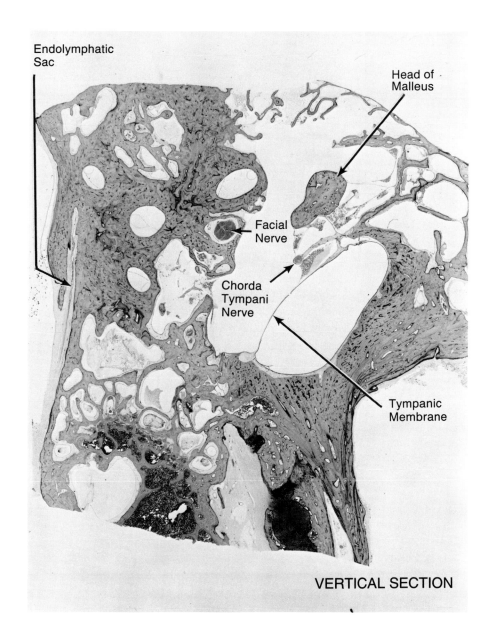

Endolymphatic
Sac

Head of
Malleus

Facial
Nerve

Chorda
Tympani
Nerve

Tympanic
Membrane

VERTICAL SECTION

FIG. 1.24: The head of the malleus is now visible in the epitympanum. The chorda tympani nerve crosses the tympanic cavity suspended in a mucosal fold. The tympanic segment of the facial nerve lies inferior to the lateral canal.

FIG. 1.25: The division of the tympanic membrane into a pars flaccida superiorly and a pars tensa inferiorly can be seen. The space superior to the lateral process of the malleus, medial to the pars flaccida, is Prussak's recess. The incus articulates with the malleus in a cog-wheel fashion.

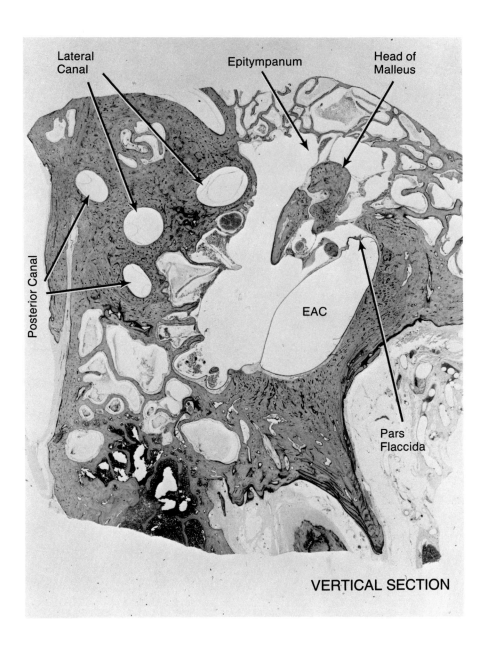

Lateral Canal

Epitympanum

Head of Malleus

Posterior Canal

EAC

Pars Flaccida

VERTICAL SECTION

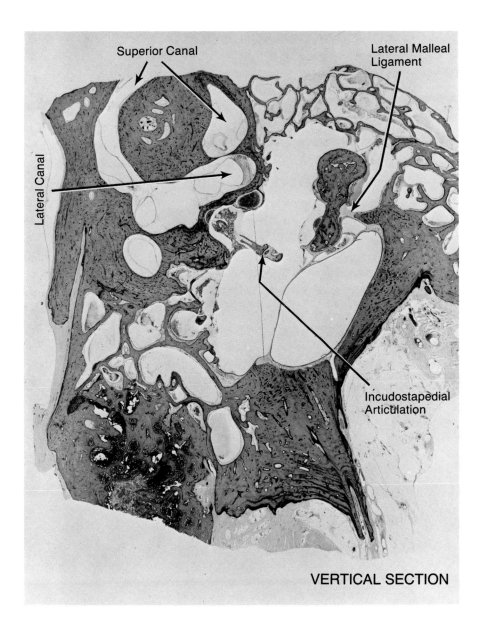

Superior Canal

Lateral Malleal Ligament

Lateral Canal

Incudostapedial Articulation

VERTICAL SECTION

FIG. 1.26: The chorda tympani nerve now is closely applied to the medial aspect of the neck of the malleus. Extending laterally from the neck of the malleus is the lateral malleal ligament. The lenticular process of the incus articulates with the head of the stapes. Within the perimeter of the superior semicircular canal one can see the petromastoid canal with its subarcuate vessels. The opening in the canal is an artifact.

FIG. 1.27: The ampulla and crista of the superior canal are visible. Inferior to the oval window niche is the bulge of the promontory.

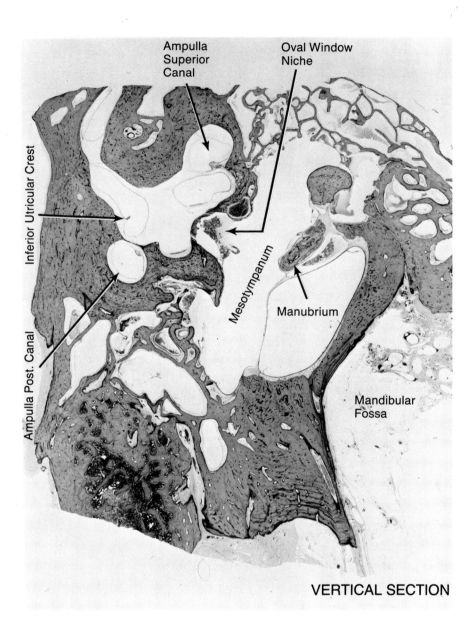

Ampulla Superior Canal

Oval Window Niche

Inferior Utricular Crest

Ampulla Post. Canal

Mesotympanum

Manubrium

Mandibular Fossa

VERTICAL SECTION

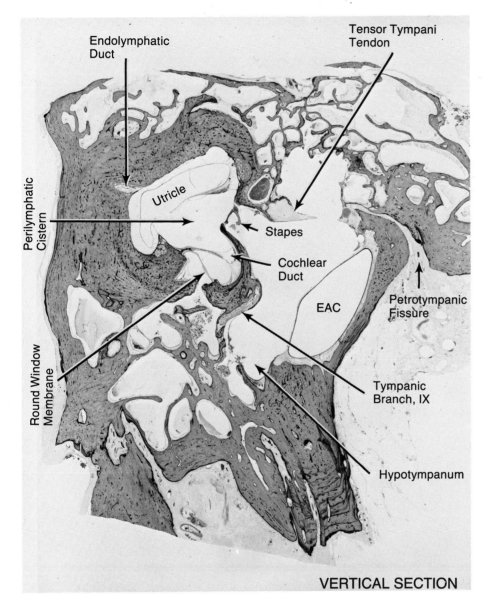

Endolymphatic Duct

Tensor Tympani Tendon

Perilymphatic Cistern

Utricle

Stapes

Cochlear Duct

EAC

Petrotympanic Fissure

Round Window Membrane

Tympanic Branch, IX

Hypotympanum

VERTICAL SECTION

FIG. 1.28: Superior to the external auditory canal (EAC) is the petrotympanic fissure. Lateral to the facial nerve, the tendon of the tensor tympani muscle lies in the concavity of the cochleariform process. The round window niche and membrane are emerging.

FIG. 1.29: The facial nerve is located just superior to the tendon of the tensor tympani muscle. The utricle and saccule now come into view. The scala vestibuli opens into the vestibule. The peaked configuration at the posterior aspect of the scala tympani is the tympanic orifice of the cochlear aqueduct. The singular canal contains the posterior ampullary nerve.

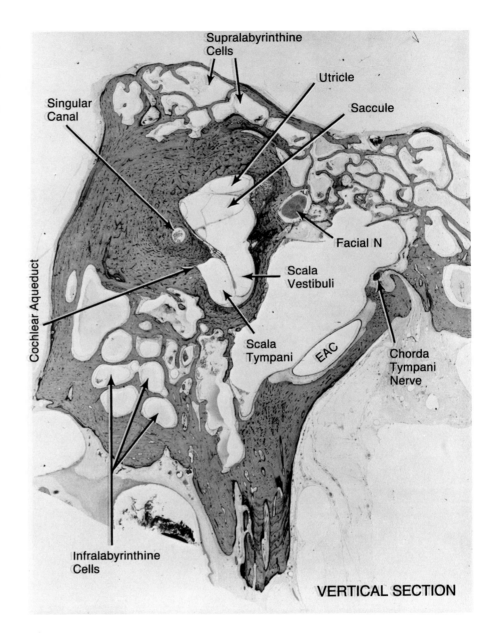

Supralabyrinthine Cells

Utricle

Saccule

Singular Canal

Facial N

Cochlear Aqueduct

Scala Vestibuli

Scala Tympani

EAC

Chorda Tympani Nerve

Infralabyrinthine Cells

VERTICAL SECTION

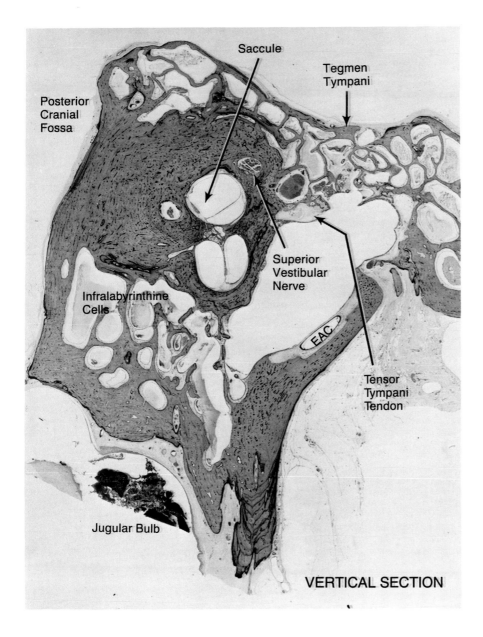

Saccule

Tegmen
Tympani

Posterior
Cranial
Fossa

Infralabyrinthine
Cells

Superior
Vestibular
Nerve

EAC

Tensor
Tympani
Tendon

Jugular Bulb

VERTICAL SECTION

FIG. 1.30: The external auditory canal (EAC) dwindles. Running medially from the scala tympani is the cochlear aqueduct. There is extensive infralabyrinthine pneumatization.

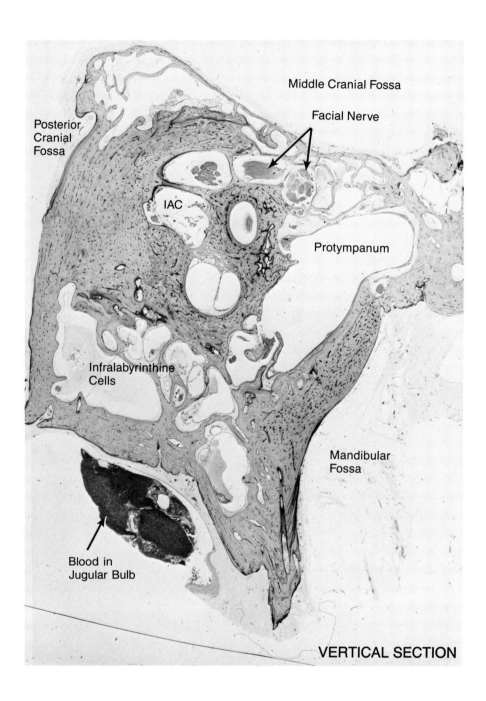

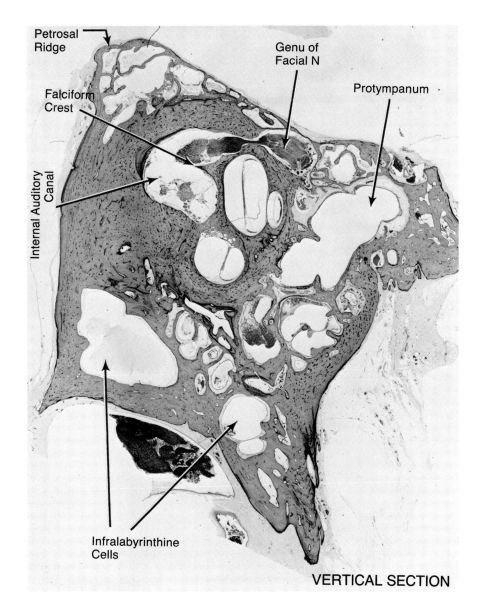

Petrosal Ridge

Falciform Crest

Internal Auditory Canal

Genu of Facial N

Protympanum

Infralabyrinthine Cells

VERTICAL SECTION

FIG. 1.32: The middle and apical turns of the cochlea are emerging as the middle ear space narrows. The falciform crest and its relationship to the cochlear and facial nerves is seen, as well as the labyrinthine segment of the facial nerve.

FIG. 1.33: The facial nerve and its geniculate ganglion lie beneath the dura of the middle cranial fossa. The facial, vestibular, and cochlear nerve trunks are seen in the internal auditory canal.

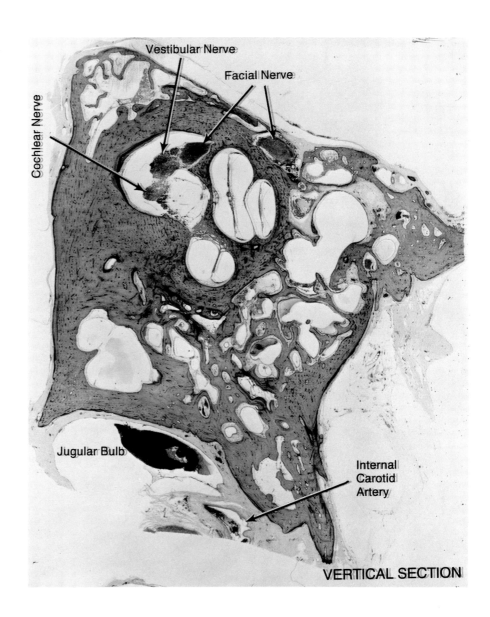

Vestibular Nerve

Facial Nerve

Cochlear Nerve

Jugular Bulb

Internal Carotid Artery

VERTICAL SECTION

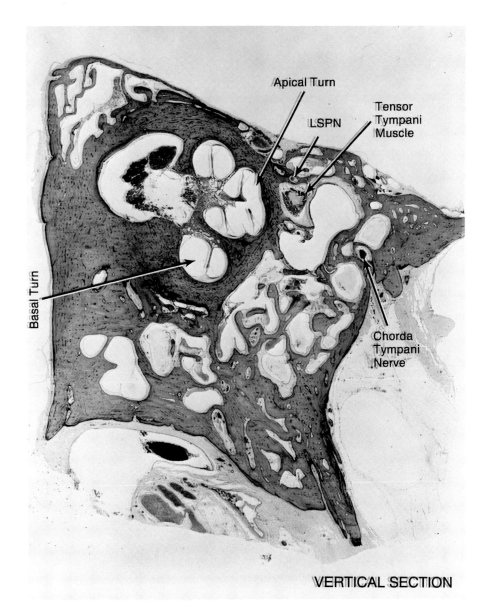

Apical Turn

LSPN

Tensor
Tympani
Muscle

Basal Turn

Chorda
Tympani
Nerve

VERTICAL SECTION

FIG. 1.34: The protympanum diminishes
in size anteriorly. The lesser superficial
petrosal nerve (LSPN) in its superior
tympanic canaliculus lies just superior
to the tensor tympani muscle. All three
turns of the cochlea and the helicotrema
are seen.

FIG. 1.35: The tensor tympani muscle lies in its semicanal just medial to the osseous part of the eustachian tube.

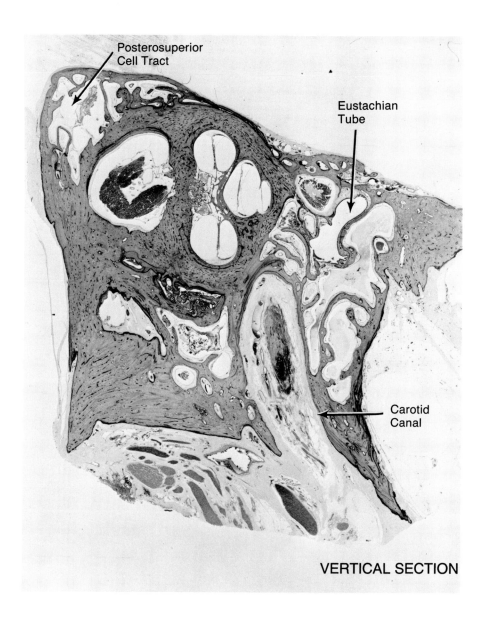

Posterosuperior
Cell Tract

Eustachian
Tube

Carotid
Canal

VERTICAL SECTION

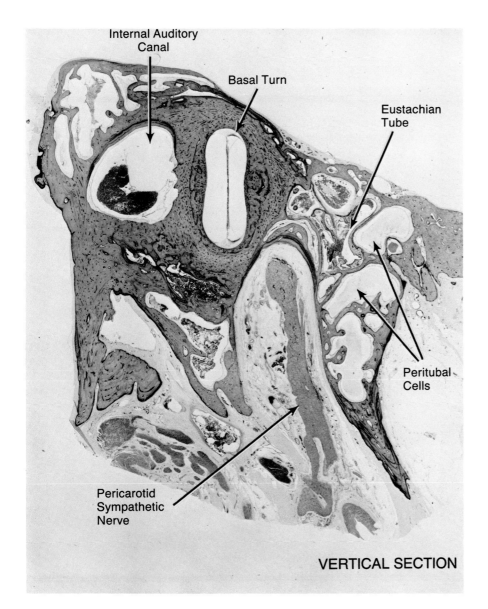

Internal Auditory
Canal

Basal Turn

Eustachian
Tube

Peritubal
Cells

Pericarotid
Sympathetic
Nerve

VERTICAL SECTION

FIG. 1.36: Progressing anteromedially, only the anterior aspect of the basal turn of the cochlea remains.

FIG. 1.37: The internal auditory canal
opens to the posterior cranial fossa. The
pericarotid and peritubal areas are well
pneumatized.

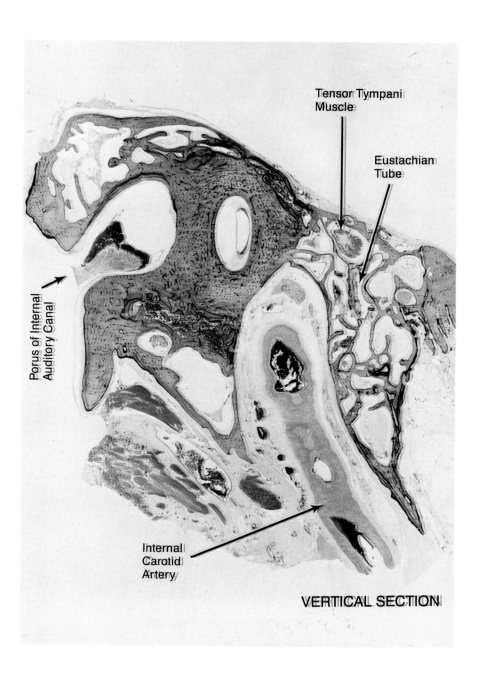

Tensor Tympani
Muscle

Eustachian
Tube

Porus of Internal
Auditory Canal

Internal
Carotid
Artery

VERTICAL SECTION

Horizontal Three-Dimensional Photographs of Celloidin-Impregnated Temporal Bones (Reels I and II)

The labeled photographs appearing in Figures 1.38 to 1.51 are matched to the stereoscopic transparencies appearing in reels I and II, and are presented only to aid in orienting the anatomic features in the stereo views. The photographs were made with a Donaldson camera from celloidin blocks during the process of sectioning. They show the three-dimensional anatomy of the temporal bone in the horizontal plane. Reel I (Figs. 1.38 to 1.44) shows a sequence of views from superior to inferior and reel II (Figs. 1.45 to 1.51) shows selected views of particular anatomic interest. We believe that these stereo views will facilitate the comprehension of ear anatomy in its three-dimensional aspect, and aid in understanding of the two-dimensional photographs in this book.

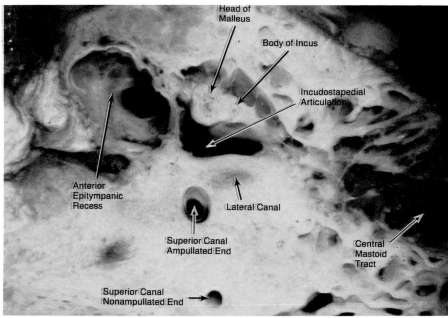

FIG. 1.38, Reel I—1: There is a large anterior epitympanic recess which opens into the mesotympanum inferiorly. The epitympanum narrows posteriorly to the aditus which in turn communicates with the mastoid air cell system. The crista is seen on the lateral wall of the ampulla of the superior canal (female, age 72 years). (Comparable to Figure 1.2.)

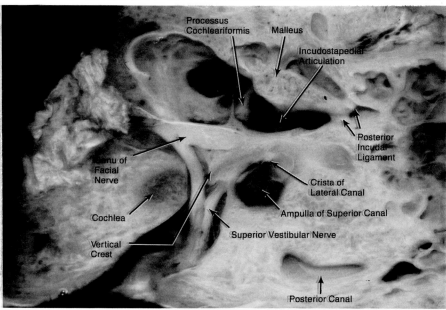

FIG. 1.39, Reel I—2: At a deeper level we see the genu of the facial nerve. It is an important landmark in the middle cranial fossa approach to the internal auditory canal. The vertical crest (also known as "Bill's bar") separates the facial nerve anteriorly from the superior vestibular nerve posteriorly. The lateral and posterior canals are both visible. The lateral part of the internal auditory canal is narrower than the mid-portion, with the cochlea located anteriorly and the ampulla of the superior canal located posteriorly. The short process of the incus is tethered to the walls of the incudal fossa by the posterior incudal ligament. (Comparable to Figure 1.4.)

FIG. 1.40, Reel I—3: Prussak's recess is seen lateral to the head and neck of the malleus. The incus articulates with the stapes by means of the lenticular process. The facial nerve is seen in its tympanic (horizontal) segment. The basal turn of the cochlea is exposed. The superior division of the vestibular nerve and its utricular branch are evident. The otoconial surface of the macula of the utricle faces medially and posteriorly. (Comparable to Figure 1.5.)

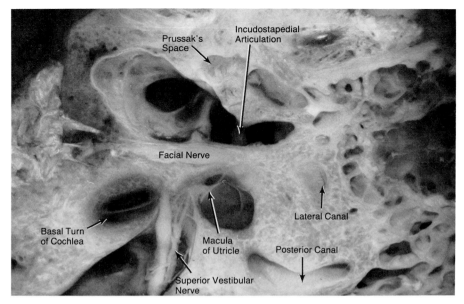

FIG. 1.41, Reel I—4: The external auditory canal (EAC) is widely opened and lies in the same plane as the internal auditory canal. The posterior pouch of von Tröltsch occupies the interval between the posterior malleal fold and the tympanic membrane. The facial nerve is seen in the beginning of its mastoid (vertical) segment. Normally the anterior crus of the stapes is straight and the posterior crus is curved, as seen here. All three turns of the cochlea are seen. Note that the apex of the cochlea points laterally, anteriorly, and inferiorly and lies medial to the cochleariform process. The saccular branch of the inferior vestibular nerve passes to the cribrose area. The tensor tympani muscle and tendon are fully exposed. (Comparable to Figure 1.11.)

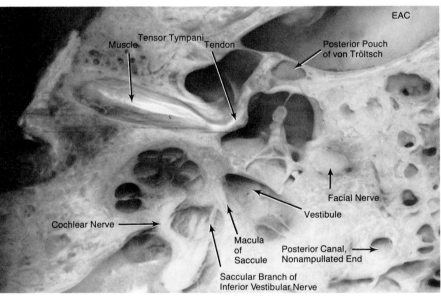

FIG. 1.42, Reel I—5: The conical shape of the pars tensa is evident. The stapedius tendon attaches to the head of the stapes. The promontory of the cochlea lies fully exposed. The posterior ampullary nerve traverses the singular canal on its way to the ampulla of the posterior canal. There is a small arachnoid cyst causing slight displacement but no atrophy of the cochlear nerve bundles in the internal auditory canal. (Comparable to Figure 1.14.)

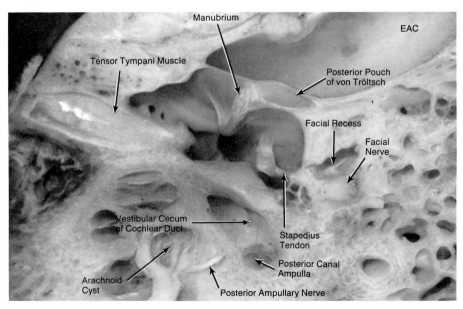

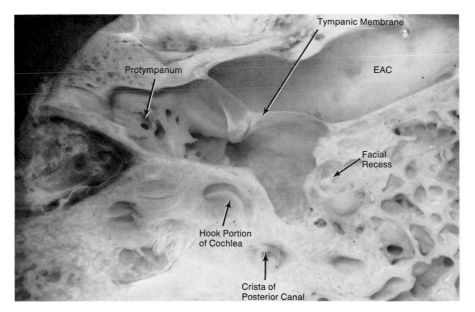

FIG. 1.43, Reel I—6: The manubrium of the malleus is visible in the region of the umbo. The protympanum and hypotympanum are seen. The facial recess lies lateral and the sinus tympani lies medial to the facial nerve. The hook portion of the cochlea is located near the ampulla of the posterior canal. Note the crista of the posterior canal. (Comparable to Figure 1.15.)

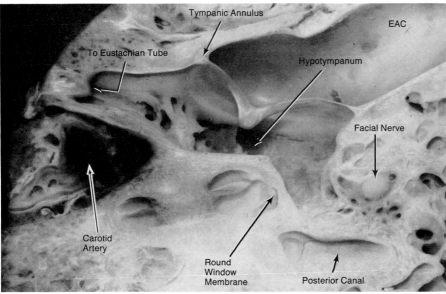

FIG. 1.44, Reel I—7: The basal turn of the cochlea and round window are seen. The protympanum leads to the tympanic orifice of the bony part of the eustachian tube. (Comparable to Figure 1.19.)

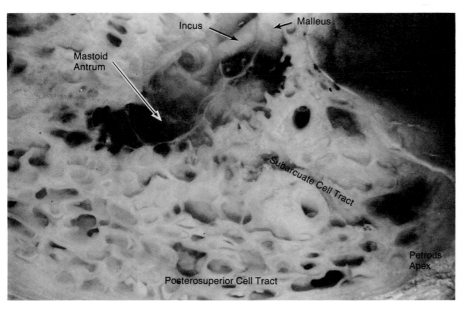

FIG. 1.45, Reel II—1: There is extensive pneumatization of the temporal bone. The posterosuperior cell tract leads to the pneumatized petrous apex. The subarcuate tract passes through the arch of the superior canal, also leading to the petrous apex. Note that the semicircular duct hugs the outer wall of the bony canal (female, age 67 years).

Serial Photographs of Sections of the Temporal Bone   31

FIG. 1.46, Reel II—2: This view shows Koerner's (petrosquamosal) septum which marks the junction of the lateral or squamous part and the medial or petrous part of the mastoid. The crista of the lateral canal and the ampullated end of the superior canal are visualized (male, age 67 years).

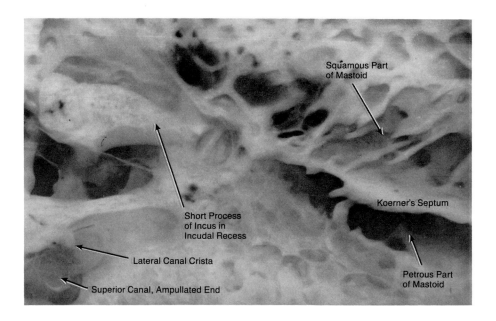

FIG. 1.47, Reel II—3: The anterior inferior cerebellar artery (AICA) loops deeply into the internal auditory canal (IAC). The facial nerve is seen in the internal auditory canal and in its tympanic segment. The superior division of the vestibular nerve and its utricular branch, as well as the utricular macula are seen (male, age 87 years).

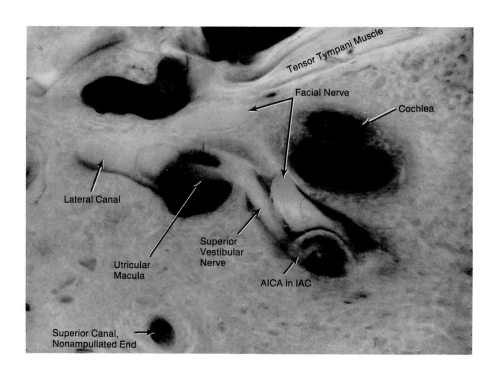

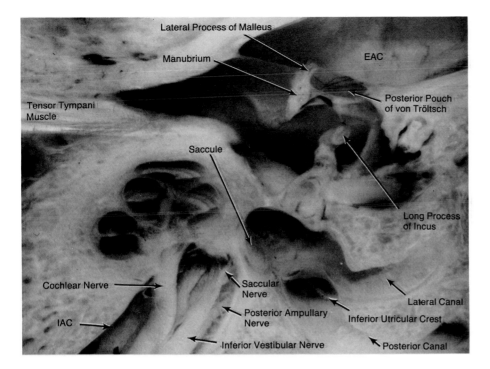

Lateral Process of Malleus

Manubrium

EAC

Posterior Pouch
of von Tröltsch

Tensor Tympani
Muscle

Saccule

Long Process
of Incus

Cochlear Nerve

Saccular
Nerve

IAC

Posterior Ampullary
Nerve

Lateral Canal

Inferior Utricular Crest

Inferior Vestibular Nerve

Posterior Canal

FIG. 1.48, Reel II—4: The cochlear nerve and the inferior division of the vestibular nerve with its two branches, the posterior ampullary and saccular nerves, are seen. The inferior utricular crest marks the boundary between the nonampullated end of the lateral semicircular duct and the utricle. The modiolus, osseous spiral lamina, limbus, organ of Corti, and spiral ligament can be seen. The saccule narrows inferiorly to the ductus reuniens (female, age 68 years).

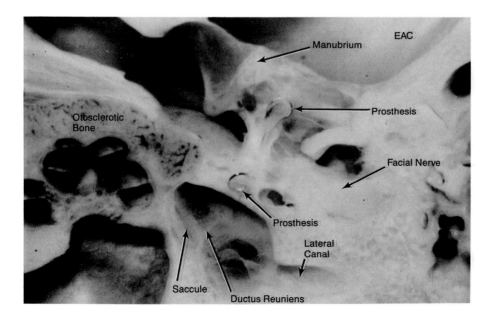

EAC

Manubrium

Otosclerotic
Bone

Prosthesis

Facial Nerve

Prosthesis

Lateral
Canal

Saccule

Ductus Reuniens

FIG. 1.49, Reel II—5: This is the right ear of a 62-year-old male who underwent stapedectomy for otosclerosis 2 years before death. A gelfoam-wire prosthesis was implanted and attached to the incus. Hearing was improved. The prosthesis is partially enveloped in fibrous tissue. The ductus reuniens is seen passing from the saccule to the cochlear duct.

FIG. 1.50, Reel II—6: This photograph shows the sinus tympani as it lies medial to the facial nerve, separated from the round window niche by the subiculum. Medially lies the ampullated end of the posterior canal. The carotid canal is located close to the basal turn of the cochlea (male, age 69 years).

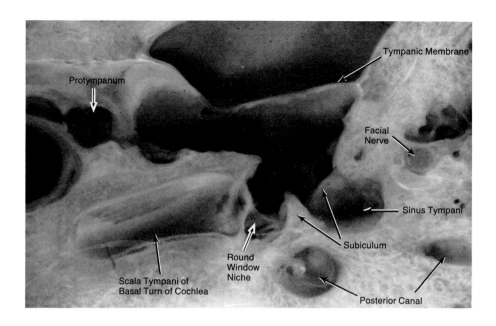

FIG. 1.51, Reel II—7: The protympanum is that portion of the middle ear space anterior to a coronal plane passing through the anterior margin of the tympanic annulus. It leads into the eustachian tube. Note the hook end of the cochlear duct and the utricular opening into the ampulla of the posterior canal (female, age 68 years).

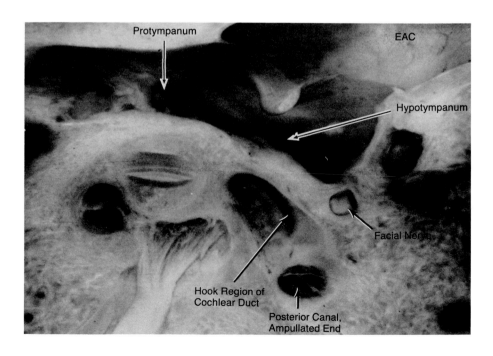

2. The Pinna and External Auditory Canal

The Pinna

In vernacular parlance, the term "ear" evokes an image of that bilaterally symmetric, cartilage-framed, cranial appendage known as the pinna or auricle. This structure acts to focus and localize sound; otoplasty (surgical correction of lop ears), if not properly done, can increase the error in the latter function from 4° to 20° (Pye & Hinchcliffe, 1976). The pinna normally rests at an angle of 30° to the sagittal plane of the head, while the concha lies at an angle of 90° (plus or minus 15°) to the bony cortex of the mastoid (Rogers, 1974). The pinna's growth parallels overall body growth until approximately 9 years of age; in general, the left ear is smaller than the right (Rogers, 1974). This text is not concerned with auricular congenital deformities and diseases. Suffice it to say that, due to the multi-component nature of its embryologic development, the pinna manifests a wide variety of configurations. Despite this variability, there are certain relatively constant features that can be recognized in the human ear.

The topography of the visualized pinna is determined almost solely by the contour of its underlying cartilaginous frame. The flange-like pinna has a convex medial surface which attaches to the head at its medial one-third; the lateral surface is concave. The major concavity of the lateral aspect of the pinna is the concha (Fig. 2.1). Anteriorly, the tragus delimits the concha as it extends over the orifice of the external auditory canal. Superiorly and posteriorly the concha is bounded by the anthelix and its anterior crus. The inferior extent of the concha is determined by the antitragus, which is separated from the anthelix posteriorly by the posterior auricular sulcus, and from the tragus anteriorly by the intertragic incisura. The concha is partitioned at the crus of the helix into a superior cymba concha and an inferior cavum concha; the latter depression points to the meatus of the external auditory canal. Anteroinferiorly, the crus of the helix is separated from the tragus by the anterior incisure. The helix, with its furled edge, sweeps superiorly and posteriorly from the crus of the helix to end at the lobule; a projection, the Darwinian or auricular tubercle, occasionally exists at its posterosuperior aspect. There are two additional depressions of note. As it curves anterosuperiorly, the anthelix bifurcates into two crura, between which lies a depression known as the triangular fossa. The scaphoid fossa is a trench-like groove separating the helix from the anthelix. Lop ears lack an anthelix, with the consequence that the helix assumes an outstanding position; therefore in a surgical correction an anthelix must be created.

The medial aspect of the pinna is a negative relief model of the lateral aspect. The scaphoid, conchal and triangular eminences correspond to the respective fossae on the lateral surface. Similarly, depressions of the medial aspect (i.e., the transverse sulcus of the anthelix, the sulcus of the crus of the helix, and the fossa of the anthelix) correspond to elevations of the lateral surface of the pinna and are hidden by the cranial attachment of the pinna.

The framework of the pinna consists of elastic cartilage, the contours of which determine its topography; the cartilage measures 0.5 to 2 mm in thickness (Senturia et al., 1980). It consists of two furled plates of cartilage separated by the terminal incisure. The larger plate supports the major bulk of the pinna; the lesser underlies the tragus and is connected to the larger by a narrow isthmus. While the cartilage features much the same topography as the surface of the pinna, there are additional elements which are obscured by its mantle of skin and subcutaneous tissue. Anteriorly, from that portion of the helix just superior to the crus, arises the spine of the helix. Inferiorly, the antitragohelicine fissure separates the tail of the helix (cauda helicis), the posteroinferior terminus of the helix, from the antitragus.

The pinna is attached to the cranium by its skin, cartilage, and a complex of muscles and ligaments. There are three extrinsic ligaments and three extrinsic muscles, both sets referred to as superior, anterior, and posterior. The superior ligament links the superior aspect of the bony external auditory canal to the spine of the cartilaginous helix, the anterior ligament connects the zygoma to the helix and tragus, and the posterior ligament attaches the eminence of the concha to the mastoid process.

The three extrinsic muscles originate from the galea aponeurotica of the scalp. The superior auricular muscle inserts upon the eminence of the triangular fossa, the anterior auricular muscle inserts upon the spine of the helix, and the posterior auricular muscle inserts upon the eminence of the cavum concha.

The six intrinsic auricular muscles show great individual variability in their extent of development and are poorly represented in man; four are found on the lateral surface and two on the medial surface. On the lateral surface the helicis major extends from the spine of the helix to attach tangentially to the anterosuperior curve of the helix. The helicis minor hugs the crus of the helix. The tragicus overlies the tragus, and the antitragicus spans the antitragohelicine fissure between the tail of the helix and the inferior aspect of the antitragus. On the medial surface the transverse auricular muscle links the eminence of the scaphoid fossa and the cavum concha. The oblique auricular muscle connects the eminence of the triangular fossa and the cymba concha.

The skin and subcutaneous tissue reproduce the irregular contours of the cartilaginous frame; the skin of the medial aspect is only loosely attached, while on the lateral surface it is snugly secured by subcutaneous areolar tissue. The usual skin adnexal structures are present, including sebaceous and sudoriferous (sweat) glands, and hair. The sebaceous glands

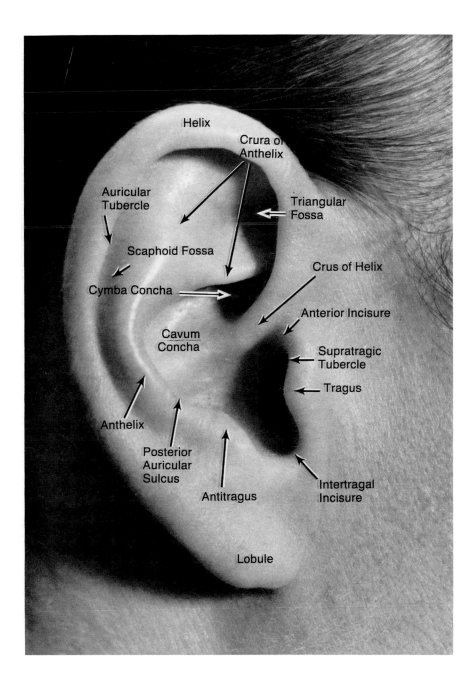

Helix

Crura of
Anthelix

Auricular
Tubercle

Triangular
Fossa

Scaphoid Fossa

Crus of Helix

Cymba Concha

Anterior Incisure

Cavum
Concha

Supratragic
Tubercle

Tragus

Anthelix

Posterior
Auricular
Sulcus

Antitragus

Intertragal
Incisure

Lobule

FIG. 2.1: The right auricle (pinna) of the co-author (AJG) showing the principal anatomic features of its lateral surface.

are distributed both medially and laterally, especially in the regions of the concha and triangular fossa (Anson & Donaldson, 1981). Sudoriferous glands are sparse. A rudimentary type of hair is in abundance over the entirety of the pinna; in elderly male persons, the hairs may be long and large, especially over the tragus and antitragus.

The lobule, the inferior appendage of the pinna, is essentially a fibrofatty nodule. While the lobule has no known physiologic function, its adipose tissue serves as a reservoir for autogenous tissue grafts and its convenient anatomical site serves admirably as a tethering base for ornamentation.

The External Auditory Canal

NORMAL ANATOMY

The external auditory canal is approximately 2.5 cm in length and serves as a channel for sound transmission to the middle ear. It also functions to protect the middle and inner ears from foreign bodies and fluctuations in environmental temperature (Pye & Hinchcliffe, 1976). Its lateral one-third is bolstered by elastic cartilage oriented in an upward and backward fashion; its anterior aspect is pierced by two or three variably present vertical fissures known as the fissures of Santorini (Fig. 2.6); these fissures are a potential route for spread of infections or neoplasms between the external auditory canal and the parotid gland.

The medial one-third of the external auditory canal is osseous and is oriented in a downward and forward direction. Because of the different angulations of the fibrocartilaginous and bony canal walls, the adult auricle must be pulled upward and posteriorly to achieve alignment during otoscopic examination.

The narrowest portion of the external auditory canal or isthmus is located just medial to the junction of the bony and fibrocartilaginous canals. The inferior tympanic recess is a depression in the inferior aspect of the osseous canal. Because of the angulation of the tympanic membrane, the canal is approximately 6 mm longer anteroinferiorly than posterosuperiorly, thus creating an acute angle between the tympanic membrane and anteroinferior bony canal wall (Fig. 2.2). Although the condition is unusual, our collection contains several examples of pneumatization of the anterior wall of the external auditory canal (Fig. 2.3).

The skin of the osseous canal is much thinner than that of the fibrocartilaginous portion (Fig. 2.4), measuring about 0.2 mm in thickness (Senturia et al., 1980), and is continuous with the skin of the tympanic membrane. The subcutaneous layer has no glands or hair follicles. The bony

Fig. 2.2: This horizontal section demonstrates the anatomy of the normal osseous external auditory canal. The anterior wall of the canal forms an acute angle with the tympanic membrane. An excessive convexity of the anterior wall can impair otoscopic visualization of the anterior part of the tympanic membrane. Surgically created dehiscences of the anterior canal wall can result in herniation of the contents of the mandibular fossa into the external auditory canal (female, age 32 years).

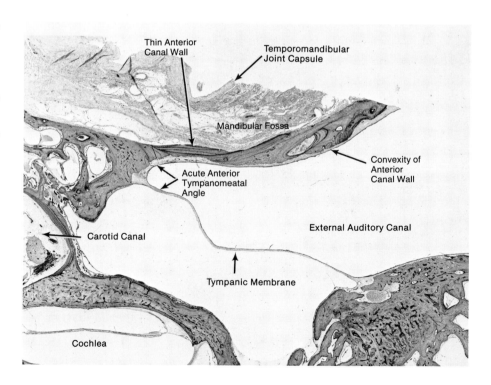

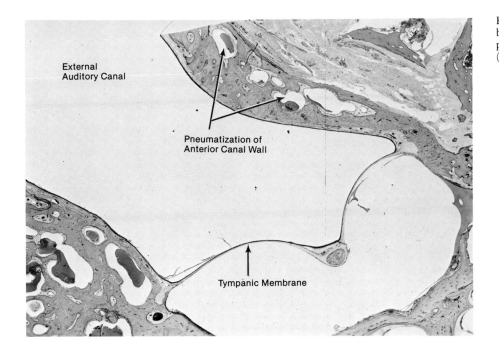

External
Auditory Canal

Pneumatization of
Anterior Canal Wall

Tympanic Membrane

FIG. 2.3: In our collection of temporal bones there are several examples of pneumatization of the tympanic bone (male, age 70 years).

posterior wall of the external auditory canal, which overlies the mastoid air cells, may be extremely thin (Fig. 2.4).

The thinness of the skin of the bony external auditory canal has the following clinical implications: 1) it is easily traumatized during manipulations such as removing cerumen, 2) it is easily torn in the course of surgical procedures such as tympanotomy, and 3) it permits thermal irritation of the periosteum and consequently the formation of exostoses caused by swimming in cold water.

The skin of the fibrocartilaginous part of the canal averages 0.5 to 1 mm in thickness (Senturia et al., 1980), with an epidermis of four layers (basal, squamous, granular, and cornified) blanketing a true subcutaneous layer. The lateral one-third of the fibrocartilaginous canal is replete with

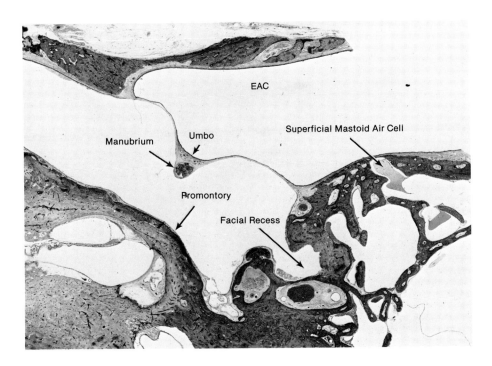

EAC

Superficial Mastoid Air Cell

Umbo

Manubrium

Promontory

Facial Recess

FIG. 2.4: Surgical enlargement of the external auditory canal (EAC) (canalplasty) is necessarily limited by the thinness of its bony walls, both anteriorly and posteriorly (female, age 67 years).

The Pinna and External Auditory Canal   39

FIG. 2.5: This schematic drawing illustrates the adnexae and secretory system of the skin of the external auditory canal. (Courtesy of Main & Lim, 1976.)

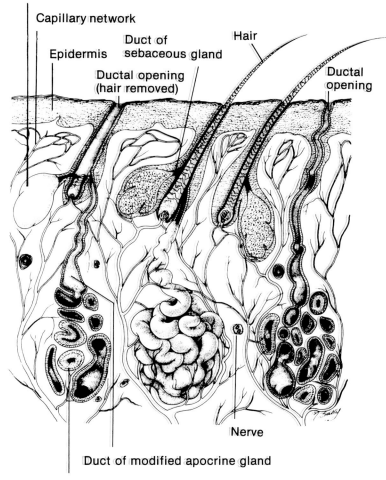

Sebaceous gland

Capillary network

Epidermis

Duct of sebaceous gland

Ductal opening (hair removed)

Hair

Ductal opening

Nerve

Duct of modified apocrine gland

Modified apocrine gland

FIG. 2.6: This photomicrograph shows the anterior wall of the fibrocartilaginous part of the external auditory canal of a three-month-old infant. The sebaceous (lipid-producing) and apocrine (ceruminous) glands are histologically distinct from the glandular tissue of the adjacent parotid gland. The fissures of Santorini in the anterior fibrocartilaginous wall facilitate the spread of bacterial and neoplastic diseases between the external auditory canal and the parotid gland. Outlined areas A and B are shown in higher magnification in Figures 2.7 and 2.8, respectively.

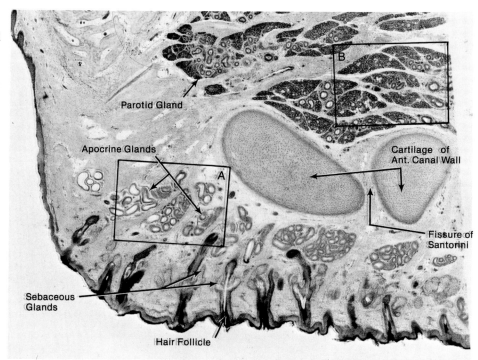

Parotid Gland

B

Apocrine Glands

A

Cartilage of Ant. Canal Wall

Fissure of Santorini

Sebaceous Glands

Hair Follicle

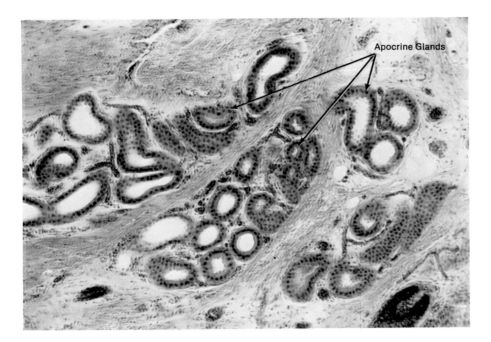

Apocrine Glands

FIG. 2.7: A higher magnification of the outlined area A in Figure 2.6 showing the cross-sectioned, coiled, secretory portion of apocrine (ceruminous) glands. These are modified sweat glands.

hair follicles, but they are less numerous in the medial part. Both sebaceous and modified apocrine (ceruminous) glands (Figs. 2.5 to 2.7) develop from the outer root sheath of hair follicles; hence their numerical distribution follows a pattern similar to that of the hair follicles. In addition, the modified apocrine glands are found mainly on the superior and inferior walls of the canal. Arrector pili muscles are not found in association with the hair follicles in any portion of the external auditory canal.

The apocrine glands are the ceruminous glands of the ear canal (Fig. 2.7). They are located in the dermis deep to the sebaceous glands and have three major components (Senturia et al., 1980): 1) a coiled secretory portion, 2) a secretory duct within the dermis, and 3) a terminal funnel. A myoepithelial cell layer is associated with the coiled secretory portion.

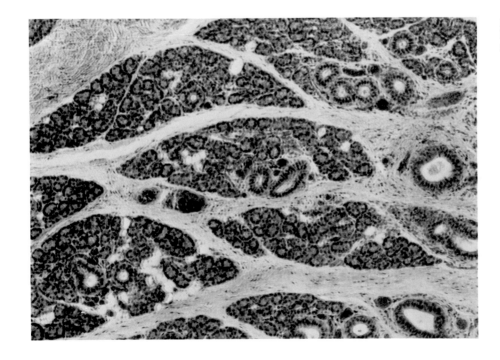

FIG. 2.8: A higher magnification of outlined area B in Figure 2.6 shows the serous cells of the parotid gland.

FIG. 2.9: This photomicrograph of the skin of the fibrocartilaginous part of the external auditory canal (EAC) demonstrates the sebaceous glands. These glands, as well as hair follicles, are most numerous at the meatus of the canal.

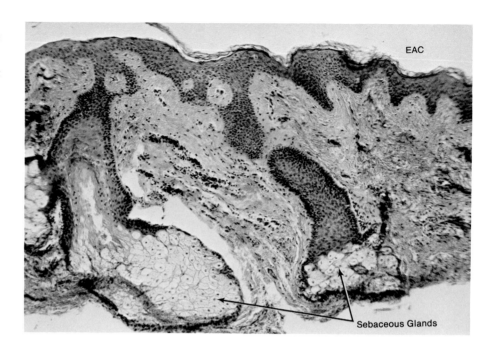

Main and Lim (1976) detected both apocrine and eccrine modes of secretion in these glands. Moreover, they found that these modified apocrine glands secreted a heterogeneous population of granules as well as secretory vesicles. The exact nature of their secreted product is unclear. They are easily differentiated from the parotid glands which consist principally of serous cells (Fig. 2.8). The sebaceous glands (Fig. 2.9) expel the combined products of several acini into the hair follicles via short excretory ducts. These sebaceous glands manifest the holocrine mode of secretion; they contain only one type of secretory granule, presumed to consist of squalene and saturated fatty acids (Main & Lim, 1976).

Acute circumscribed external otitis is a bacterial infection of a sebaceous or apocrine gland. It is an extremely painful disorder requiring aggressive antibiotic and pain therapy. A common cause is swimming in bacterially contaminated water.

Chronic external otitis is a low-grade inflammatory disorder of the skin of the external auditory canal, characterized symptomatically by itching and weeping and also by being exceptionally recalcitrant to treatment. Fibrous tissue proliferation in the subepidermal tissue may lead to stenosis requiring surgical correction.

The ear wax (cerumen) of humans, to a large extent, is the combined product of the sebaceous (lipid-producing) and apocrine (ceruminous) glands; there also is a variable component of desquamated epithelial cells. Impacted cerumen is a common cause of conductive hearing loss.

There are genetically and racially determined differences in the physical characteristics of ear wax; Caucasians and blacks tend to secrete a wet, brown wax, and Orientals a dry, gray wax (Matsunaga, 1962). These differences in appearance and consistency seem to be associated with differences in immunoglobulin and lysozyme content (Petrakis et al., 1971). The implications of these differences in relation to the role of the external auditory canal in immunocompetence is unknown and possibly irrelevant.

EXOSTOSES

Exostoses are benign bony excrescences of the external auditory canal, usually caused by refrigeration periostitis from swimming in cold water (Fig. 2.10). Histologically, they demonstrate a laminated structure (Figs. 2.11 and 2.12) consistent with a periodic growth pattern.

Exostoses remain clinically silent until they become large enough to impair the egress of epithelial debris and water from the canal, in which case there may be an associated external otitis and fluctuating hearing loss. They may also cause a hearing loss by impinging upon the tympanic membrane and/or manubrium. Symptomatic relief is attained by surgical removal and skin grafting of the epithelially denuded areas of the bony walls of the external auditory canal.

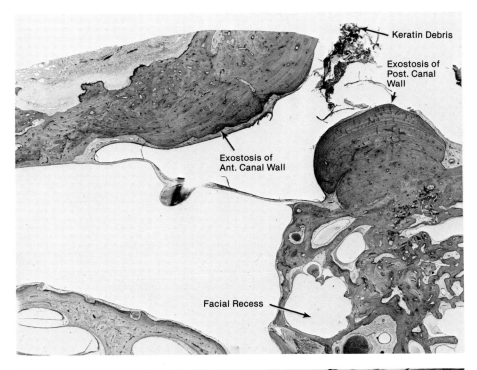

FIG. 2.10: This view shows occult (asymptomatic) exostoses of the anterior and posterior walls of the external auditory canal (male, age 75 years).

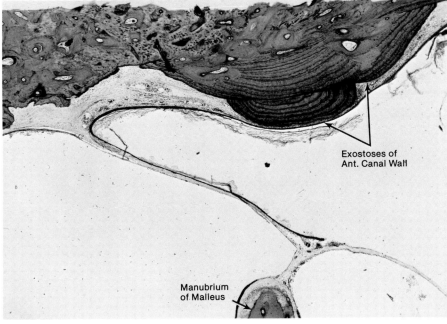

FIG. 2.11: Here we see the interesting condition in which a second exostosis appears to have formed on the surface of a pre-existing exostosis (male, age 60 years).

FIG. 2.12: This high power magnification shows the usual lamellar structure of a typical exostosis punctuated by the normal process of focal remodeling (male, age 61 years). The number of laminations may correlate with the number of cold water insults to the external auditory canal.

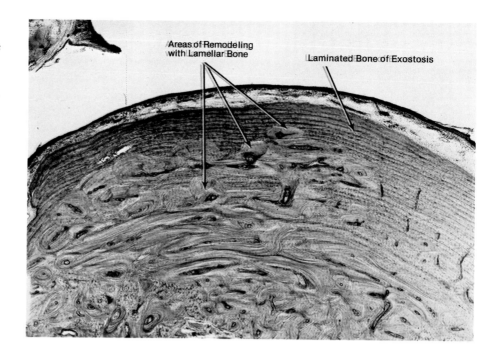

Areas of Remodeling with Lamellar Bone

Laminated Bone of Exostosis

3. The Middle Ear

The Tympanic Membrane

The tympanic membrane is irregularly round and slightly conical in shape; the apex of the cone is located at the umbo, which marks the tip of the manubrium. In the adult it is angulated approximately 140° with respect to the superior wall of the external auditory canal. The vertical diameter of the tympanic membrane as determined along the axis of the manubrium ranges from 8.5 to 10 mm, while the horizontal diameter varies from 8 to 9 mm (Wever & Lawrence, 1954). The malleal prominence (Fig. 3.1), a projection formed by the lateral process of the malleus, is located at the superior end of the manubrium. The manubrium is firmly attached to the tympanic membrane at the umbo and lateral process and is clearly visible throughout its length (the stria mallearis). The anterior and posterior tympanic striae extend from the lateral process of the malleus to the anterior and posterior tympanic spines, respectively. These striae divide the tympanic membrane into a larger pars tensa below, and a smaller, triangular pars flaccida (or Shrapnell's membrane) above.

The superior recess of the tympanic membrane is eponymically known as Prussak's space (Prussak, 1867). The pars flaccida forms the lateral border of this space as it attaches superiorly to the bony margins of the notch of Rivinus or tympanic incisura. The lateral malleal ligament limits this space anterosuperiorly as it extends from the union of the head and neck of the malleus to the periphery of the notch of Rivinus. Posteriorly, Prussak's space opens into the epitympanum. The anterior and posterior malleal folds mark the inferior limit of Prussak's space.

The thickened periphery of the pars tensa, the tympanic annulus (limbus) (Fig. 3.2), anchors the tympanic membrane in a groove known as the tympanic sulcus. The tympanic annulus and sulcus are absent superiorly in the area of the notch of Rivinus. The surgeon, when exposing the middle ear via a tympanomeatal flap approach, must elevate the tympanic annulus from the tympanic sulcus if perforation of the tympanic membrane is to be avoided.

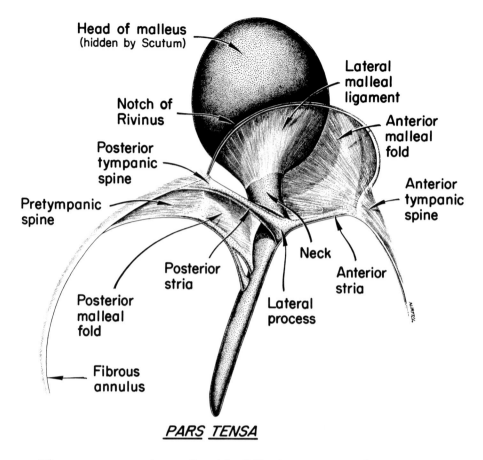

FIG. 3.1: This diagrammatic sketch illustrates the superior, anterior, and inferior boundaries of Prussak's space. Shrapnell's membrane (not illustrated) constitutes the lateral wall as it extends from the anterior and posterior tympanic striae to attach to the margins of the notch of Rivinus. (After Proctor, 1968.)

The pars tensa and pars flaccida differ in structure. The pars tensa, as its name suggests, is taut and consists of three layers: 1) a lateral epidermal layer, 2) a medial mucosal layer, and 3) an intermediate fibrous layer, the pars propria. The epidermal layer is contiguous with the skin of the external auditory canal (see Chapter 2, p. 38) and the mucosal layer is contiguous with the mucous membrane of the middle ear. The intermediate layer consists of fibrous tissue arranged in inner circular and outer radial strata. Elastic fibers are rare in the pars tensa (Lim, 1970).

FIG. 3.2: In the region of the umbo the manubrium is enveloped by the lamina propria of the tympanic membrane (see also Figure 3.19). The tympanic (fibrous) annulus is seen lodged within the tympanic sulcus. The nerves of the tympanic plexus ascend the promontory region in grooves (male, age 63 years).

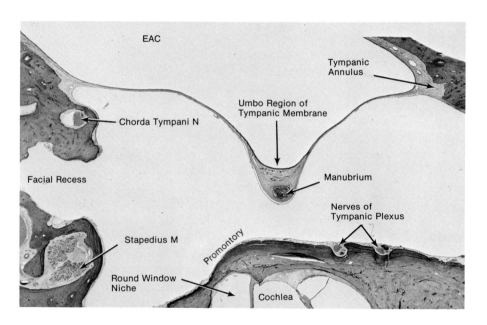

With acute infections of the middle ear, the tympanic membrane becomes acutely inflamed. It is not unusual for blebs or bullae to form at the interface between the pars propria and epidermal layers. The surgeon performing therapeutic myringotomy (incision of the ear drum) must not be misled by such a bleb and fail to incise all three layers of the membrane.

The pars flaccida, although lax, is actually thicker than the pars tensa (Lim, 1970). First described by Shrapnell (1832), it also consists of epidermal, fibrous, and mucosal layers. The epidermis is composed of 5 to 10 layers of epithelial cells, the fibrous layer consists of irregularly arranged collagen and elastic fibers, and the mucosal layer is composed of simple squamous cells, as in the pars tensa.

When the tympanic membrane is perforated by either trauma or infection, the extent of fibrous tissue proliferation determines the thickness of the healing membrane. The replacement membrane may develop a dense intermediate fibrous layer or alternately may fail to develop a fibrous layer, resulting in a thin membrane composed only of epidermal and mucosal layers (Fig. 3.3). It may vary in thickness in different areas and may have areas of hyalinization (Fig. 3.4). The replacement membrane when invaginated into the middle ear space forms a retraction pocket (Figs. 3.5 and 3.6). These pockets may be fixed by adhesions to structures in the middle ear. If not adherent, positive middle ear pressures can cause them to evert into the external auditory canal (Fig. 3.7).

For a successful functional result in myringoplasty operations (closure of perforations of the tympanic membrane), it is important to avoid postoperative fibrous obliteration (blunting) of the anterior tympanomeatal angle. Figures 3.8 and 3.9 show examples of malleus fixation caused by fibrous proliferation in this angle following myringoplasty.

The Ossicles

The ossicles serve to transmit sound energy from the tympanic membrane to the inner ear. The general size, shape, and configuration of the malleus, incus, and stapes are shown in Figure 3.10.

THE MALLEUS

The most lateral of the ossicles is the malleus. It has a head, neck, lateral process, anterior process, and manubrium. The anterior process (processus gracilis or processus Folianus) is a thin projection of bone which extends from the neck of the malleus into the petrotympanic (Glaserian) fissure, accompanied by the chorda tympani nerve (Figs. 3.11 to 3.13). It seems doubtful that the anterior process of the malleus has any important function, for in adult ears it is often found to be fractured (Fig. 3.14) or partially resorbed (Fig. 3.15) without causing hearing loss. It is held to the walls of the petrotympanic fissure by the anterior malleal ligament which, with the posterior incudal ligament, serves to establish the axis of rotation of the ossicles (Fig. 3.16). The anterior malleal ligament must not be confused with the anterior suspensory ligament of the malleus.

The dense fibrous tissue of the anterior malleal ligament is in contiguity with the periosteum of the malleus (Wolff & Bellucci, 1956) and traverses the petrotympanic fissure to reach as far as the angular spine of the sphenoid bone. On its thinner, medial aspect runs the chorda tympani nerve as it passes anteriorly to enter the iter chordae anterius at the Glaserian fissure.

FIG. 3.3: This tympanic membrane shows histologic alterations caused by chronic otitis media. Although intact, there is an anterior marginal area of fibrous thickening and a large area of replacement membrane (neomembrane). The latter area represents a site of previous perforation and is characterized by absence of the lamina propria (the fibrous layer of the tympanic membrane). The inset shows a higher magnification of the outlined area (male, age 54 years). Thin replacement membranes are frequently seen during routine otoscopic examination and, unless very large, have no effect on hearing.

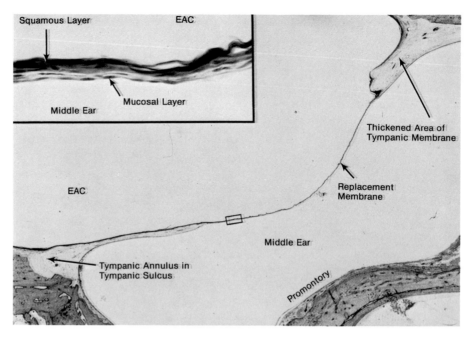

FIG. 3.4: A tympanosclerotic (hyalin) plaque is seen in the anterior part of the tympanic membrane. Otoscopically such plaques have a whitish appearance and are often erroneously termed "calcium plaques." They are the consequence of otitis media (male, age 45 years). These plaques cause no hearing loss unless they are large enough to stiffen the tympanic membrane or fix the manubrium.

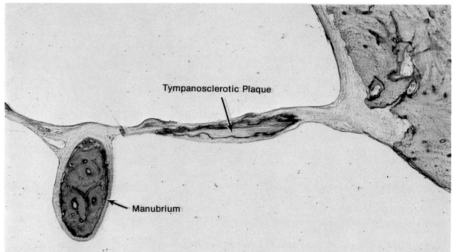

FIG. 3.5: The tympanic membrane shows a posterior retraction pocket and an anterior replacement membrane. The long process of the incus has been resorbed. Additionally, there is a healed fistulous tract leading from the mastoid to the external auditory canal (EAC). These alterations are the result of chronic otitis media and mastoiditis (female, age 48 years).

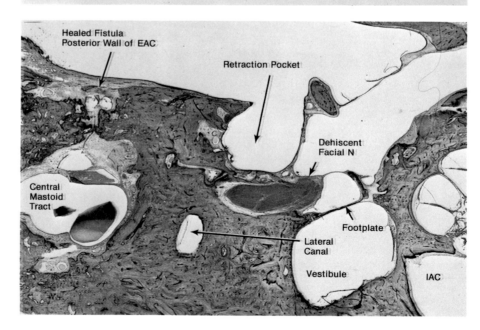

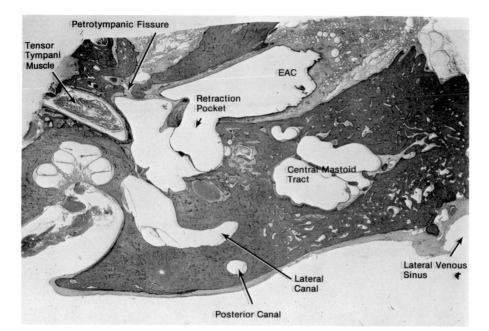

Petrotympanic Fissure

Tensor
Tympani
Muscle

EAC

Retraction
Pocket

Central Mastoid
Tract

Lateral Venous
Sinus

Lateral
Canal

Posterior Canal

FIG. 3.6: There is a deep retraction pocket in the posterior part of the tympanic membrane. The long process of the incus has been resorbed and the central mastoid tract is surrounded by sclerotic bone. These changes are the result of previous otitis media and mastoiditis (male, age 67 years).

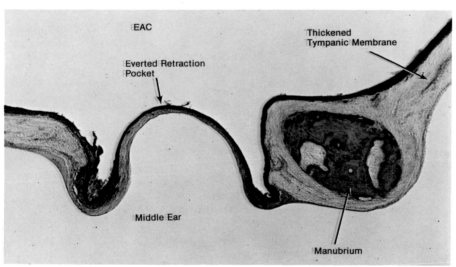

EAC

Thickened
Tympanic Membrane

Everted Retraction
Pocket

Middle Ear

Manubrium

FIG. 3.7: Retraction pockets, if not fixed to middle ear structures by adhesions, may evert or invert depending upon the state of middle ear pressure (female, age 65 years).

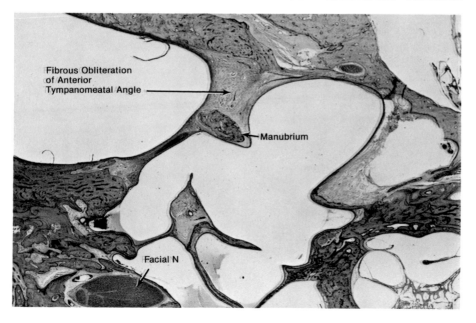

Fibrous Obliteration
of Anterior
Tympanomeatal Angle

Manubrium

Facial N

FIG. 3.8: There is fibrous fixation of the malleus and hearing loss following surgical closure (myringoplasty) of an anterior perforation of the tympanic membrane with fascia from the temporalis muscle (male, age 19 years). (See Fig. 3.9.)

The Middle Ear   49

FIG. 3.9: The opposite ear of the subject shown in Figure 3.8 demonstrates fibrous thickening of the entire tympanic membrane with hearing loss following myringoplasty for an anterior perforation (male, age 19 years). Such untoward results can be avoided by the proper use of skin grafts.

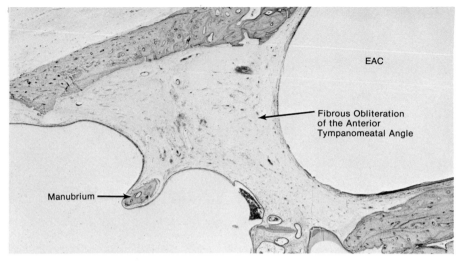

FIG. 3.10: This sketch shows the articulated ossicles and the form and dimensions of the stapes. (After Anson & Donaldson, 1967.)

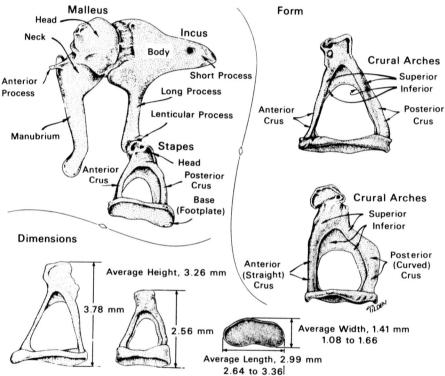

FIG. 3.11: Mesenchyme is still present in the middle ear cavity. The long anterior process of the malleus (processus gracilis or Folianus) is demonstrated in its normal configuration (male, age 5 months).

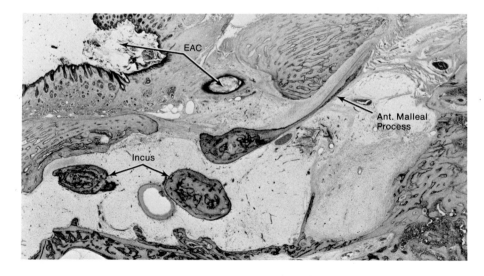

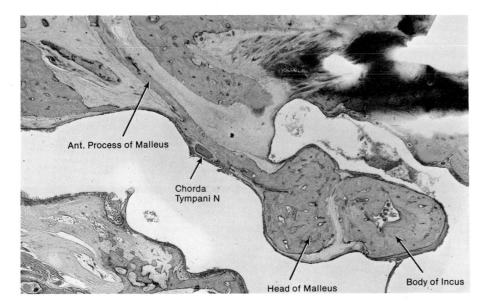

Ant. Process of Malleus

Chorda
Tympani N

Head of Malleus

Body of Incus

FIG. 3.12: The anterior process of the malleus is believed to develop in membrane bone and to fuse secondarily with the enchondral bone of the remainder of the malleus (male, age 39 years).

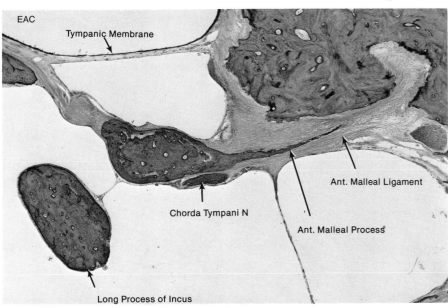

EAC

Tympanic Membrane

Chorda Tympani N

Ant. Malleal Ligament

Ant. Malleal Process

Long Process of Incus

FIG. 3.13: The anterior process of the malleus and the anterior malleal ligament constitute the anterior pole of the axis of ossicular rotation. The anterior malleal ligament may reach as far as the angular spine of the sphenoid bone (male, age 65 years).

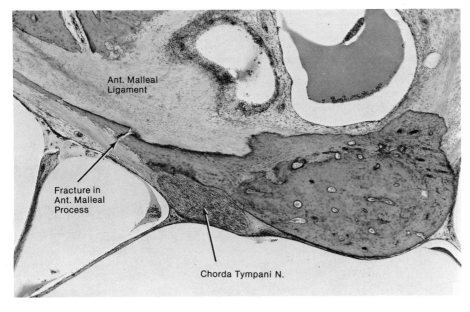

Ant. Malleal
Ligament

Fracture in
Ant. Malleal
Process

Chorda Tympani N.

FIG. 3.14: In the adult temporal bone the anterior process of the malleus frequently shows fractures (female, age 85 years).

Fig. 3.15: In this ear, the anterior process of the malleus has undergone partial resorption. The chorda tympani nerve frequently lies in a groove on the medial surface of the malleus near the base of the anterior process (female, age 85 years).

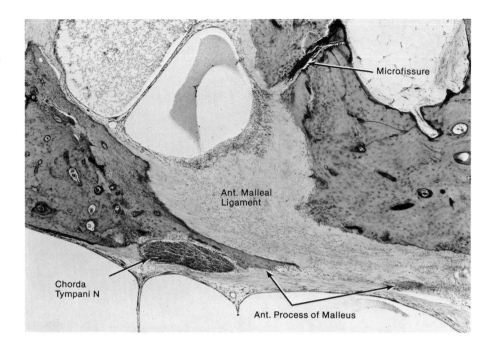

The lateral process of the malleus contains a cartilaginous cap attached to the pars tensa of the tympanic membrane (Figs. 3.17 and 3.18). The inferior end of the manubrium is firmly attached to the tympanic membrane as the pars propria splits to envelop it (the umbo) (Fig. 3.19). In surgical procedures the tympanic membrane can be readily separated from the malleus except at the umbo.

Midway between the lateral process and umbo, the manubrium, because of its gentle medial curvature, may separate slightly from the pars propria so that its only attachment is a fold of mucous membrane, the plica mallearis (Fig. 3.20). Prostheses clamped to the manubrium in the region midway between the lateral process and umbo therefore may have little or no contact with the pars propria of a normal tympanic membrane.

Fig. 3.16: The anterior suspensory ligament, shown here, lies superior to the anterior malleal ligament seen in Figures 3.13 to 3.15. Apparently the suspensory ligaments do not interfere with the process of sound transmission even though they are outside the axis of rotation (male, age 47 years).

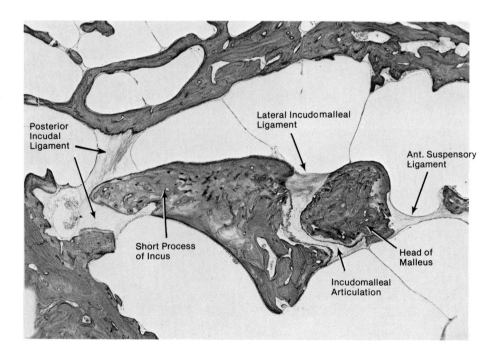

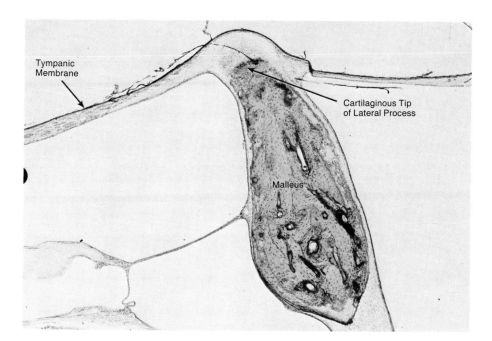

Tympanic Membrane

Cartilaginous Tip of Lateral Process

Malleus

FIG. 3.17: Although the lateral process of the malleus is firmly adherent to the tympanic membrane, surgical separation without perforation is readily accomplished (male, age 28 years).

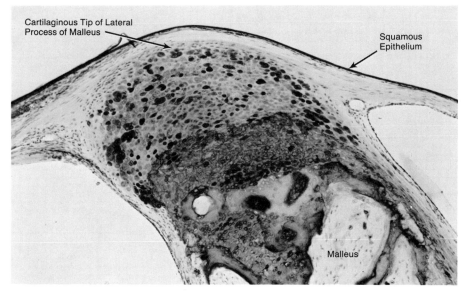

Cartilaginous Tip of Lateral Process of Malleus

Squamous Epithelium

Malleus

FIG. 3.18: The lateral process of the malleus has a cartilaginous cap which facilitates separation of the malleus from the tympanic membrane in this region (male, age 72 years).

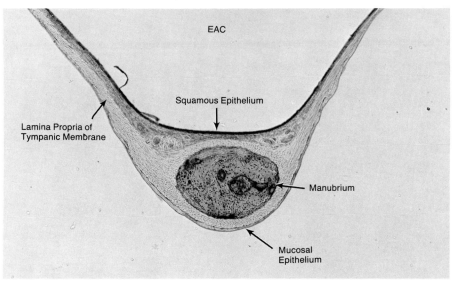

EAC

Squamous Epithelium

Lamina Propria of Tympanic Membrane

Manubrium

Mucosal Epithelium

FIG. 3.19: At the umbo the lamina propria splits to envelop the manubrium of the malleus, making it difficult to separate the malleus from the tympanic membrane without perforation (male, age 28 years).

The Middle Ear   53

FIG. 3.20: At its mid-portion, the manubrium is normally separated from the
tympanic membrane by a mucosal fold
(the manubrial fold or plica mallearis)
(male, age 63 years).

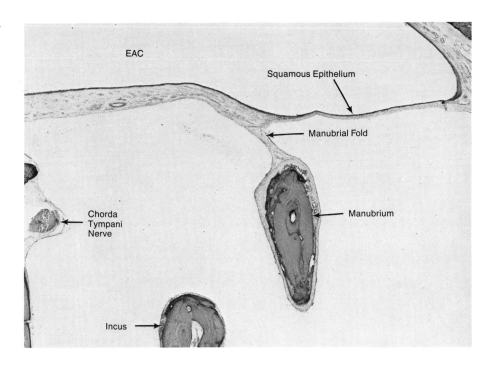

Usually the manubrium lies midway between the anterior and posterior
borders of the tympanic membrane (Fig. 3.21), but may occupy a more
anterior position (Fig. 3.22). The surgical significance of an anteriorly located manubrium is the difficulty it may cause in the repair of an anterior
perforation of the tympanic membrane, as well as in the removal of exostoses and stenoses of the external auditory canal. Surgical procedures on
the tympanic membrane and external auditory canal are especially difficult
when an anteriorly located malleus is associated with convexity of the
anterior canal wall.

The cross-sectional ovoid configuration of the manubrium (Figs. 3.23
and 3.24) is an important determinant in the design of prostheses that
attach to it (Figs. 3.25 and 3.26).

FIG. 3.21: In the anteroposterior dimension the manubrium is normally located
near the middle of the tympanic membrane (male, age 87 years).

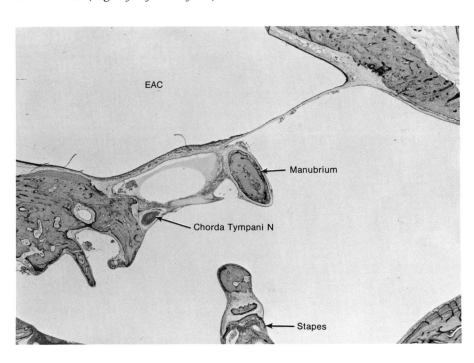

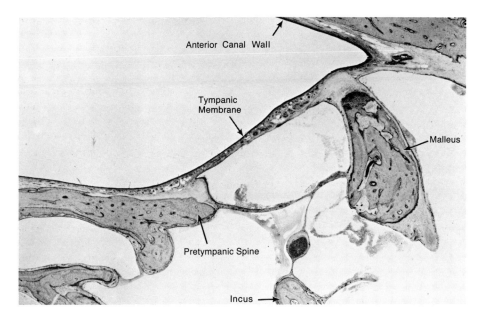

Anterior Canal Wall

Tympanic
Membrane

Malleus

Pretympanic Spine

Incus

FIG. 3.22: In this ear the manubrium is positioned anteriorly in the tympanic membrane. While this anatomical variant is compatible with normal hearing, it increases the risk of fibrous fixation of the malleus following myringoplasty (male, age 79 years). (See Figs. 3.8 and 3.9.)

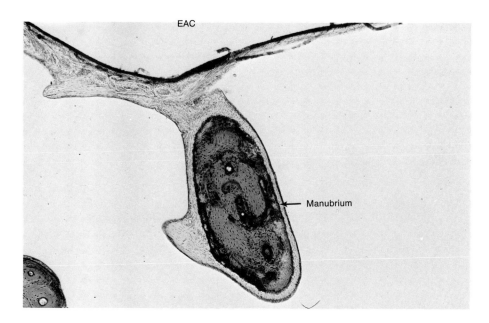

EAC

Manubrium

FIG. 3.23: Except at the umbo the manubrium is oval-shaped, an anatomical feature that must be considered in the design of prostheses that attach to it (male, age 28 years).

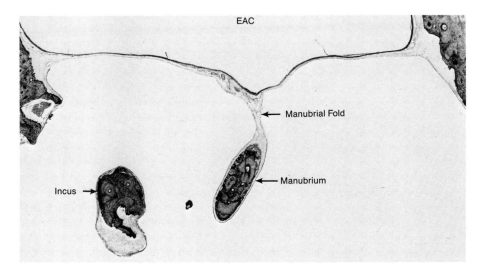

EAC

Manubrial Fold

Manubrium

Incus

FIG. 3.24: Midway between the lateral process and umbo the manubrium is separated from the tympanic membrane with only the manubrial fold of mucous membrane joining them. This is the ideal location for attachment of prostheses (female, age 60 years).

The Middle Ear 55

FIG. 3.25: Attachment of a prosthesis (e.g., teflon wire piston) to the oval-shaped manubrium requires a longer loop than is needed for the circular-shaped long process of the incus. The fabrication of such a loop is illustrated in this figure. The black semicircles represent the jaws of a small forceps. (Schuknecht, 1971.)

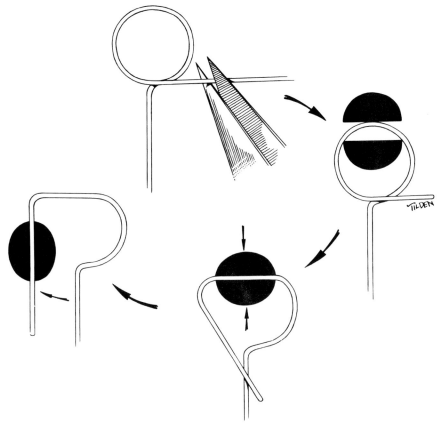

FOR WRAP-AROUND MALLEUS LOOP

The malleus is held in place by five ligaments, one articulation, the tensor tympani tendon, and the tympanic membrane. Three of the five ligaments are well outside the axis of rotation and have a suspensory function; they are: 1) the anterior suspensory ligament which lies superior to the anterior malleal ligament and attaches the head of the malleus to the anterior wall of the epitympanum (Fig. 3.16), 2) the lateral suspensory ligament (Figs. 3.27 and 3.28) which attaches the neck of the malleus to the

FIG. 3.26: The metallic prosthesis is firmly attached to the manubrium in a wrap-around manner. A loose attachment invariably results in traumatic osteitis and extrusion of the prosthesis. (Schuknecht, 1971.)

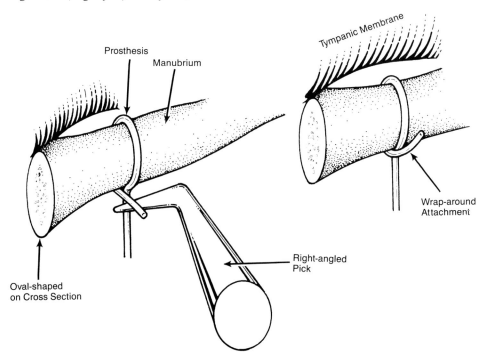

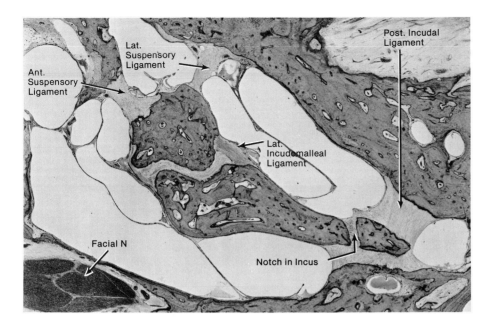

Fig. 3.27: The anterior and lateral suspensory ligaments of the malleus are shown. The notch in the short process of the incus, originally described by Lempert and Wolff (1945), is well visualized; its derivation and function (if any) is not known (male, age 77 years).

bony margins of the tympanic notch (the notch of Rivinus), and 3) the superior suspensory ligament which bridges the gap between the head of the malleus and the tegmen of the epitympanum. These ligaments apparently do not interfere with sound transmission because of the small movement of the ossicles. They may be useful in damping the response of the ossicles to low frequency stimuli of high intensity and in resisting ossicular displacement with large changes in middle ear pressures. The anterior malleal ligament, in concert with the anterior process of the malleus, is in the axis of ossicular rotation. The posterior malleal ligament (Fig. 3.29) is the thickened inferior margin of the posterior malleal fold and stretches from the neck of the malleus to the pretympanic spine. The tympanic membrane attaches the manubrium to the tympanic sulcus.

Additionally the malleus is tethered by the capsule of the incudomalleal articulation which features two thickenings known as the medial and lateral incudomalleal ligaments and by the capsule of the incudostapedial articulation.

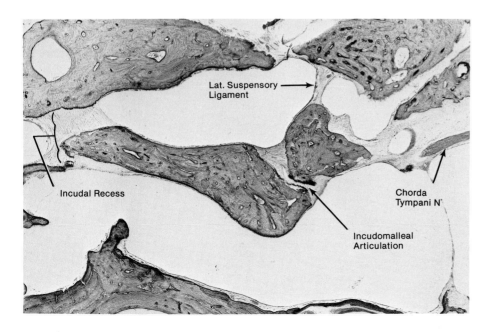

Fig. 3.28: The lateral suspensory ligament of the malleus extends from the neck of the malleus to the bony margin of the notch of Rivinus (male, age 65 years).

The Middle Ear   **57**

FIG. 3.29: The thickened, inferior portion of the posterior malleal fold forms
the posterior malleal ligament. It
stretches from the neck of the malleus
to the pretympanic spine (female, age
64 years).

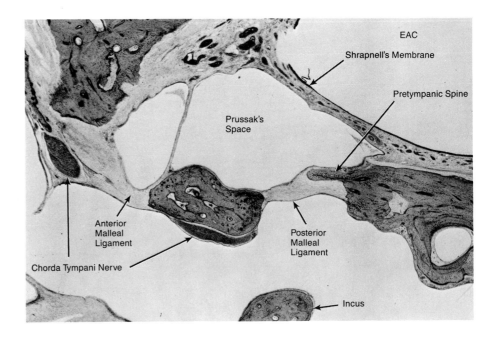

The tendon of the tensor tympani muscle extends laterally from the
cochleariform process to attach to the neck and manubrium of the malleus.
Often some of its fibers pass anterior to the manubrium to reach the tympanic membrane (Figs. 3.30 to 3.32). The function of the tensor tympani
muscle is to pull the manubrium medially and thus exert tension on the
tympanic membrane.

Normally the pull of the tensor tendon is opposed by the elasticity of
the pars propria. With a large perforation of the tympanic membrane the
unopposed pull of the tensor tendon causes a medial displacement of the
inferior end of the manubrium (Figs. 3.33 and 3.34). In some cases the
manubrium may eventually reach the promontory. In surgical reconstructive procedures, such as myringoplasty, it may be prudent to section the
tensor tendon prior to manipulating the manubrium back into its normal
position.

FIG. 3.30: In this ear the tensor tympani
tendon attaches to the tympanic bone as
well as to the neck of the malleus
(male, age 81 years).

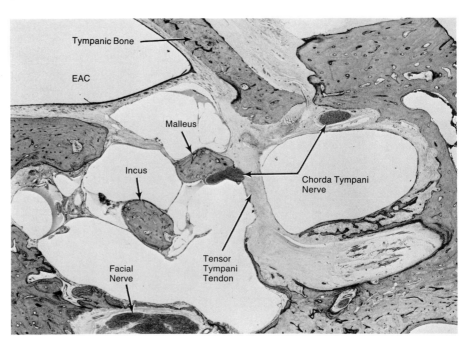

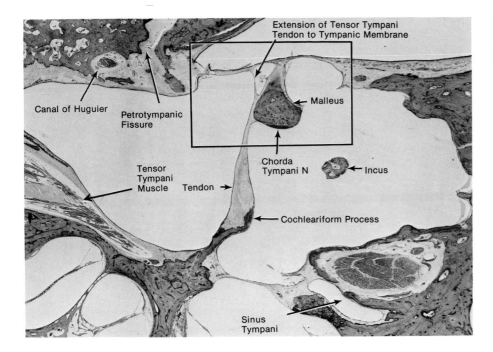

Canal of Huguier · Petrotympanic Fissure · Extension of Tensor Tympani Tendon to Tympanic Membrane · Malleus · Tensor Tympani Muscle · Tendon · Chorda Tympani N · Incus · Cochleariform Process · Sinus Tympani

FIG. 3.31: In addition to inserting into its normal position on the posterior aspect of the neck of the malleus, a small slip of the tensor tendon extends laterally to the tympanic membrane. Anteriorly, the canal of Huguier transmits the chorda tympani nerve as it leaves the petrotympanic (Glaserian) fissure. A stapedectomy for otosclerosis had been performed (male, age 72 years). (See Fig. 3.32.)

Frequently there are projections of bone from the anterior and superior walls of the epitympanum which approximate the head of the malleus. In some instances only a thin layer of loose fibrous tissue separates them (Figs. 3.35 to 3.40). Davies (1968) reasoned that developmental failure of the normal epitympanic expansion and inadequate absorption of bony spicules by the tympanic epithelium might result in restricted epitympanic clearance for the head of the malleus. Fusion of the malleus to the epitympanic wall is normally seen in a number of mammals, such as the flying fox or the fruit bat (Pye & Hinchcliffe, 1976).

We have found ankylosis of the head of the malleus in 15 of 1200 temporal bones which had no other evidence of middle ear abnormality or disease. Malleus ankylosis can be diagnosed clinically by pneumatic otoscopy or by palpation and is thus differentiated from stapes fixation which it mimics functionally (Goodhill, 1966a, 1966b; Guilford & Anson, 1967; Schuknecht, 1974) (Figs. 3.41 to 3.43).

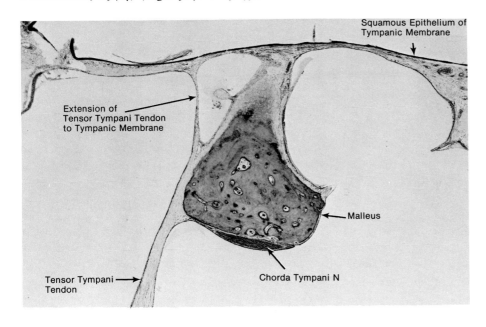

Squamous Epithelium of Tympanic Membrane · Extension of Tensor Tympani Tendon to Tympanic Membrane · Malleus · Tensor Tympani Tendon · Chorda Tympani N

FIG. 3.32: High power view of outlined area of Figure 3.31.

The Middle Ear   59

FIG. 3.33: This subject had a long history of recurrent otorrhea. There is a perforation of the tympanic membrane and displacement of the manubrium towards the promontory (male, age 35 years).

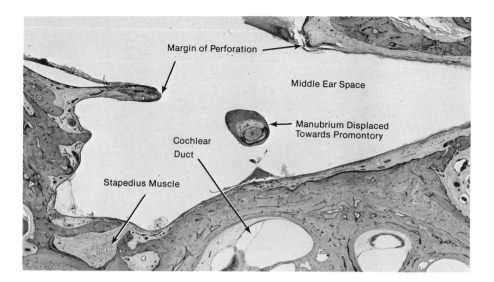

FIG. 3.34: With a large perforation of the tympanic membrane, the tensor tympani muscle acts with diminished opposition which eventually results in medial displacement of the manubrium (female, age 74 years).

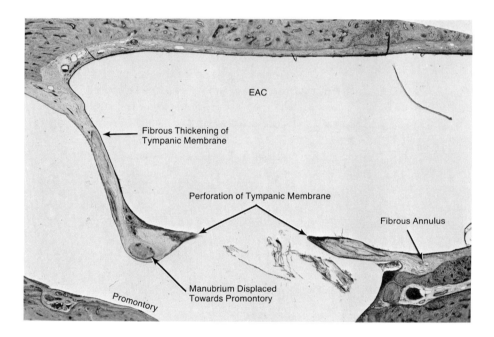

FIG. 3.35: A bony spur extends from the lateral wall of the epitympanum to approximate the lateral aspect of the head of the malleus, causing no apparent hearing loss (female, age 22 years).

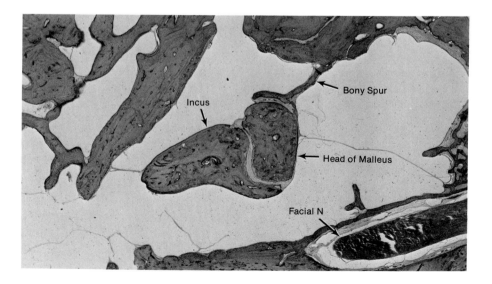

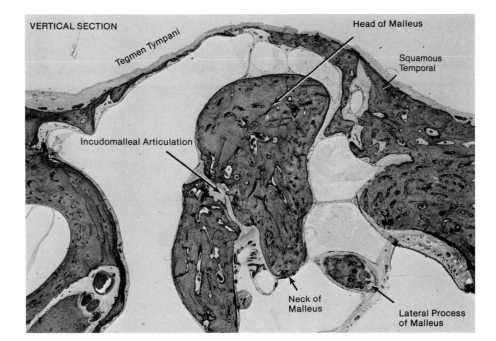

VERTICAL SECTION

Tegmen Tympani

Head of Malleus

Squamous Temporal

Incudomalleal Articulation

Neck of Malleus

Lateral Process of Malleus

FIG. 3.36: A vertical section through the epitympanum illustrates a close proximity of the head of the malleus to the squamous part of the temporal bone. Note the normal thinness of the tegmen tympani (female, age 55 years).

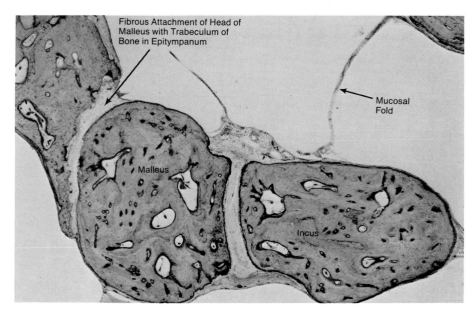

Fibrous Attachment of Head of Malleus with Trabeculum of Bone in Epitympanum

Mucosal Fold

Malleus

Incus

FIG. 3.37: There is a fibrous attachment of the head of the malleus with a bony spur extending from the anterior wall of the epitympanum (squamous temporal). There was no documented hearing loss (male, age 77 years).

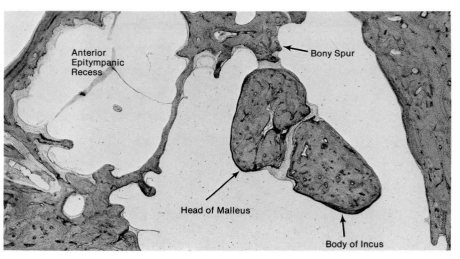

Anterior Epitympanic Recess

Bony Spur

Head of Malleus

Body of Incus

FIG. 3.38: There is a fibrous attachment of the head of the malleus to a bony spur arising from the lateral wall of the epitympanum causing no effect on hearing (female, age 22 years).

The Middle Ear 61

FIG. 3.39: A bony spur projects from the lateral epitympanic wall to make a fibrous attachment to the lateral aspect of the head of the malleus. We propose that these fibrous attachments may, in some instances, lead to bony ankylosis and fixation of the malleus (male, age 36 years).

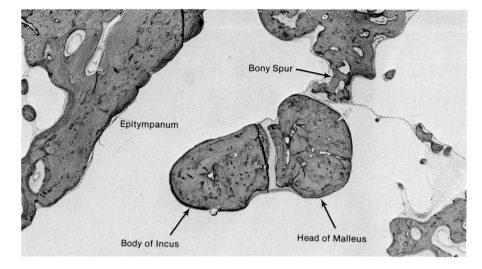

FIG. 3.40: A vertical section illustrates that the superior aspect of the head of the malleus is in fibrous union with the tegmen tympani. There was no documented hearing loss. There is an exceptionally large vein in the fallopian canal, an anatomical variant probably representing a persistent lateral capital vein (female, age 87 years).

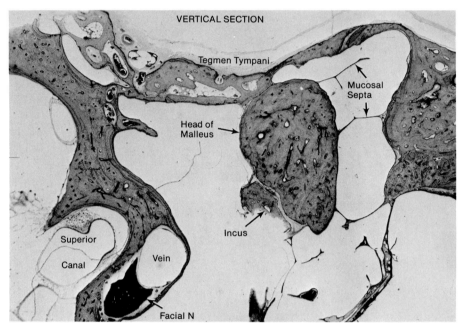

FIG. 3.41: In this ear with chronic otitis media there is bony fixation of the malleus to the anterolateral wall of the epitympanum. There was a mild conductive hearing loss (female, age 64 years).

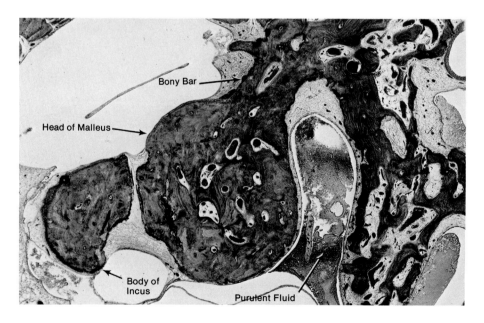

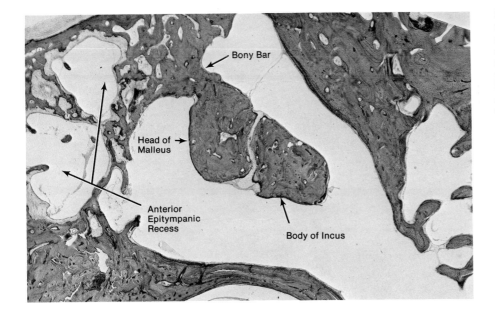

FIG. 3.42: This horizontal section through the epitympanum of the left ear of a 60-year-old female with otosclerosis and conductive hearing loss shows the head of the malleus fixed by a trabeculum of lamellar (not otosclerotic) bone which reaches from the anterior epitympanic wall to the anterior aspect of the head of the malleus.

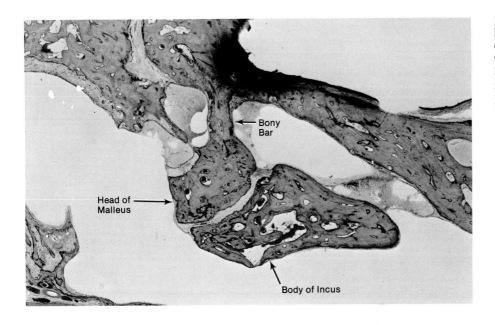

FIG. 3.43: There is ankylosis of the head of the malleus to the lateral epitympanic wall by lamellar (not otosclerotic) bone. Otosclerosis was also present and stapedectomy 13 years before death had resulted in excellent hearing improvement (female, age 82 years).

THE INCUS

The incus, the largest of the auditory ossicles, consists of a body, short process, long process, and lenticular process. The body of the incus rests in the epitympanum in association with the head of the malleus. Movement of the incus is closely geared to that of the malleus by virtue of their cog-type, saddle articulation (see p. 71); this gearing is responsible for the "secondary incus effect" (Goodhill, 1966a, 1966b) in which malleal fixation also interferes with the transfer of sound energy through the incus.

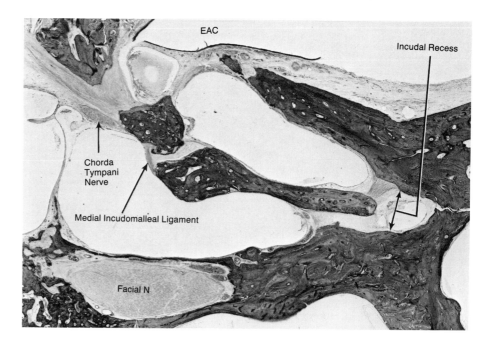

The short process of the incus extends posteriorly, occupying the posterior incudal recess (fossa incudis) (Fig. 3.27); in some cases the short process may be long and slender (Fig. 3.44). The long process reaches inferiorly, paralleling the manubrium, to end in the lenticular process; the convex surface of this process articulates with the concave surface of the head of the stapes in the diarthrodial incudostapedial articulation (Fig. 3.45). The horizontal, cross-sectional configuration of the long process of the incus is circular (Figs. 3.46 and 3.47), in contradistinction to the ovoid shape of the manubrium of the malleus. These differing shapes are taken into consideration in the design of prostheses (Fig. 3.48).

Three ligaments anchor the incus in place. The posterior incudal ligament secures the short process in the posterior incudal recess. Anteriorly the medial and lateral incudomalleal ligaments secure the body of the incus

FIG. 3.45: The head of the stapes articulates with the lenticular process of the incus and also acts as a site of attachment for the stapedius tendon. There is partial resorption of the long process of the incus presumably caused by osteoporosis (male, age 71 years).

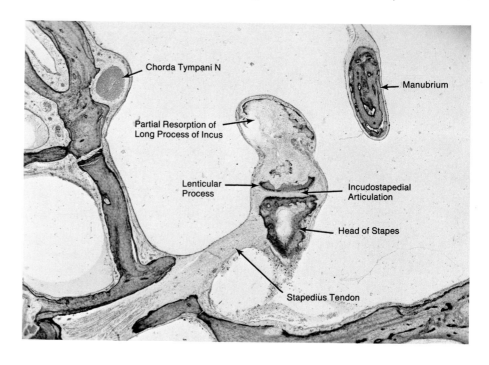

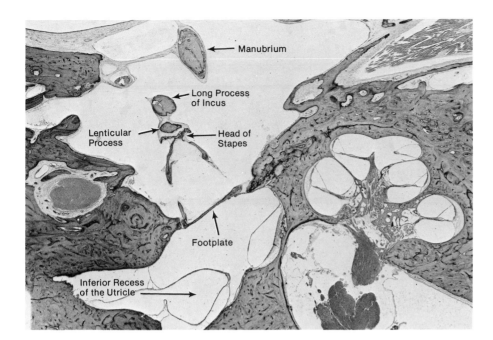

FIG. 3.46: The anatomic relationships of the long process of the incus, the lenticular process, and the head of the stapes are shown (male, age 63 years).

to the head of the malleus (Figs. 3.27 and 3.49). Calcification of the posterior incudal ligament has been noted on histopathological examination of the temporal bone; however, its effect on sound conduction is unknown. A superior incudal ligament has been mentioned (Anson & Donaldson, 1981); however, we have not been able to identify such a structure.

The long process of the incus is highly susceptible to osteitic resorption caused by chronic otitis media (Fig. 3.45).

In newborn infants both the malleus and incus have large marrow spaces (Fig. 3.50) which may persist into adulthood.

It is common for the long process to show slight pneumatization in the form of a pit (Fig. 3.51). Highly pneumatized incudes are rare (Figs. 3.52 and 3.53), but in such cases the long process would be vulnerable to fracture during surgical manipulation.

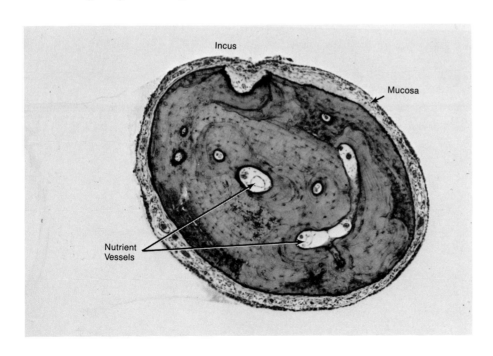

FIG. 3.47: The long process of the incus is roughly circular in cross section. There are numerous nutrient vessels within the bone as well as in the surface mucosa (female, age 54 years).

FIG. 3.48: The round cross-sectional configuration of the long process of the incus permits a simple, crimp-on prosthesis as is schematically illustrated. (Schuknecht, 1971.)

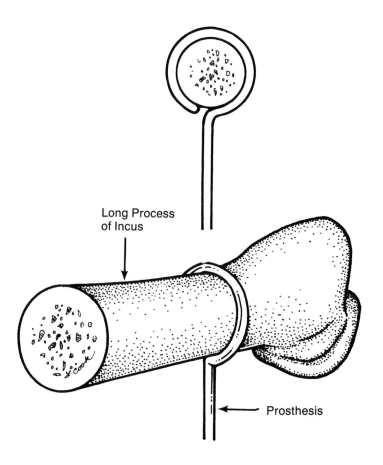

Long Process of Incus

Prosthesis

FIG. 3.49: The embryologic derivation and purpose of the consistently present notch in the short process of the incus, first described by Lempert and Wolff (1945), is not known. In this ear the chorda tympani nerve lies in a groove on the medial aspect of the base of the anterior process of the malleus (female, age 53 years).

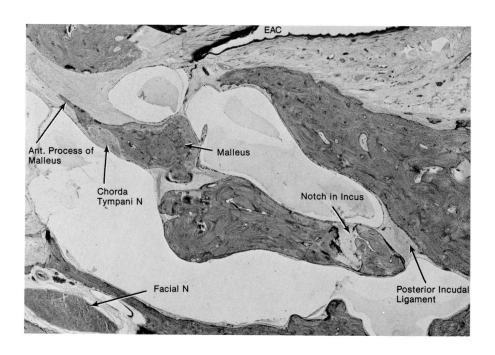

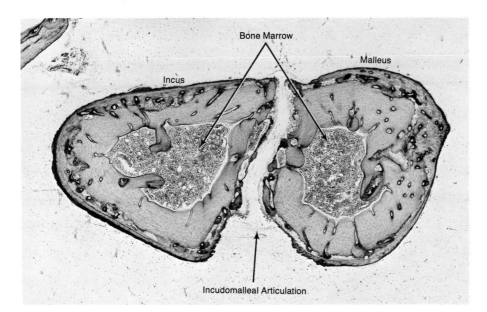

Bone Marrow

Malleus

Incus

Incudomalleal Articulation

FIG. 3.50: In infancy the malleus and incus normally contain a central core of bone marrow (female, age 25 days).

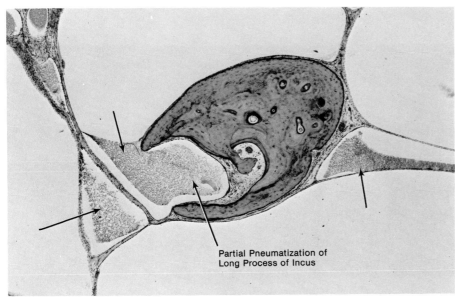

Partial Pneumatization of Long Process of Incus

FIG. 3.51: There is a pneumatized pit in the long process of the incus. These excavations in the incus are seen in the course of otologic surgery. Fluid with proteinaceous precipitate (arrows) occupies the pneumatized spaces. Fluid collections in the tympanomastoid compartment sometimes occur as a terminal event in patients in coma and/or circulatory failure (male, age 77 years).

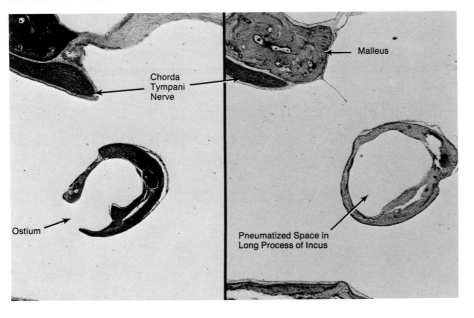

Chorda Tympani Nerve

Malleus

Ostium

Pneumatized Space in Long Process of Incus

FIG. 3.52: There is extensive pneumatization of the bony long process and body (see Fig. 3.53) of the incus. The ostium (left view) is located on its anteromedial aspect approximately 2 mm from its inferior tip. As the pneumatized area extends superiorly (right view), only a shell of bone remains (female, age 44 years).

The Middle Ear **67**

FIG. 3.53: Same ear as Figure 3.52
showing the pneumatization extending
into the body of the incus (female, age
44 years).

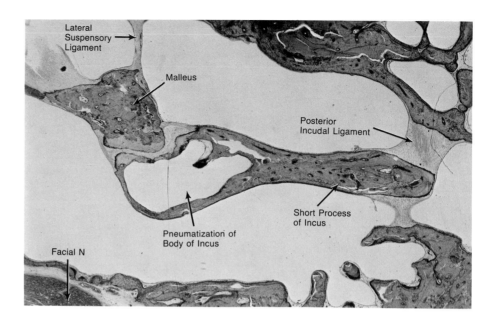

THE STAPES

The stapes is the smallest and the most medial link of the ossicular chain; it consists of a head, footplate (the basis stapedis), and two crura or legs (Anson & Donaldson, 1981). The anterior crus is straighter and more delicate than the posterior (Figs. 3.10 and 3.54). There is an irregular area near the superior aspect of the posterior crus to which the stapedius tendon variably attaches. The area delimited by the concave arches of the crura is the obturator foramen, sometimes bridged by a veil of mucous membrane.

The footplate, in association with the annular ligament, seals the oval window (Figs. 3.55 and 3.56). The shape, thickness, and curvature of the footplate are inconstant. On its lateral surface it has a variably present longitudinal ridge known as the crista stapedis. The vestibular surface may be flat, slightly convex, or slightly concave. The head articulates with the lenticular process of the incus at its fovea (see articulations, p. 71), and it may have a muscular process for the attachment of the stapedius tendon.

The relative thickness and curvature of the crura varies among individuals, as does the locale for attachment of the stapedius tendon. Both the external configuration and the degree of internal excavation may vary in

FIG. 3.54: This cross-sectional view of the stapes shows the crura and head; the stapes has no neck. An expanding otosclerotic focus at the anterior margin of the footplate has caused jamming of the posterior edge of the footplate against the margins of the oval window, resulting in mild conductive hearing loss (female, age 86 years).

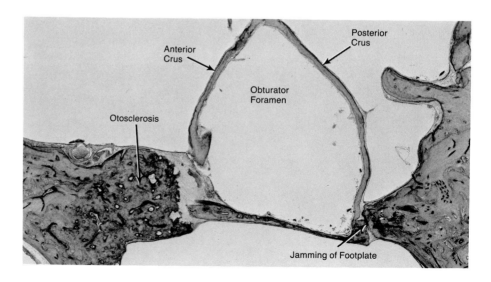

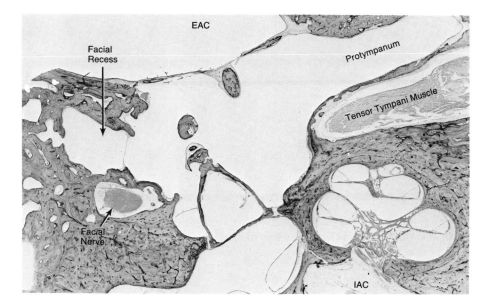

FIG. 3.55: The normal stapes is seen in relation to the adjacent anatomic structures. The posterior crus is normally more curved than the anterior one. Posterior tilting is caused by the unopposed pull of the stapedius muscle and is routinely observed in postmortem specimens (male, age 45 years). IAC—internal auditory canal, EAC—external auditory canal.

the head and crura. The depth of the fovea for the lenticular process of the incus and the presence of a muscular process on the head are variable. The obturator foramen is embryologically related to the stapedial artery which at one time passes through the blastema of the stapes (see embryology, Chapter 9). Presumably failure of normal interaction between these two structures causes occasional columellar formation of the stapes (Fig. 3.57). In cretins the stapes shows a consistent anomaly (Fig. 3.58). The Mondini anomaly may be associated with defects in the footplate, leading to cerebrospinal fluid otorrhea and meningitis (Schuknecht, 1980).

The most dependable method for removing the stapes without fracturing it is to cut its tendon and rock it forward by gentle pressure on the posterior surface of its head, keeping the stress in the plane of the crura.

The Ossicular Articulations (Joints)

The ossicular articulations are true articulations in the sense of uniting two bones. The articulating surfaces are lined by cartilage and there may or

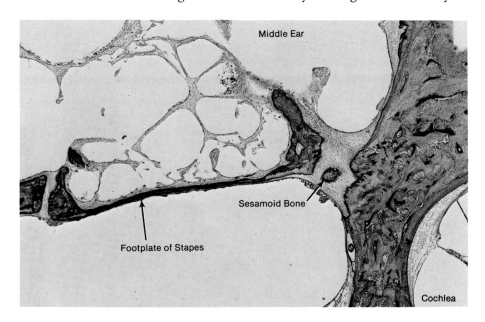

FIG. 3.56: An infrequent finding is that of a sesamoid bone in the anterior aspect of the stapediovestibular articulation (male, age 78 years).

FIG. 3.57: The left ear of this 30-year-old man with conductive hearing loss demonstrates congenitally malformed crura. The capitulum is well developed, but the crural arch is replaced by a single thick columella making fibrous contact with the promontory immediately inferior to the oval window. The footplate was also deformed and fixed.

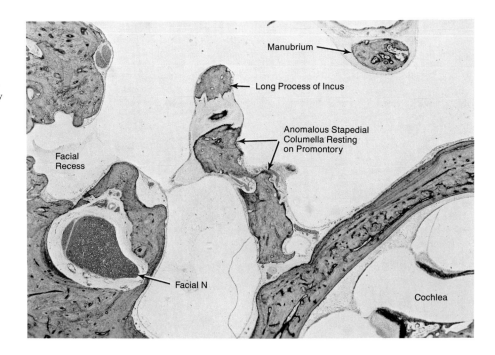

FIG. 3.58: This right ear of a 43-year-old congenitally deaf female shows the classical middle ear anomalies of cretinism. The stapedius muscle and tendon are absent, as are the pyramidal eminence and facial recess. The head of the stapes and the lenticular process of the incus rest against the posterior wall of the tympanic cavity. The facial nerve is widely dehiscent.

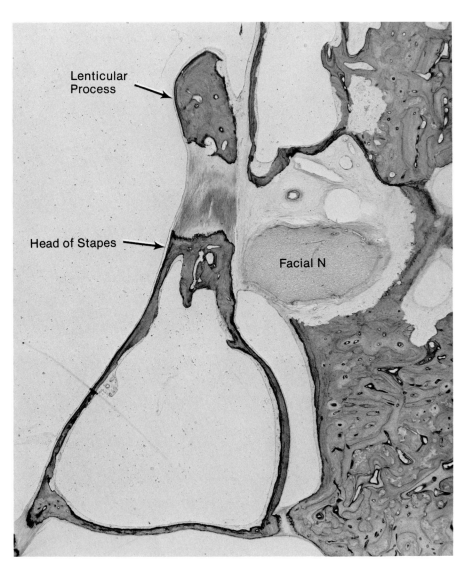

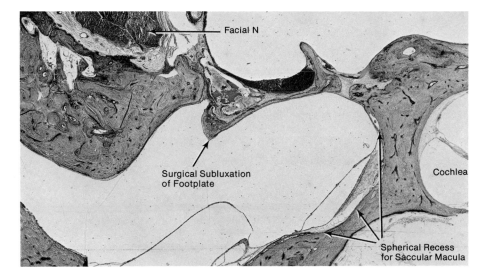

Facial N

Surgical Subluxation
of Footplate

Cochlea

Spherical Recess
for Saccular Macula

FIG. 3.59: Here is shown a surgically induced inward subluxation of the posterior margin of the footplate of the stapes. A modified radical mastoidectomy had been performed 14 years before death. The membranous labyrinth appears normal and there was no postoperative sensorineural hearing loss (female, age 60 years).

may not be an interarticular disc. Each articulation has a true capsule composed of ligamentous fibers originating from the periosteum of the linked bones and lined by a synovial membrane.

While the ossicular articulations are sufficiently strong to withstand physiologic stresses, they are easily torn by direct trauma to the middle ear, fracture of the temporal bone, or surgical manipulation (Fig. 3.59). The ossicles may be partially luxated in which case only part of the capsule is torn and ossicular displacement is partial, or luxated in which case the entire capsule is torn and total disarticulation occurs.

THE INCUDOMALLEAL ARTICULATION

The incudomalleal articulation is a non-weight-bearing, synovial, diarthrodial articulation linking the malleus and incus (Fig. 3.60). It is generally described as saddle-shaped, although Wolff and Bellucci (1956) point out that in vertical sections the opposing joint surfaces appear to present interlocking jaw-like surfaces (Fig. 3.61). A capsule of elastic tissue surrounds the articular margin and there is an interarticular disc. The capsule is trilaminar with: 1) the synovial membrane lining the cavity, 2) the mucous membrane of the middle ear, and 3) an intervening fibrous layer. The capsule is not uniform in structure. At superior levels the medial aspect of the capsule shows greater length and density of the fibrous layer and is known as the medial incudomalleal ligament (Figs. 3.62 to 3.64). At inferior levels the lateral part of the capsule is thicker and is known as the lateral incudomalleal ligament. These regional variations in fiber length, density, and thickness all interact to control the interdigitation of the two ossicles.

The articular cartilage is bilaminar. The deep layer, adjacent to ossicular bone, demonstrates enchondral bone formation as well as direct osseous transformation of its cartilaginous matrix. This latter process is characteristic of secondary or chondroid cartilage which derives from membrane bone (Gussen, 1971). The superficial layer is of primitive cartilage, a product of and maintained by the synovial membrane; it is considered analogous to epiphyseal cartilage.

The Middle Ear **71**

FIG. 3.60: The normal incudomalleal articulation is shown here (male, age 10 weeks).

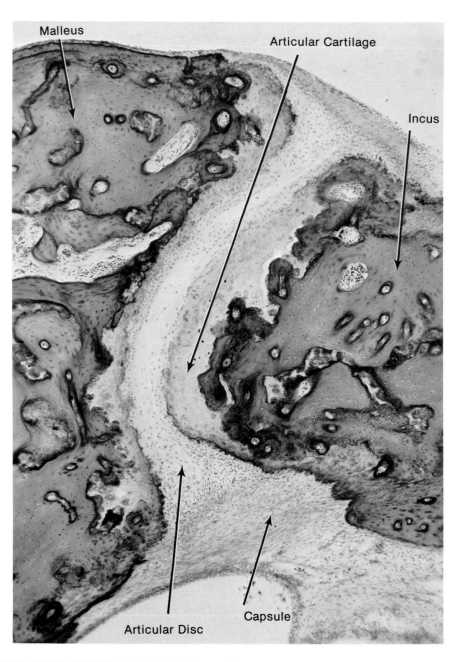

Malleus

Articular Cartilage

Incus

Articular Disc

Capsule

THE INCUDOSTAPEDIAL ARTICULATION

The incudostapedial articulation (Fig. 3.65), also a non-weight-bearing, synovial, diarthrodial articulation, joins the convex lenticular process of the incus (Fig. 3.66) and the concave surface of the head of the stapes. The lenticular process may exist as an accessory bone. There is a joint space, but an interarticular cartilage is not usually present. The fibers of the capsule are longer than those of the incudomalleal articulation, but are of similar thickness and variability of thickness (Wolff & Bellucci, 1956). At the inferior aspect of the articulation, the posterior capsular fibers sometimes merge with those of the tendon of the stapedius muscle with the effect that contraction of the stapedius muscle, in addition to pulling the head of the stapes posteriorly, also draws the long process of the incus posteriorly.

In surgical procedures for otosclerosis the head and crura of the stapes are usually removed preparatory to fenestrating the fixed footplate. The

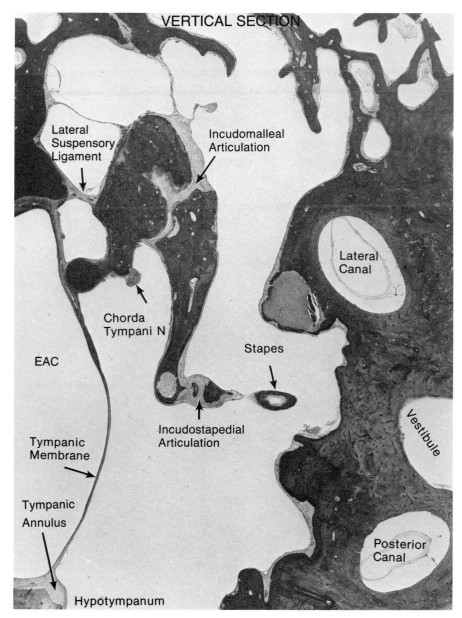

VERTICAL SECTION

Lateral Suspensory Ligament

Incudomalleal Articulation

Lateral Canal

Chorda Tympani N

Stapes

EAC

Vestibule

Incudostapedial Articulation

Tympanic Membrane

Tympanic Annulus

Posterior Canal

Hypotympanum

FIG. 3.61: Both the incudomalleal and incudostapedial articulations (joints) are seen in this vertical section. The space inferior to the lateral malleal ligament is Prussak's space (male, age unknown).

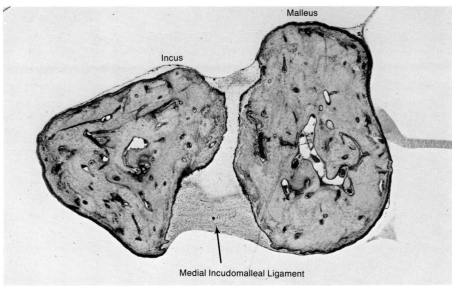

Malleus

Incus

Medial Incudomalleal Ligament

FIG. 3.62: The capsule of the incudomalleal articulation is thickened on its medial side to form the medial incudomalleal ligament (male, age 9 years).

The Middle Ear **73**

FIG. 3.63: At a level slightly inferior to that of Figure 3.62 the capsule is thickened to form the lateral incudomalleal ligament (male, age 9 years).

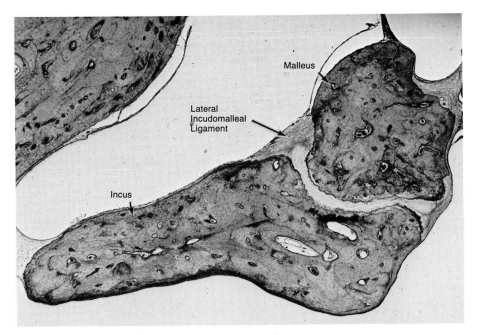

FIG. 3.64: The anterior suspensory ligament of the malleus is located superior to the anterior malleal ligament. Mucosal folds from the lateral epitympanic wall transmit the vascular supply for the ossicles (male, age 81 years).

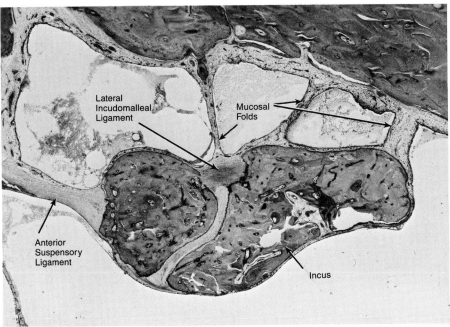

incudostapedial articulation is fragile enough that downward pressure on the head in the direction of the promontory causes separation of the joint without luxating the incus; thus fracture-dislocation of the head and crura is easily performed.

THE STAPEDIOVESTIBULAR ARTICULATION

The stapediovestibular articulation is the junction between the stapes footplate and the oval window. This articulation is one of the sites of predilection for otosclerosis and has been the focus of detailed study. It has been variously labeled as a syndesmosis, an amphiarthrosis, and a "half-joint". The annular ligament holds the footplate of the stapes in the oval window; peripherally its connective tissue fibers fuse with periosteum and endosteum. Wolff and Bellucci (1956) have identified fibers which span the

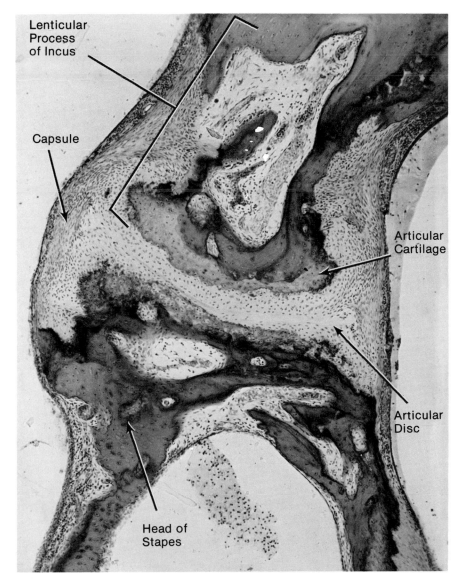

Lenticular
Process
of Incus

Capsule

Articular
Cartilage

Articular
Disc

Head of
Stapes

FIG. 3.65: The incudostapedial articulation of a 10-week-old male infant is shown here. The articular facet of the lenticular process is convex and that of the head of stapes is concave. The lenticular process normally contains islands of fibrous tissue; perhaps this fibrous component underlies the susceptibility of the lenticular process to resorption in chronic otitis media.

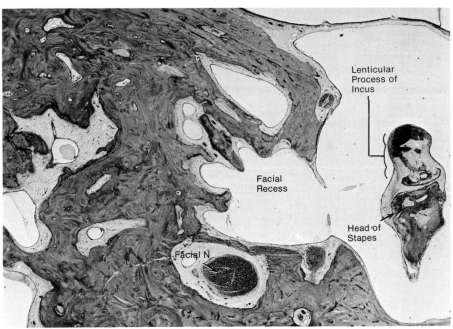

Lenticular
Process of
Incus

Facial
Recess

Head of
Stapes

Facial N

FIG. 3.66: The lenticular process of the incus is shown as it rests in the concavity of the head of the stapes. The facial recess is located directly posterior to the incudostapedial articulation (male, age 58 years).

The Middle Ear **75**

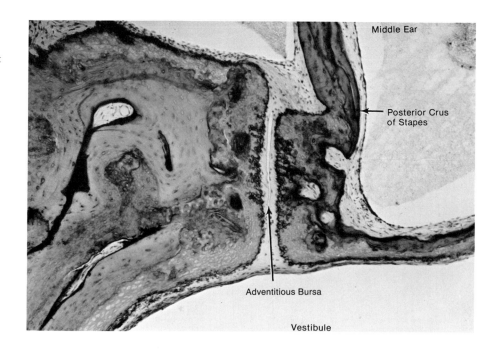

Middle Ear

Posterior Crus of Stapes

Adventitious Bursa

Vestibule

entire distance from the endosteal surface of the footplate to the periosteum of the tympanic aspect of the bony labyrinth; moreover, they have documented that "posteroinferiorly, . . . endosteal ligamentous fibers are continuous with those of the spiral ligament of the basal turn of the cochlea."

Spaces within the stapediovestibular articulation (Fig. 3.67) were recognized as long ago as 1873 (Brunner) but later were attributed to artifact (Gussen, 1969). In a more recent study of the morphology of the stapediovestibular articulation, Bolz and Lim (1972) found such spaces in 70% of adult temporal bones, usually in the posterior pole of the articulation. Because no such spaces were found in the temporal bones of children, they hypothesized that these spaces represent adventitious bursae developing in response to friction, pressure, or trauma.

Changes of Aging in the Articulations

Both the incudomalleal and incudostapedial joints show pathologic changes of aging in which chondroid cartilage undergoes a change to a chondro-osseous matrix (Gussen, 1971).

Etholm and Belal (1974) describe three grades of degenerative change. Grade I shows fraying (Fig. 3.68), vacuolization, and fibrillation of the articular cartilage. Grade II changes show narrowing of the joint space, rarefaction and calcification of the articular cartilage, and hyaline deposition in the capsule and disc (Figs. 3.69 and 3.70). Grade III changes include obliteration of the joint space, as well as calcification of the articular cartilage, capsule, and disc (Figs. 3.71 to 3.73).

Fibrous fixation or bony ankylosis of the incudomalleal and/or incudostapedial articulations appears to have little or no effect on hearing (Etholm & Belal, 1974), and therefore is of minor pathologic significance.

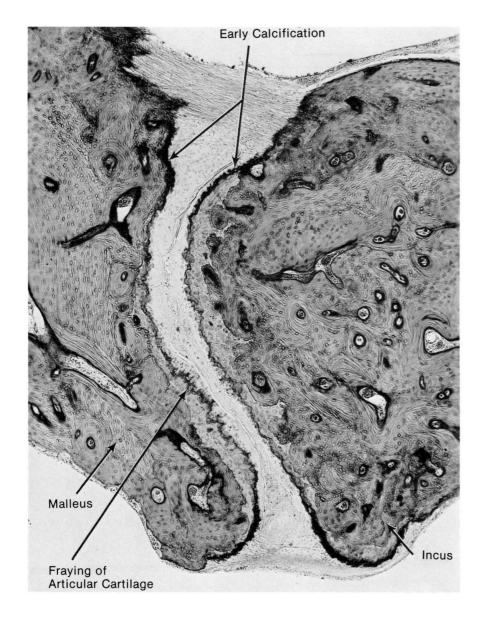

Early Calcification

Malleus

Fraying of
Articular Cartilage

Incus

FIG. 3.68: The incudomalleal articulation of a 16-year-old female illustrates grade I changes of aging.

The Middle Ear 77

FIG. 3.69: The incudomalleal articulation of this 34-year-old female shows narrowing of the joint space, hyalinization of cartilage, and deposition of hyalin within the articular cartilage characteristic of grade II changes of aging.

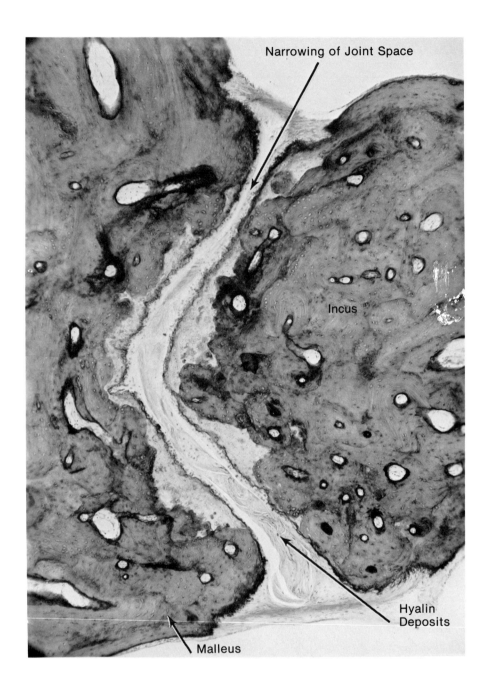

Narrowing of Joint Space

Incus

Hyalin Deposits

Malleus

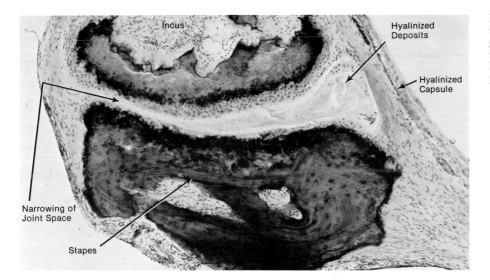

Incus

Hyalinized
Deposits

Hyalinized
Capsule

Narrowing of
Joint Space

Stapes

FIG. 3.70: The incudostapedial articulation of this 59-year-old man shows grade II changes consisting of hyalinization of the joint capsule, as well as hyalinized deposits and narrowing of the joint space.

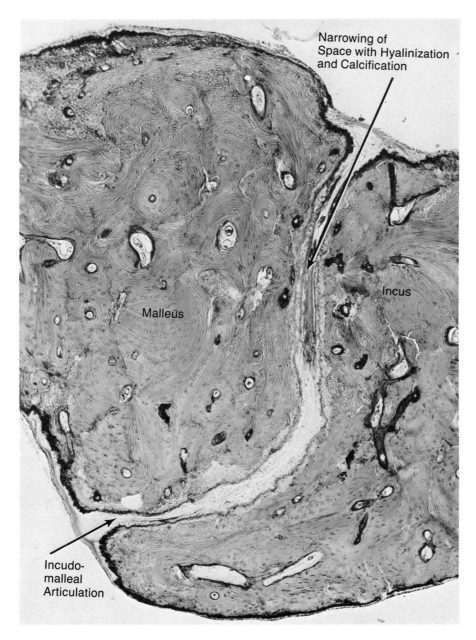

Narrowing of
Space with Hyalinization
and Calcification

Incus

Malleus

Incudo-
malleal
Articulation

FIG. 3.71: The incudomalleal articulation of this 60-year-old female demonstrates grade II changes with narrowing of the joint space, calcification, and hyalinization.

The Middle Ear   **79**

FIG. 3.72: The incudomalleal articulation of this 65-year-old male shows severe (grade III) arthritic changes. The joint space is obliterated laterally, while medially there are scattered calcium deposits. There is irregular thinning and calcification of the articular cartilage. The joint capsule shows atrophic changes.

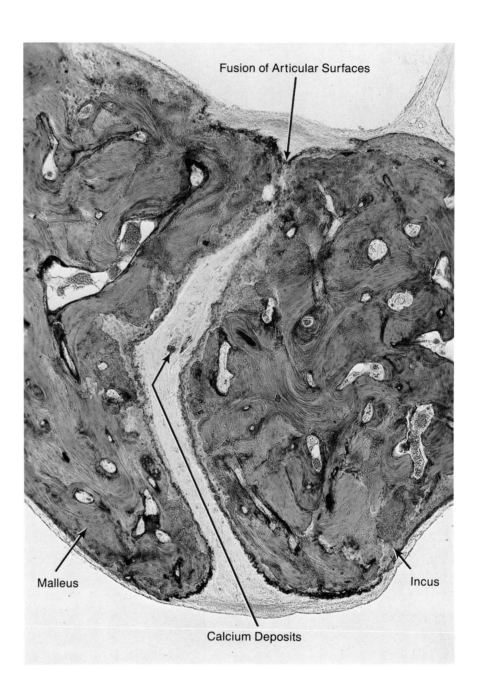

Fusion of Articular Surfaces

Malleus

Incus

Calcium Deposits

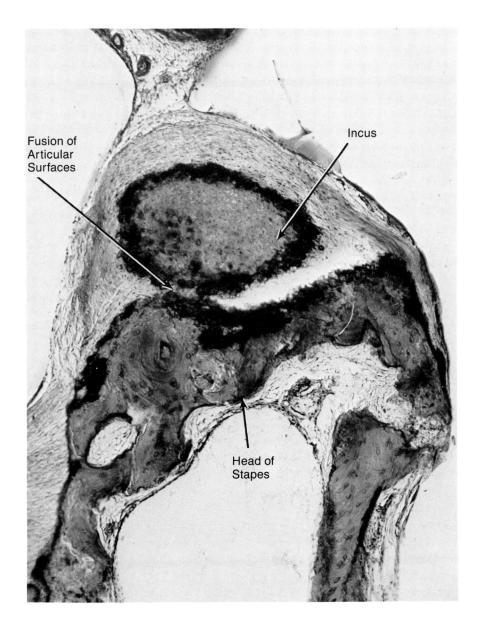

Fusion of
Articular
Surfaces

Incus

Head of
Stapes

FIG. 3.73: The incudostapedial articulation shows fusion of the articular surfaces (grade III changes). Audiometric tests showed no conductive hearing loss (female, age 96 years).

The Muscles

THE STAPEDIUS MUSCLE

The stapedius muscle, the smallest of the skeletal muscles, lies in a bony sulcus adjacent to the facial canal in the posterior wall of the tympanic cavity. This penniform muscle is a mixture of striated and non-striated fibers that converge into a tendon which emerges from the orifice of the pyramidal eminence into the tympanic cavity. It variably attaches to the head and/or posterior crus of the stapes (Anson & Donaldson, 1981) (Figs. 3.74 to 3.76). The stapedius muscle receives its innervation from the facial nerve. Its contraction draws the anterior border of the footplate laterally and the posterior border medially. This tilting of the stapes stretches the annular ligament, thus fixing the footplate and damping its response to acoustic stimulation.

FIG. 3.74: The stapedius tendon normally attaches to the head of the stapes and to the capsule of the incudo-stapedial articulation (female, age 5 years).

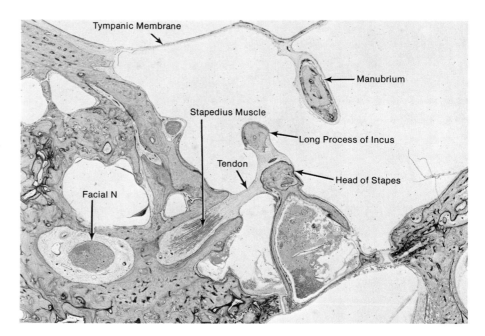

FIG. 3.75: The stapedius tendon emerges from the pyramidal eminence to attach to the head of the stapes (male, age 44 years).

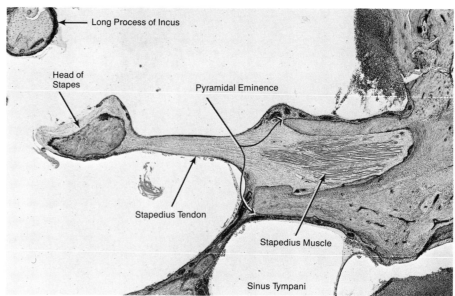

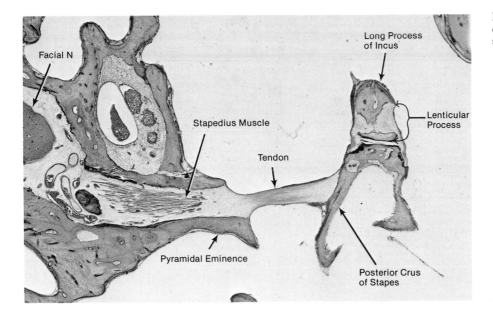

FIG. 3.76: In this case the stapedius tendon attaches to the posterior crus of the stapes (female, age 73 years).

THE TENSOR TYMPANI MUSCLE

The tensor tympani muscle, in concert with the stapedius muscle, acts to modify the movements of the ossicular chain. The tensor tympani muscle (Fig. 3.77) arises from the cartilage of the eustachian tube, the walls of its enveloping semicanal, and the adjacent portion of the greater wing of the sphenoid bone. A bony sheath, the semicanal, houses the muscle for the majority of its 2-cm length. The fibers converge to form a central fibrous core which, proceeding posteriorly, forms the tendon of the muscle. The most medial fibers of the tendon attach to the concave surface of the cochleariform (spoon-shaped) process, at which point the main body of the tendon turns laterally to attach to the medial and anterior surfaces of the neck and the manubrium of the malleus. It should be observed that the cochleariform process does not function mechanically in the same fashion as a pulley.

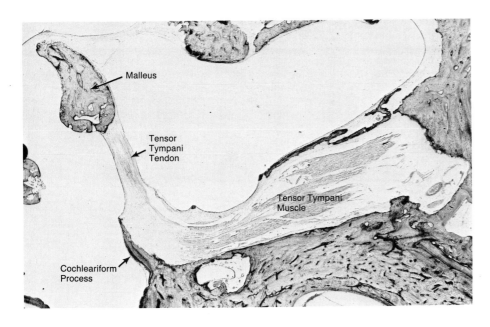

FIG. 3.77: The tensor tympani tendon makes a nearly right-angled turn at the cochleariform (spoon-shaped) process on its way to the neck of the malleus (male, age 45 years).

The Middle Ear 83

FIG. 3.78: This illustration shows the probable derivation of the tensor tympani muscle from the tensor palatini muscle. (Courtesy of Lupin, 1969.)

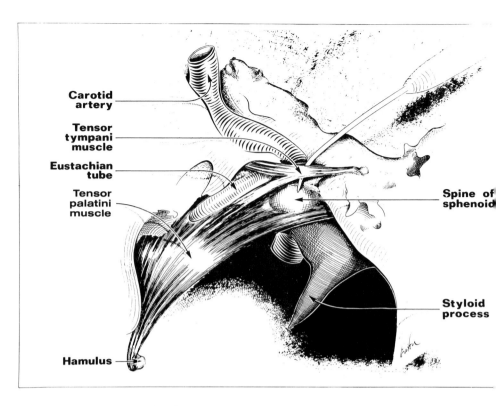

Lupin (1969), on the basis of anatomic dissections, suggests that the tensor tympani muscle represents a continuation of the muscle fibers of the tensor veli palatini muscle (Fig. 3.78). Its innervation is from the trigeminal nerve via the nerve to the medial pterygoid muscle. Histologically, striated as well as non-striated muscle fibers can be observed. The muscle bundles and tendinous fibers are surrounded by varying amounts of adipose tissue (Fig. 3.79). This tissue may facilitate their adaptation to the confines of the bony semicanal upon contraction. The action of the tensor tympani muscle is to draw the manubrium medially, thus tensing the tympanic membrane.

Spontaneous contractions of this muscle may cause a clicking or fluttering tinnitus in the ear and/or vertigo. Cutting the tendon has been advocated for the relief of these symptoms (Epley, 1981).

FIG. 3.79: Normally there is adipose tissue surrounding the bundles of the tensor tympani muscle. Presumably this yielding tissue facilitates contraction of the muscle within its bony semicanal. The muscle consists predominantly of striated fibers (inset) (male, age 66 years).

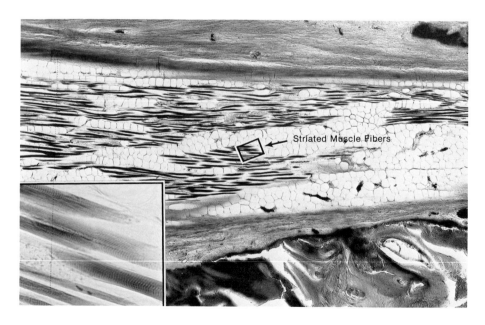

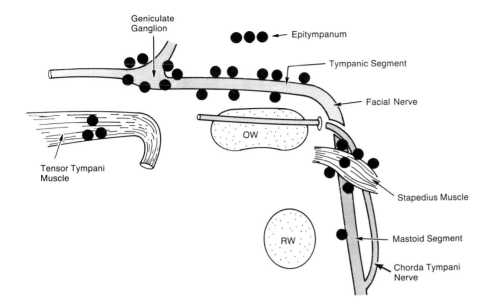

FIG. 3.80: The black dots in this sketch show the location of ectopic muscle bundles in 25 of 500 ears studied by Wright and Etholm (1973). OW—oval window, RW—round window.

ECTOPIC AND ANOMALOUS MUSCLES

Wright and Etholm (1973) found a total of 28 ectopic or anomalous muscles in a study of 500 temporal bone specimens (Fig. 3.80). In no case was the muscle anomaly bilateral and in three ears there were two separate anomalies. Ectopic muscle was most frequent along the course of the facial nerve, either within or close to the fallopian canal. They attributed this anomaly to the persistence of mesenchymal rests along the hyostapedial ligament (interhyale—see embryology, Chapter 9) which in the seven-week embryo connects the primordial stapes to the laterohyale of Reichert's cartilage origin.

In three temporal bones they found the tensor tympani muscles split into medial and lateral bundles. The lateral bundles followed the normal path of the tensor tympani muscle to the cochleariform process. In two of three cases the medial bundles pursued aberrant courses within the fallopian canals and terminated by joining with the stapedius muscles. In certain mammals the tensor tympani may show a double origin—one from the semicanal and one from the medial wall of the middle ear (Pye & Hinchcliffe, 1976).

Wright and Etholm (1973) observed anomalies of the stapedius muscle in six ears. In two cases the stapedius tendons, muscles, and pyramidal eminences were rudimentary, in two the stapedius tendons were absent, and in two there was duplication of the muscles. In one of the latter cases, the duplicate muscle bundle was located superior to the normal muscle (Fig. 3.81) and the associated tendon failed to gain access into the tympanic cavity. The authors suggested that premature separation of the interhyale from the stapes due to an aberration of development was responsible for these anomalies. They noted that anomalies of the stapes bone were frequently associated with muscle anomalies. Hoshino and Paparella (1971) found absent stapedius muscles, unassociated with any other congenital anomaly, in approximately 1% of ears undergoing surgical procedures. The presence of ectopic muscle in the middle ear appears to be of no clinical importance.

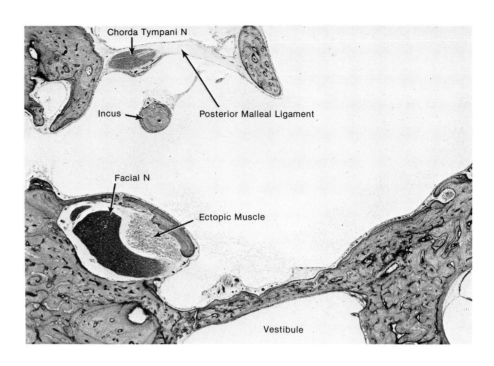

The Middle Ear Spaces

The tympanic cavity is a cleft in the sagittal plane measuring about 15 mm in the vertical and anteroposterior dimensions; in its transverse dimension it expands superiorly to 6 mm and inferiorly to 4 mm from a central constriction of 2 mm (Fig. 3.82). It is pneumatized via the eustachian tube which links it with the nasopharynx; posteriorly the mastoid antrum connects the tympanic cavity with the mastoid air cells. It is traversed by the ossicular system and is lined by mucous membrane.

The floor of the tympanic cavity (jugular wall) is comprised principally of the jugular bulb, the surface of which may show irregularities due to overlying pneumatized cells (Fig. 3.83). In the posterior part of the floor is the root of the styloid process which gives rise to the *styloid eminence*.

FIG. 3.82: Schematic view of the middle ear cleft. (After Deaver, 1901–1903; Brödel, 1946.)

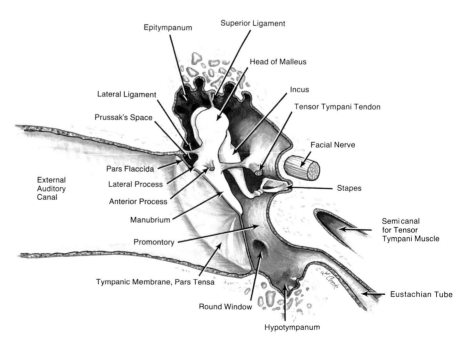

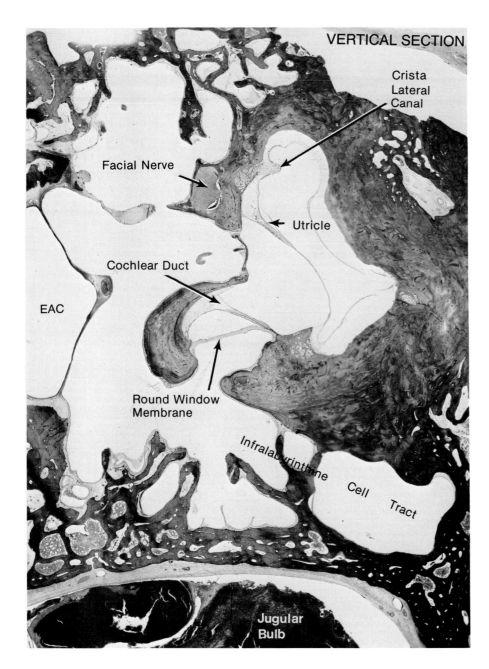

VERTICAL SECTION

Crista
Lateral
Canal

Facial Nerve

Utricle

Cochlear Duct

EAC

Round Window
Membrane

Infralabyrinthine Cell Tract

Jugular
Bulb

FIG. 3.83: This vertical section depicts the relative positions of the oval and round windows. The facial nerve runs in the medial wall of the middle ear at the boundary of the mesotympanum and epitympanum. The hypotympanum is normally studded with trabeculations. The infralabyrinthine cell tract can be the site of extension for cholesteatomas and neoplasms (male, age unknown).

The posterior wall (mastoid wall) of the tympanic cavity narrows inferiorly and features numerous anatomic structures. At its inferior aspect, tympanic air cells are surmounted by the *pyramidal eminence* from which the tendon of the stapedius muscle emerges. The *chordal eminence* is lateral to the pyramidal eminence and medial to the posterior rim of the tympanic membrane; there is a foramen in this eminence, known as the iter chordae posterius (or the apertura tympanica canaliculi chordae tympani), through which the chorda tympani nerve gains access to the middle ear. The facial recess is interposed between the chordal eminence laterally and the pyramidal eminence medially. Acting as the superior limit of the facial recess is the incudal fossa, in which the short process of the incus is held in place by the posterior incudal ligament. More superiorly, the epitympanic recess opens into the mastoid antrum. There are three ridges connecting the

FIG. 3.84: The tympanic sinus is one of the three major depressions of the medial wall of the tympanic cavity. The ponticulus limits this space superiorly, while the subiculum limits it inferiorly. Its extension posteriorly is variable and may amount to several millimeters. (After Donaldson et al., 1968.)

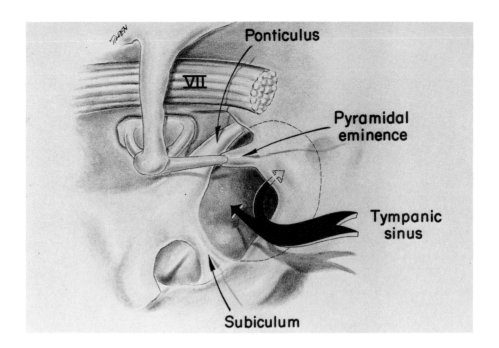

three eminences of the posterior tympanic wall: the *chordal ridge* links the chordal eminence to the pyramidal eminence, the *styloid ridge* connects the styloid prominence to the chordal eminence, and the *pyramidal ridge* joins the styloid prominence to the pyramidal eminence (Proctor, 1969).

The anterior wall of the middle ear (carotid wall) narrows inferiorly where it is formed by the thin bony shell of the carotid canal which is often covered by pneumatized cells. Located more superiorly in the anterior wall is the orifice of the eustachian tube and above it the tensor tympani muscle lies in its semicanal.

The roof (tegmental wall, tegmen tympani) separates the tympanic cavity from the cranial cavity. In an autopsy series, 6% of cases showed dehiscences in this wall (Jahrsdoerfer et al., 1981).

The lateral boundary (membranous wall) is composed of the tympanic membrane, the bony tympanic ring, and a layer of bone from the squama—the scutum or shield of Leidy (Proctor et al., 1981). Erosion of the scutum is a classical radiologic sign of cholesteatoma of the epitympanum.

The medial wall (labyrinthine wall) of the tympanic cavity is marked by three main depressions—the sinus tympani, the round window niche, and the oval window niche (Fig. 3.84). The sinus tympani lies between the ponticulus which bridges the gap between the pyramidal eminence and the promontory superiorly, and the subiculum (subiculum promontorii), a ridge stretching inferiorly between the styloid eminence to the posterior lip of the round window niche (Platzer, 1961). The round window niche is located anteroinferior to the subiculum and posteroinferior to the promontory; the latter structure is the bulge of the bone overlying the basal turn of the cochlea. The oval window niche is anterosuperior to the ponticulus and the cochleariform process of the tensor tympani muscle is even more anteriorly and superiorly located. Located posterosuperiorly is the prominence of the facial canal as it traverses the medial wall and then descends along the mastoid wall of the tympanic cavity.

It is useful in descriptions of disease or surgery to divide the middle ear space into four regions: 1) The *mesotympanum* (middle ear proper) is that area located medial to the tympanic membrane and the bony tympanic annulus. 2) The *epitympanum* is that area which lies superior to a horizontal plane drawn through the most superior level of the tympanic membrane (Anson & Donaldson, 1981). It is approximately one-third the vertical dimension of the entire tympanic cavity, and houses the head of the malleus as well as the body and short process of the incus. 3) The *protympanum* lies anterior to a frontal plane drawn through to the anterior margin of the tympanic annulus. It leads to the tympanic orifice of the eustachian tube. 4) The *hypotympanum* is that part of the middle ear located inferior to a horizontal plane through the most inferior part of the tympanic annulus.

Otologic surgeons are aware of variability in the depth of the hypotympanum. This variability may be ascribed to its tripartite origin (Spector & Ge, 1981) from the tympanic bone, the otic capsule, and the petrosa. A shallow hypotympanum is usually associated with a superiorly located jugular bulb and can be an undesirable anatomic feature in tympanoplasty surgery where one of the objectives is to preserve or attain a pneumatized hypotympanic space. Otologic surgeons are required to have an intimate knowledge of the normal and variant anatomy of the middle ear if removal of disease (granulations, cholesteatoma, etc.) and preservation of function are to be realized.

THE ANTERIOR EPITYMPANIC RECESS

The anterior epitympanic recess is located anterior to the head of the malleus. Its boundaries include the middle cranial fossa superiorly, the petrous apex and middle cranial fossa anteriorly, the tympanic bone laterally and inferiorly, and the facial nerve and geniculate ganglion medially. Posteriorly it communicates with the epitympanum (Figs. 3.85 to 3.87). Also known as the "sinus epitympani" (Wigand & Trillsch, 1973), this recess varies greatly in size; it may be quite large, in which case it may be partly walled off from the epitympanum by a perforate septum.

It is common for cholesteatoma of the epitympanic space to extend into the anterior epitympanic recess. Surgeons must be aware that the facial nerve and geniculate ganglion may be dehiscent in its medial wall.

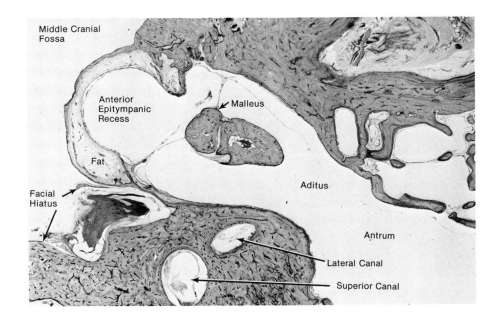

FIG. 3.85: In this ear the anterior epitympanic recess bulges into the middle cranial fossa. This configuration renders it susceptible to perforation during surgical procedures in the middle cranial fossa (male, age 46 years).

FIG. 3.86: The anterior epitympanic recess may be partly isolated from the epitympanum by a bony septum (female, age 75 years).

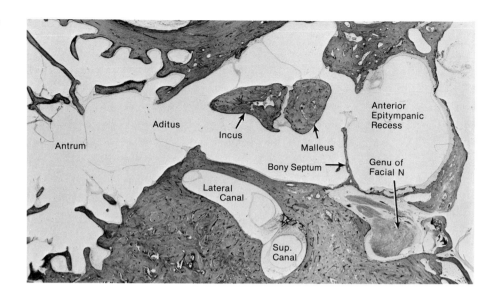

FIG. 3.87: In this ear the genu of the facial nerve lies immediately beneath the dura of the middle cranial fossa (male, age 50 years).

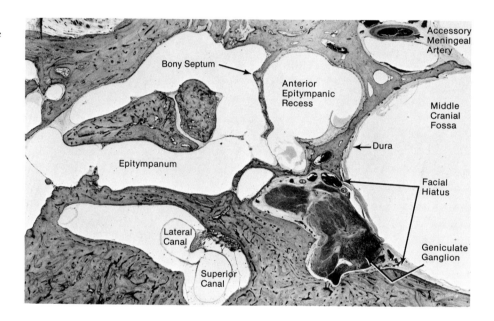

THE OVAL WINDOW NICHE

The oval window niche is located in the medial wall of the posterior part of the mesotympanum and harbors the stapes (Figs. 3.84 and 3.88). It is bounded superiorly by the facial nerve and inferiorly by the promontory. Located anteriorly is the cochleariform process and posteriorly the ponticulus, sinus tympani, and pyramidal eminence.

With the advent of tympanoplasty surgery for chronic infections, stapes operations for otosclerosis, labyrinth operations for Ménière's disease, and reconstructive surgery for congenital anomalies of the middle ear, the oval window area has become an important anatomic site. The stapes is vulnerable to fracture or subluxation, and the facial nerve, which may be dehiscent and bulging from its canal, can be injured. Some of the spatial relationships concerning the middle ear and oval window are seen in Figure 3.89.

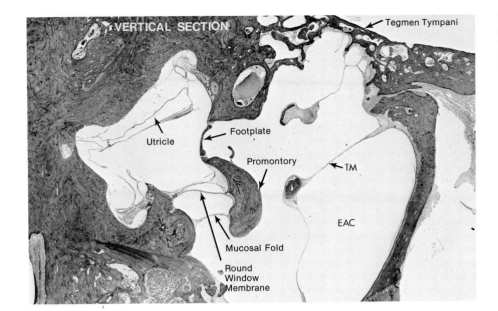

FIG. 3.88: This vertical section depicts the anatomical relationships of inner and middle ear structures (male, age 47 years). TM—tympanic membrane, EAC—external auditory canal.

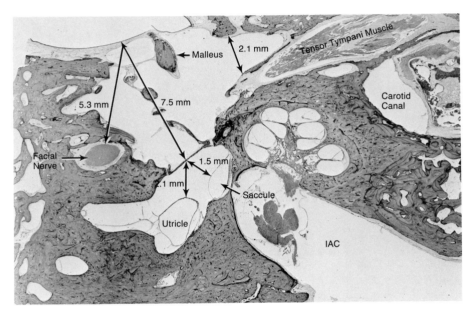

FIG. 3.89: The measurements shown here are average normal for the adult ear. (Anson & Donaldson, 1981.)

THE ROUND WINDOW NICHE

The round window niche (fossula fenestra cochleae) is a depression of variable depth located in the posteroinferior aspect of the medial wall of the tympanic cavity (Figs. 3.84 and 3.90). A bony ridge of bone, the subiculum, separates the round window niche from the sinus tympani posterosuperiorly. The round window niche is delimited anterosuperiorly by the promontory and inferiorly by the hypotympanum (Fig. 3.91).

Ultrastructural studies of the round window membrane in guinea pigs (Kawabata & Paparella, 1971; Richardson et al., 1971; Schachern et al., 1984) reveal that it is composed of three layers. In the external layer, facing the tympanic cavity, there are four distinct types of cells: osmiophilic, osmiophobic, dark granulated, and goblet. Numerous microvilli stud the free epithelial surface, the cells of which are flat and mostly non-ciliated. The internal layer, facing the scala tympani, consists of a single layer of thin cells having long, thin, cytoplasmic extensions into the scala tympani, a

FIG. 3.90: The subiculum is shown in relation to the round window niche and sinus tympani. The microfissure extending from the round window niche to the ampulla of the posterior canal is normally present in adult temporal bones. The posterior part of the tympanic membrane is pathologically thin and retracted medially, probably as a consequence of previous otitis media (male, age 83 years).

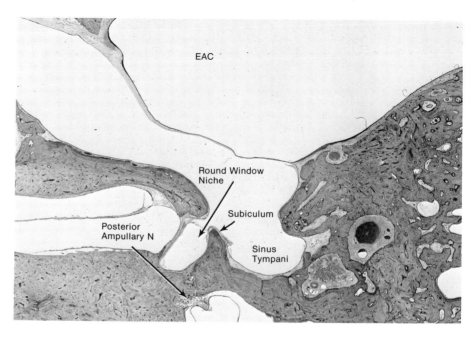

cytoarchitectural pattern very similar to that of the perilymphatic surface of Reissner's membrane. An intermediate layer consists of a dense lattice-work of fibrocytes interspersed with large intercellular spaces containing collagen and elastic fibers, blood vessels, and myelinated as well as unmyelinated nerve fibers.

The round window membrane functions as a yielding area of the bony labyrinth, permitting movement of the inner ear fluids associated with movement of the stapedial footplate. Conductive hearing loss associated with congenital absence of the round window has been successfully treated by surgical fenestration (Ombredanne, 1968). The round window membrane is believed to be a route by which toxic substances (bacterial exotoxins, chemical solutions) may enter the inner ear to cause sensorineural hearing loss.

The round window niche is angulated posteroinferiorly with respect to the external auditory canal. The membrane lies mostly in the horizontal plane, but assumes a more vertical orientation as it curves anteriorly to-

FIG. 3.91: The tympanic ostium of the cochlear aqueduct is located just medial to the semilunar crest of the round window. The inferior cochlear vein provides the principal venous drainage for the inner ear (male, age 68 years).

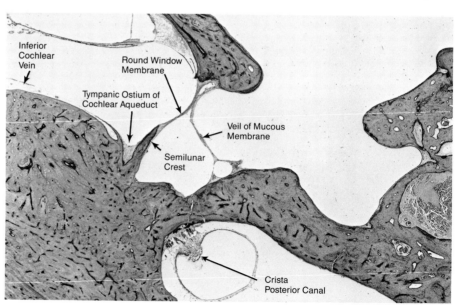

wards the scala tympani. It frequently lies partly hidden behind an incomplete curtain of mucosa which bridges the mouth of the niche (Fig. 3.91).

Goodhill et al. (1973) have implicated rupture (fistulization) of the round window membrane as a cause of sudden sensorineural hearing loss occurring in association with barotrauma or head injury. When a surgical exploration is done for a suspected round window fistula, the mucous membrane fold must not be mistaken for the round window membrane. The bony lip of the round window niche will usually have to be removed if the round window membrane is to be visualized. Patency of the niche is essential for efficient acoustic transmission. In tympanoplasty surgery the objective is to achieve a pneumatized round window niche behind a protective tympanic membrane.

Section of the posterior ampullary nerve has been advocated for relief of benign paroxysmal positional vertigo (Gacek, 1974). The singular canal which contains this nerve lies immediately inferior to the posterior attachment of the round window membrane. This membrane and the ampulla of the posterior canal are vulnerable to injury in the surgical approach to the posterior ampullary nerve.

THE SINUS TYMPANI

The sinus tympani is one of the three depressions in the medial wall of the posterior part of the mesotympanum (Fig. 3.92), the other two are the round and oval windows. Superiorly it is bounded by the ponticulus and lateral semicircular canal, posteriorly by the posterior semicircular canal, and inferiorly by the subiculum, styloid eminence, and jugular wall (Saito et al., 1971). It is bounded medially by the bony labyrinth and laterally by the pyramidal eminence and facial nerve. It extends for variable distances in a posterior direction, medial to the facial nerve (Figs. 3.93 to 3.95).

The sinus tympani may harbor diseased tissue such as cholesteatoma, and is not directly visible by the usual surgical approaches to this area (Cheatle, 1907; Ballance, 1919; Dworacek, 1960). Visualization may be facilitated by the use of mirrors, and access to its depths may be afforded by 3- or 4-mm right-angled picks and small, curved, metal suction tubes. Partial removal of the bony tympanic annulus is often necessary to gain access to the sinus tympani.

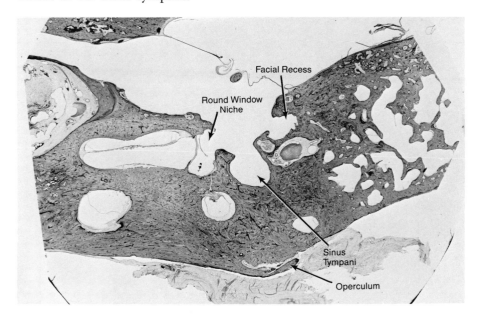

FIG. 3.92: Located lateral to the facial nerve is the facial recess and medial to it is the sinus tympani. The subiculum separates the round window niche from the sinus tympani. The operculum is a scale of bone that partly overlies the endolymphatic sac (male, age 47 years).

FIG. 3.93: The sinus tympani may extend for several millimeters medial and posterior to the facial nerve as seen in this ear. Invariably there is a bony partition between the sinus tympani and mastoid air cells due to their different routes of pneumatization (male, age 49 years).

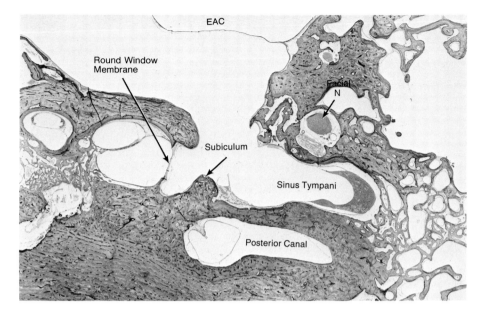

FIG. 3.94: The ponticulus (little bridge), which forms the superior boundary of the sinus tympani, stretches from the pyramidal eminence to the promontory. The facial recess lies lateral to the facial nerve and is used by otologic surgeons as a route from the mastoid to the middle ear (the posterior tympanotomy approach) (male, age 9 years).

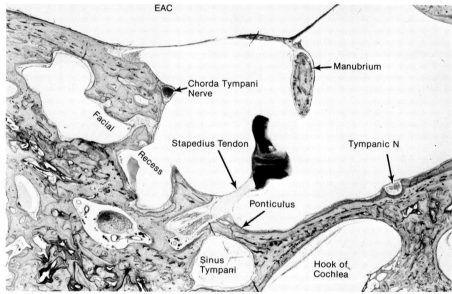

FIG. 3.95: The sinus tympani and round window niche are seen in relationship to the subiculum. The posterior ampullary nerve, located in the singular canal, is surgically accessible by an approach through the middle ear (male, age 40 years).

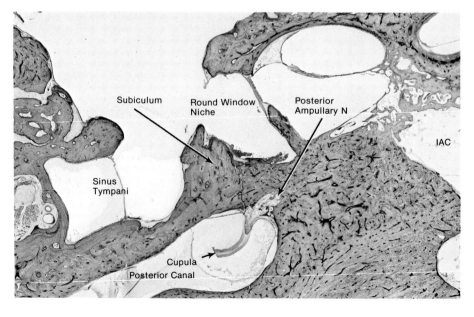

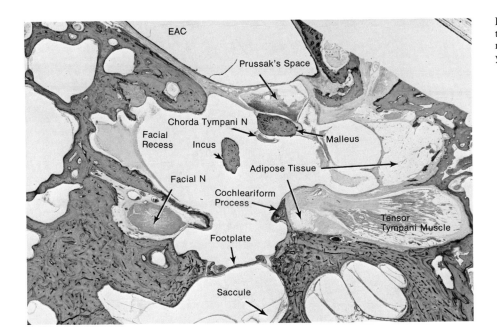

FIG. 3.96: This photomicrograph shows the anatomical relationships of several middle ear structures (female, age 60 years).

THE FACIAL RECESS

The facial recess is a depression of variable depth in the posterior wall of the middle ear. It is bounded medially by the facial canal and styloid complex and laterally by the tympanic bone (Fig. 3.96). The styloid complex (Proctor, 1969) is the term used to describe the derivatives of the superior portion of the second branchial arch; once ossified, it gives rise to three projections present in all adult temporal bones—the pyramidal, styloid, and chordal eminences. The facial recess, like the sinus tympani, is a potential site for the sequestration of disease, such as cholesteatoma.

The surgeon will find that the facial nerve is occasionally dehiscent in the medial wall of the facial recess, making it vulnerable to surgical injury (Fig. 3.97). In intact-canal-wall tympanoplasty, the route from the mastoid to the middle ear is via the facial recess, a surgical maneuver commonly known as posterior tympanotomy.

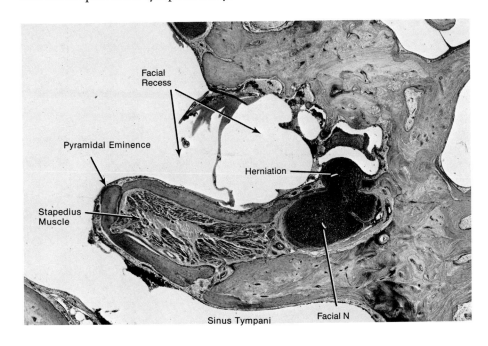

FIG. 3.97: In this ear the mastoid segment of the facial nerve bulges into the facial recess (male, age 61 years).

The Middle Ear 95

The Eustachian Tube

The eustachian tube, a mucosally lined pathway between the nasopharynx and the middle ear, permits ventilation of the pneumatized spaces of the temporal bone while safeguarding against bacterial contamination of these spaces. The posterolateral one-third is bony while the anteromedial two-thirds is fibrocartilaginous; these two sections are joined at the tubal isthmus. The overall length of the eustachian tube in the adult varies from 31 to 38 mm (Proctor, 1967, 1973).

THE BONY EUSTACHIAN TUBE

The bony part of the eustachian tube lies lateral to the internal carotid artery (Fig. 3.98); the thin bone separating these structures has dehiscences permitting the passage of the caroticotympanic arteries. The tubal isthmus marks a region of structural transition, with cartilage forming its anterolateral and superior walls and bone forming its posteromedial and inferior limits (Fig. 3.99). The lining mucosa is a low columnar ciliated epithelium with abundant goblet cells on a tunica propria of basement membrane and loose connective tissue. The tympanic ostium of the eustachian tube is in the anterior wall of the middle ear cavity, about 4 to 6 mm superior to the inferior wall of the hypotympanum. Here, the lumen is triangular, measuring 3 to 5 mm in diameter. As the osseous part of the tube heads anteriorly and inferiorly to the isthmus, its vertical diameter shrinks to 2 to 3 mm and its horizontal diameter to 1 to 1-1/2 mm.

THE FIBROCARTILAGINOUS EUSTACHIAN TUBE

This part of the tube in cross section resembles a shepherd's crook. The lumen is maintained by a larger medial cartilaginous lamella and a smaller lateral one (Fig. 3.100). The salpingopharyngeal fascia stretches between the inferior edge of the medial lamella and the free edge of the lateral lamella. The tubal incisura is a groove in the middle one-third of the inferior margin of the medial lamella which accommodates the levator veli palatini muscle.

FIG. 3.98: The next four photomicrographs are from vertical sections in the coronal plane of the eustachian tube of a 1-month old infant presented serially from posterior to anterior. This section at the tympanic orifice shows the thin bony shell separating the internal carotid artery from the cartilage of the eustachian tube. (Courtesy of Doyle & Rood.)

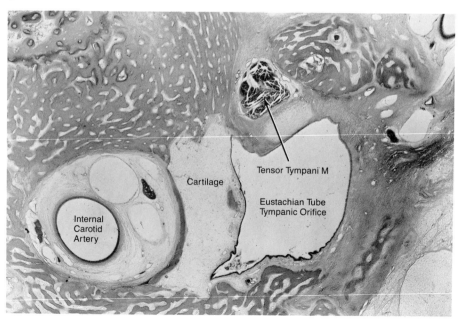

Cartilage

Tensor Tympani M

Eustachian Tube Tympanic Orifice

Internal Carotid Artery

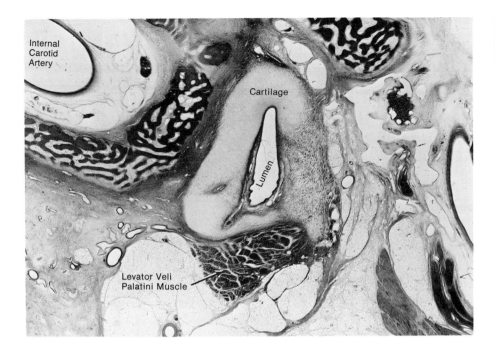

FIG. 3.99: This section shows the eustachian tube at the junction of the cartilaginous and bony portions (the isthmus tubae). (Courtesy of Doyle & Rood.)

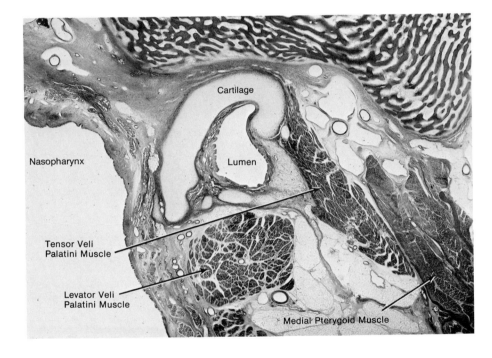

FIG. 3.100: This section shows the classical shepherd's crook (Hirtenstabkrümmung) configuration of a cross section of the cartilage of the eustachian tube. The anatomic relationships of the levator veli palatini, tensor veli palatini, and medial pterygoid muscles are shown. (Courtesy of Doyle & Rood.)

The histology of the tubal cartilage varies with age; in the newborn it is entirely hyaline, while in the adult an elastic component can be found concentrated at the inner aspect of the junction of the medial and lateral lamellae.

In the adult the nasopharyngeal orifice lies some 15 mm inferior to the tympanic ostium (Fig. 3.101). At rest the orifice is a vertical slit measuring about 8 by 4 mm. The posterior lip of the pharyngeal orifice is the mobile portion which forms the torus tubarius. The fossa of Rosenmüller is located posterior to the torus.

A series of photomicrographs showing the anatomical features of the eustachian tube of an adult is seen in Figures 3.102 to 3.105.

FIG. 3.101: The nasopharyngeal orifice of the eustachian tube is seen in this section. (Courtesy of Doyle & Rood.)

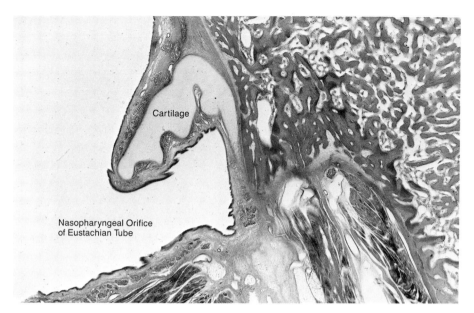

Cartilage

Nasopharyngeal Orifice
of Eustachian Tube

FIG. 3.102: The next four photomicrographs are from vertical sections in the coronal plane of the eustachian tube of an adult presented serially from posterior to anterior. A thin bony partition separates the bony eustachian tube (ET) from the internal carotid artery. (Courtesy of Sando.)

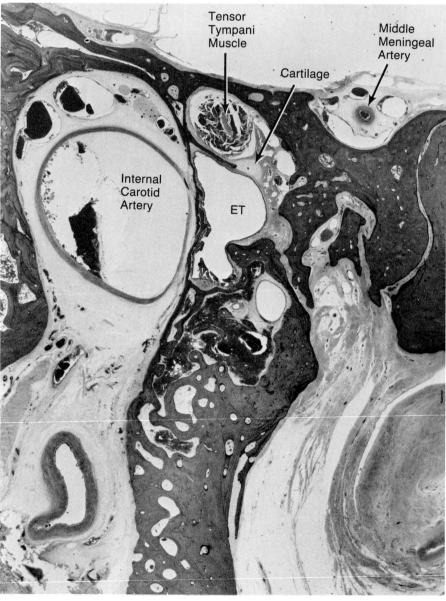

Tensor
Tympani
Muscle

Middle
Meningeal
Artery

Cartilage

Internal
Carotid
Artery

ET

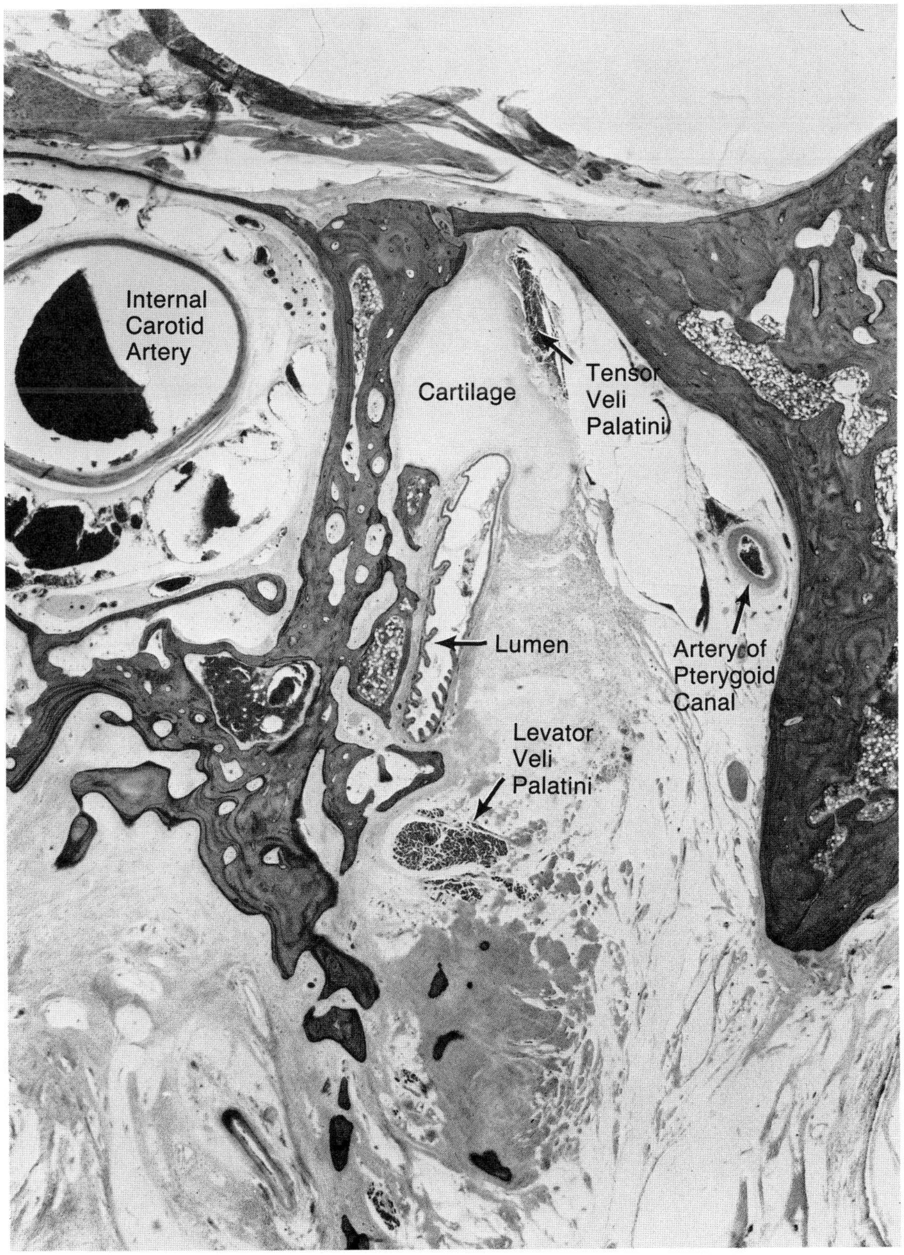

FIG. 3.103: This section of the eustachian tube, taken at its isthmus, shows its lumen and cartilage as well as adjacent structures. (Courtesy of Sando.)

THE LINING MEMBRANE

The lining (mucosal) membrane is composed of a pseudostratified, ciliated columnar epithelium interspersed with goblet cells that are most abundant at the pharyngeal orifice (Figs. 3.106 to 3.108). The supporting lamina propria is of variable thickness and can be divided into three layers: 1) a basement membrane directly beneath the epithelium, 2) a sheet of lymphoid tissue, the thickness of which varies inversely with the age of the individual, and 3) a layer of compound tubo-alveolar glands. The mucosa of the eustachian tube consists of pseudostratified ciliated columnar cells mixed with a cuboidal ciliated epithelium and goblet cells (Lim, 1974). Some authors (Eggston & Wolff, 1947; Aschan, 1955) believe that lymphatic tissue of the nasopharynx never reaches up to, or into, the pharyngeal orifice of the eustachian tube but occurs as a distinct extra-tubal lymphoid mass (the so-called Gerlach's tubal tonsil).

FIG. 3.104: The relationship of the cartilaginous part of the eustachian tube to the tensor and levator veli palatini muscles is shown. (Courtesy of Sando.)

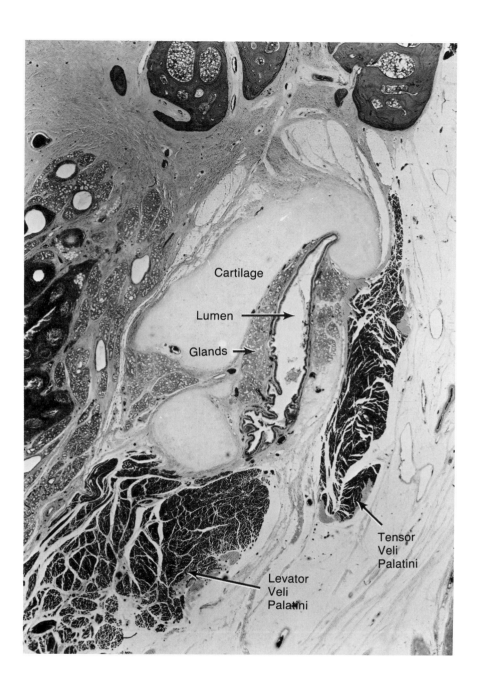

Cartilage

Lumen →

Glands →

Tensor Veli Palatini

Levator Veli Palatini

THE PALATAL MUSCLES

The tensor veli palatini muscle arises from the spine of the sphenoid bone, the scaphoid fossa, the lateral lamina of the tubal cartilage, and the salpingopharyngeal fascia (Graves & Edwards, 1944) to run a course nearly parallel to the slit-like lumen of the tube. Anteroinferiorly, it forms a tendon which sweeps around the hamulus of the medial pterygoid plate and inserts medially into the soft palate. Its crucial role in tubal opening is to draw the lateral lamella of the tubal cartilage inferiorly. Some of its fibers are thought to be continuous with those of the tensor tympani muscle (Lupin, 1969; see p. 84 and Fig. 3.78). Its innervation is derived from the mandibular division of the trigeminal nerve.

The levator veli palatini muscle arises from the inferior aspect of the petrous bone anterior to the carotid canal, as well as from the medial cartilaginous lamina of the eustachian tube. The belly of this muscle de-

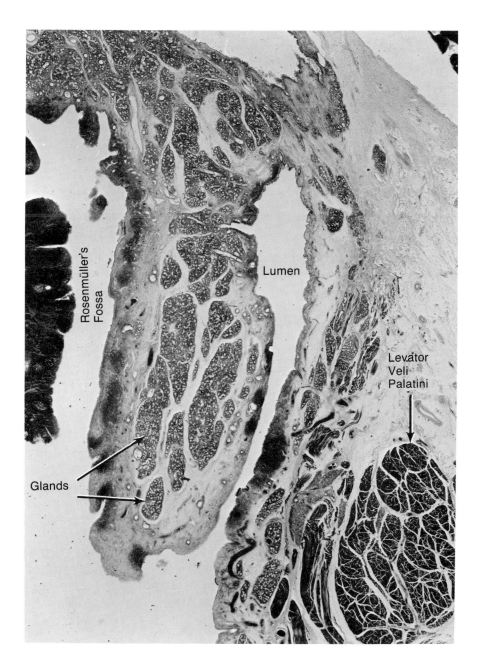

Rosenmüller's Fossa

Lumen

Levator Veli Palatini

Glands

FIG. 3.105: The pharyngeal orifice of the eustachian tube is seen in this view. Also shown are Rosenmüller's fossa and the levator veli palatini muscle. (Courtesy of Sando.)

scends parallel to the tube to insert into the soft palate. Upon stimulation through the pharyngeal plexus of the vagus, the levator veli palatini muscle shortens and thickens, thus elevating the eustachian tube and widening its lumen (Fig. 3.100).

The salpingopharyngeus muscle originates from the inferior aspect of the medial cartilaginous lamella of the eustachian tube and divides inferiorly to insert into the posterior wall of the pharynx and onto the superior horn of the thyroid cartilage. It also is innervated by the vagus nerve.

In its resting position, the eustachian tube is closed due to a combination of passive mechanisms including the elasticity of the cartilage, pressure from surrounding tissues, and the capillary force of apposed moist mucous membranes (Aschan, 1955). With deglutition or yawning, the tensor veli palatini, the levator veli palatini, and the salpingopharyngeus muscles act in concert to open the tube (Aschan, 1955; Proctor, 1967, 1973).

FIG. 3.106: This photomicrograph and the following two magnified views from the outlined areas A and B, are from horizontal sections of a newborn infant.

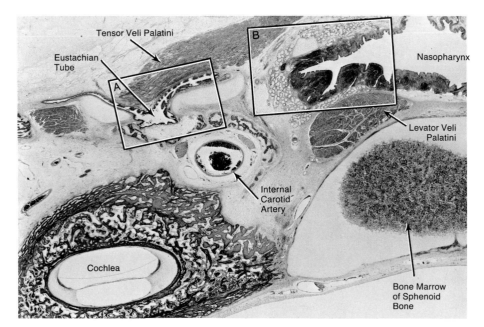

FIG. 3.107: This magnified view of area A in Figure 3.106 shows the respiratory epithelium of the fibrocartilaginous part of the eustachian tube.

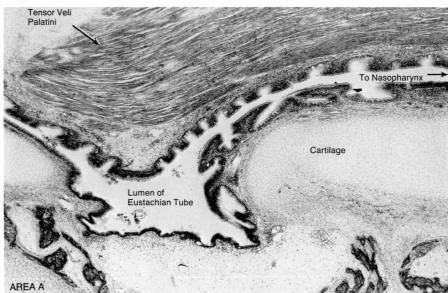

FIG. 3.108: This magnified view of area B in Figure 3.106 shows the mucous glands and lymphoid tissue at the naso-pharyngeal orifice of the eustachian tube.

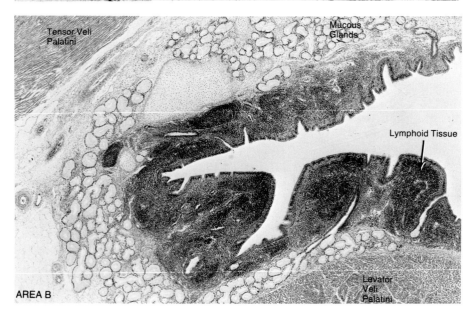

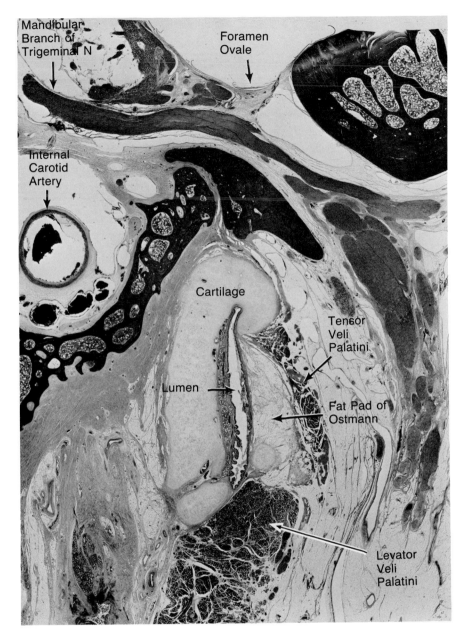

Mandibular Branch of Trigeminal N

Foramen Ovale

Internal Carotid Artery

Cartilage

Tensor Veli Palatini

Lumen

Fat Pad of Ostmann

Levator Veli Palatini

FIG. 3.109: This photo shows the mid-portion of the eustachian tube and adjacent anatomic structures. (Courtesy of Sando et al., in press.)

Dysfunctions of the mechanisms controlling tubal function cause: 1) serous otitis (otitis media with effusion) when the tube fails to open on swallowing and 2) the patulous tube syndrome (autophony) when it fails to close. Another dysfunction of this mechanism is palatal myoclonus in which clonic spasms of the levator palatini and/or tensor tympani muscles cause an annoying clicking sensation in the ear. The function of the eustachian tube is affected by the amount of peritubal adiposity (fat pad of Ostmann) (Ostmann, 1893) (Fig. 3.109). Obesity may lead to eustachian tube obstruction, while loss of body weight may cause tubal patency.

The Middle Ear Mucosa

HISTOLOGY

A knowledge of the structure of the normal mucosa of the human middle ear, mastoid, and eustachian tube will help in understanding the mechanisms involved in otitis media and middle ear effusions (Fig. 3.110).

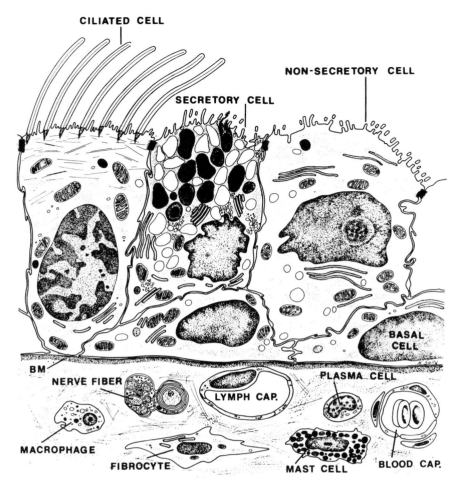

In electron microscopic observations, Hentzer (1970) distinguished five types of cells in the middle ear mucosa: 1) nonciliated without secretory granules, 2) nonciliated with secretory granules, 3) ciliated, 4) intermediate, and 5) basal. He analyzed the distribution of these five types of cells within the middle ear, mastoid, and eustachian tube and divided them into seven regions: 1) The mastoid contained ciliated cells and nonciliated cells without secretory granules. 2) The posterior part of the middle ear had a thicker epithelium with two additional types of cells—nonciliated cells with secretory granules and basal cells. Simple squamous epithelium without cilia could also be found. 3) The epitympanic recess was lined with epithelium similar to that of the posterior part of the middle ear; however, simple nonciliated squamous epithelium could also be found. 4) In the area of the promontory, pseudostratified ciliated columnar epithelium predominated over ciliated cuboidal epithelium. Goblet cells as well as intraepithelial and submucosal glands were seen. Simple nonciliated squamous epithelium no longer appeared. 5) At the tympanic orifice of the eustachian tube the epithelium was similar to that of the promontory, save for less frequent glands and more nonciliated cells with secretory granules. 6) The pars flaccida possessed a simple nonciliated epithelium. 7) The epithelium of the pars tensa varied in height from pseudostratified, ciliated columnar to simple, nonciliated cuboidal. Mature goblet cells were not found on the tympanic membrane.

Hentzer (1970) concluded that the mucosa of the middle ear represents a modified respiratory mucosa. He proposed that the nonciliated cell was its sole secretory structure which, in its most active secretory phase, resembled a goblet cell.

THE MUCOCILIARY TRANSPORT SYSTEM

The secretions produced by the glands and goblet cells produce a mucous blanket and the ciliated cells mobilize this blanket to create the mucociliary transport system. Studies by Shimada and Lim (1972), Lim et al. (1973), and Lim (1974, 1979) have demonstrated that the distribution of the ciliated cells corresponds to that of the secretory cells. Metachronal motion (coordinated beating) of the cilia is responsible for propelling the mucous blanket. By using 6 power or higher magnification, ciliary activity can frequently be observed in the anterior part of the hypotympanum through a perforation of the tympanic membrane. Light reflections in the mucous sheath will be observed to be shimmering.

Lim (1979) describes three distinct mucociliary tracts in the tympanic cavity: 1) a hypotympanic tract commencing in the hypotympanum and leading into the eustachian tube, 2) an epitympanic tract from the epitympanum to the eustachian tube, and 3) a promontory tract leading from the promontory to the eustachian tube (Lim, 1979). The eustachian tube likewise possesses a mucociliary transport system; its lining cells are believed to secrete a surface-active agent (like a surfactant) which reduces surface tension, thus facilitating tubal opening (Birken & Brookler, 1973). The mastoid air cells do not appear to have a mucociliary transport system.

Blockage of the eustachian tube in children characteristically results in a seromucinous fluid in the tympanomastoid compartment, whereas in adults the fluid is serous. The difference is probably related to an associated inflammatory reaction in children, causing hyperactivity of the mucous producing goblet cells and glands.

A perforation of the tympanic membrane in association with a blocked eustachian tube may cause a mucoid otorrhea, especially in children.

THE IMMUNE SYSTEM OF THE MIDDLE EAR

Another defense mechanism in the middle ear involves the secretion of immunoglobulin-A (IgA) and the antibacterial enzyme, lysozyme, by the mucosal epithelium (Liu et al., 1975). Tissue macrophages are also seen in normal human middle ear mucosa (Lim, 1974). Acid phosphatase, a cytochemical marker for lysosomes (Novikoff & Essner, 1962), has been found in the epithelium of normal mucosa, although its exact cellular location is undetermined (Hiraide & Paparella, 1972; Lim et al., 1972). Possibly some of the lysosomal enzymes are integrated into the enzymatic defense of the middle ear by the mucosal secretory cells. Tracer studies (Lim & Hussl, 1975) have documented pinocytosis of tracer particles by the surface epithelium; these particles then either enter the blood or lymphatic circulation or are acted upon by the tissue macrophages of the submucosa.

Thus, the submucosa also participates in middle ear defense. This thin connective tissue layer consists of fibroblasts and fibrocytes with their associated collagen fibers. Scattered wandering tissue phagocytes, occasional plasma cells and lymphocytes, as well as sporadic clumps of mast cells are also present in the submucosa; it is permeated by a multitude of blood and lymph capillaries, and there is an abundance of nerve fibers. Plasma cells producing immunoglobulins A, E, G and M have been detected in the submucosa by immunohistochemical methods; in contrast, only IgA-stain-

FIG. 3.111: This view shows the tympanic membrane and ossicular anatomy at the level of the lateral process of the malleus. The posterior pouch of von Tröltsch is bounded medially by the posterior malleal fold (male, age 63 years).

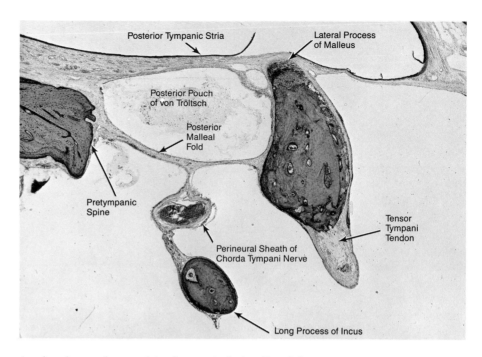

FIG. 3.111: This view shows the tympanic membrane and ossicular anatomy at the level of the lateral process of the malleus. The posterior pouch of von Tröltsch is bounded medially by the posterior malleal fold (male, age 63 years).

ing has been observed in the epithelial cells of the mucosa (by immunofluorescence techniques; Sainte-Marie, 1962). These immunoglobulins are believed to play a role in local immunocompetency (Tomasi, 1976).

THE MUCOSAL FOLDS

The middle ear is completely lined by a mucous membrane that is continuous with the mucosa of the eustachian tube and the mastoid antrum (for histology see p. 104). It also extends from the walls of the tympanic cavity to envelop the middle ear structures such as the ossicles with their various ligaments and the tendons of the intratympanic muscles. In doing so, the mucosa forms several folds and pouches. As the mucosa drapes over the anterior process and anterior ligament of the malleus, as well as the closely associated chorda tympani nerve, it forms the *anterior malleal fold*. This fold extends from the notch of Rivinus to the head and neck of the malleus and, in conjunction with the anterior tympanic stria (see tympanic membrane, p. 45), encloses a blind pouch, the anterior pouch of von Tröltsch. The *posterior malleal fold* envelops the posterior segment of the chorda tympani nerve as the latter stretches from the pretympanic spine to the neck of the malleus. The posterior pouch of von Tröltsch lies between the posterior malleal fold and the posterior tympanic stria. In Figure 3.111, Prussak's space communicates with the posterior pouch of von Tröltsch. As the mucosa descends from the roof of the tympanic cavity to cover the body and short process of the incus, it forms the *incudal fold*. The stapes, including the obturator foramen, is sheathed by an extension of mucosa from the posterior tympanic wall referred to as the *stapedial fold*.

Proctor (1964) produced an exhaustive description of the genesis of these folds as well as detailed diagrams of their anatomy. Their constancy is related to the development of the tubotympanic recess as an outpouching of the nasopharynx (see embryology, Chapter 9). By approximately 28 weeks' gestation, four buds known as primary sacs or pouches invade the middle ear cavity: 1) The saccus anticus, the smallest of the four, forms the anterior pouch of von Tröltsch as it extends superiorly, anterior to the tendon of the tensor tympani muscle. 2) The saccus medius also reaches superiorly, forming the attic; it then sprouts three saccules. The anterior

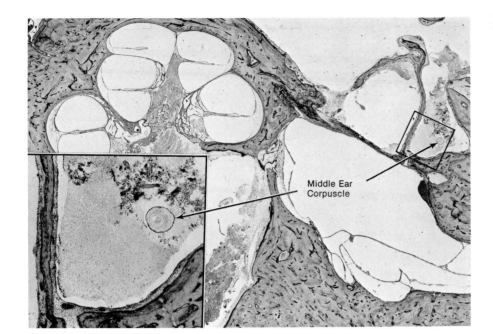

Fig. 3.112: Middle ear corpuscles may be of variable size and are found scattered throughout the middle ear and mastoid. They have not been found in ears having previous otitis media or in children less than 6 years of age (male, age 65 years). Their function, if any, is unknown.

Middle Ear
Corpuscle

saccule gives rise to the anterior compartment of the attic, while the medial saccule develops into the superior incudal recess. The posterior saccule is responsible for the pneumatization of the petrous part of the mastoid air cell system. 3) The saccus superioris forms the posterior pouch of von Tröltsch and the inferior incudal recess as it expands posterolaterally between the manubrium and the distal aspect of the long process of the incus. With continued posterior expansion, the saccus superioris also extends medially, entering the antrum and eventually pneumatizing the pars squamosa of the temporal bone. 4) The saccus posticus courses in the hypotympanum and forms the round window niche, the sinus tympani, and the majority of the oval window niche. Mucosal folds, carrying the vessels which supply the ossicles (much like the abdominal mesentery), develop where these four major sacs come into contact with each other.

According to Proctor (1964), the various compartments of the ear defined by these folds limit, at least in early stages, the extent of disease processes such as cholesteatoma, and also designate probable routes of extension of disease. Proctor believes that as long as the mucosal folds are intact, it is possible to remove a cholesteatoma and its lining epithelium and still preserve the integrity of the particular middle ear compartment involved and the blood supply of the ossicles. Clinical observations indicate, however, that these folds have minimal influence on the location or magnitude of advanced disease in the tympanomastoid compartment.

THE MIDDLE EAR CORPUSCLES

The presence of a small "oval body" near the tympanic membrane was first noted in 1859 by von Tröltsch (cited by Kessel, 1870); he considered it a pathologic entity, having seen it in the ear of an elderly woman with hearing loss. Politzer (1869) and Kessel (1870) described similar structures tethered by connective tissue in the middle ear, antrum, and mastoid; they thought that these structures were physiologic rather than pathologic (Fig. 3.112).

Gussen (1970) studied 77 adult human temporal bones, all without evidence of infection, and found "Pacinian corpuscles" (her terminology) in the middle ears of all specimens examined. She emphasized that their

Fig. 3.113: In this sketch each black dot represents the location of a middle ear corpuscle as found in 151 temporal bones by Lim et al. (1975).

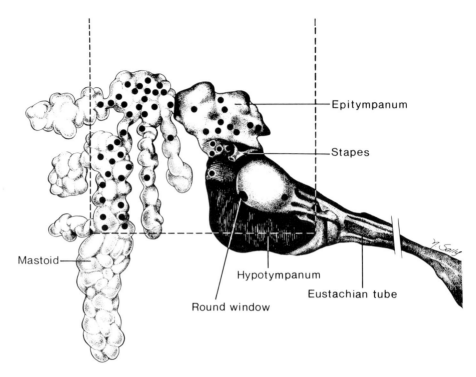

Fig. 3.113: In this sketch each black dot represents the location of a middle ear corpuscle as found in 151 temporal bones by Lim et al. (1975).

suspension from mucosal-mesentery folds was consistently in relation to either of the three ossicles or to the stapedius or tensor tympani tendons. She hypothesized that they have a kinesthetic receptor capacity of maintenance and coordination of the movements of the ossicles.

Lim et al. (1975) disputed these findings. They studied 124 temporal bones by light microscopy and an additional 27 temporal bones with the electron microscope. While the middle ear corpuscles are most commonly located in the mastoid antrum and epitympanic recess, they also occur throughout the mastoid cavity (Fig. 3.113). There was great variability in size, ranging from 0.8 to 10 mm in length and 0.4 to 2.5 mm in diameter. Histologic study showed these round or elliptical bodies (Fig. 3.114) to consist of an encircling mucous membrane, an outer capsule of concentri-

Fig. 3.114: This cross section of a middle ear corpuscle shows its multilaminar structure. There is a distinct central core surrounded by a laminated capsule, all enveloped in a surface lining of mucous membrane (male, age 47 years).

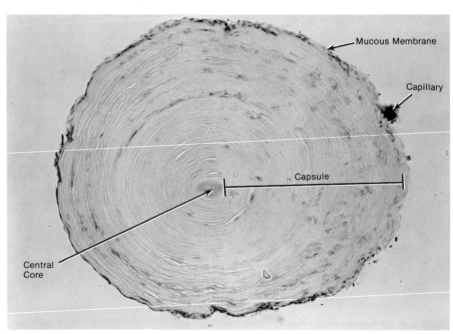

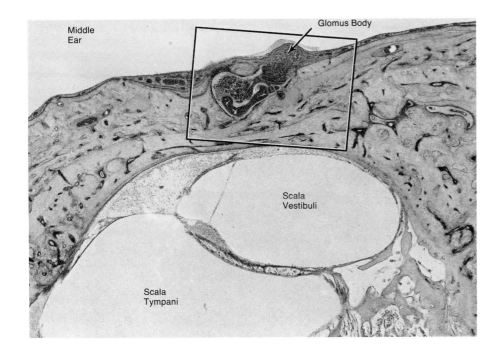

Middle Ear

Glomus Body

Scala Vestibuli

Scala Tympani

FIG. 3.115: There is a normal glomus body on the promontory of the cochlea in association with the tympanic branch of the glossopharyngeal nerve (female, age 68 years). (See Fig. 3.116.)

cally laminated collagen fibers and fibrocytes, and a central core. Electron microscopic study of the central core failed to reveal any nerve fibers— only homogeneous ground substance was found. These bodies were not found in specimens from patients less than 6 years old or from those with a history of chronic otitis media, otitis media with effusion, or mastoiditis. Although this study did not reveal the functional nature of these middle ear corpuscles, it provided evidence which invalidates the concept of their being Pacinian corpuscles. While they have no known physiologic function, they may be viewed with some curiosity by the otologic microsurgeon seeing them for the first time.

GLOMUS BODIES

Glomus bodies occurring in the middle ear were first described by Guild (1941) as glomus jugulare (glomus jugularis) formations. Glomus formations may be found anywhere along the course of Arnold's nerve (tympanic branch of the vagus) as far distally as the intersection with the descending portion of the facial nerve, and also along Jacobson's nerve (the tympanic branch of the glossopharyngeal nerve) (Figs. 3.115 and 3.116). Guild (1953) determined that just over 50% of the glomus formations were situated in the region of the jugular fossa accompanying either of the above-mentioned nerves or in the adventitia of the jugular bulb. Less frequently they are found in the tympanic canaliculus or in the mastoid segment of the facial canal.

The glomus body tumor is the most commonly found neoplasm in the middle ear (Spector et al., 1973). This relatively benign neoplasm is also known as carotid body-like tumor (Rosenwasser, 1945), glomus jugulare tumor (Winship et al., 1948), nonchromaffin paraganglioma (Lattes & Waltner, 1949), chemodectoma (Mulligan, 1950), receptoma (Gaffney, 1953), and glomerocytoma (Zettergren & Lindstrom, 1951). The most commonly recognized appellation is that of glomus tumor. The term "glo-

FIG. 3.116: Here is a higher magnification of the outlined area in Figure 3.115 showing details of the glomus body (female, age 68 years).

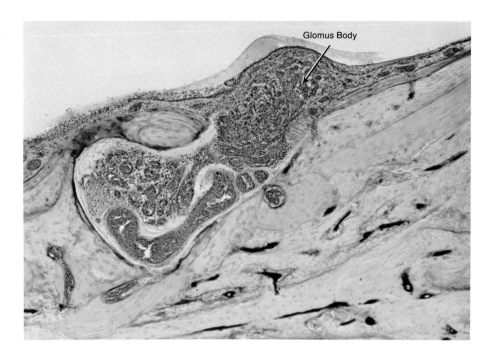

mus tympanicum" is reserved for those tumors arising in the mesotympanum, while those arising in the hypotympanum are designated as glomus jugulare (Alford & Guilford, 1962).

Glomus jugulare neoplasms tend to extend into the infralabyrinthine cells, an area that is demonstrated in Figure 3.83. In well pneumatized temporal bones the growth will then extend anteriorly into the petrous apex and pericarotid areas (Fig. 4.1) and occasionally into the mastoid and jugular vein. Surgical removal requires careful planning of the surgical approach to prevent or minimize hearing loss.

4. Pneumatization

The extent of pneumatization of the normal human temporal bone is variable (Hagens, 1934; Meltzer, 1934; Tremble, 1934; Lindsay, 1940, 1941). The growth pattern is thought to be controlled by heredity, environment, nutrition, bacterial infections, and the adequacy of ventilation as determined by eustachian tube function.

Hug and Pfaltz (1981) conducted a planimetric study of temporal bone pneumatization by x-ray examination in 73 children, evaluating normal ears as well as those with middle ear disease. They found that both otitis media with effusion and recurrent suppurative otitis media had an inhibitory effect upon the pneumatization process. They also presented data indicating that after infection is controlled, pneumatization again proceeds. They noted, however, that in no case could they observe a normal-sized air cell system once the pneumatization process had been inhibited.

The reader's understanding of the three-dimensional anatomy of the pneumatization of the temporal bone will be enhanced by the study of stereo views of celloidin blocks (Reels I and II) as well as stereo views of surgical dissection (Reels III through VI).

The pneumatized spaces of the temporal bone may be divided into five regions which are further subdivided into areas. A diagrammatic sketch showing most of the regions, areas, and tracts is seen in Figure 4.1, and the complete classification appears below (Allam, 1969).

PNEUMATIZED SPACES OF THE TEMPORAL BONE

A. Middle Ear Region
1. Mesotympanic area
2. Epitympanic area
3. Hypotympanic area
4. Protympanic area
5. Posterior tympanic area

B. Mastoid Region
1. Mastoid antrum area
2. Central mastoid tract
3. Peripheral mastoid areas
   (a) Tegmental cells
   (b) Sinodural cells
   (c) Sinal cells
   (d) Facial cells
   (e) Tip cells

C. Perilabyrinthine Region
1. Supralabyrinthine area
2. Infralabyrinthine area

D. Petrous Apex Region
1. Peritubal area
2. Apical area

E. Accessory Region
1. Zygomatic area
2. Squamous area
3. Occipital area
4. Styloid area

F. Tracts of Pneumatization
1. Posterosuperior tract
2. Posteromedial tract
3. Subarcuate tract
4. Perilabyrinthine tracts
5. Peritubal tracts

FIG. 4.1: Two vertical planes, one passing through the plane of the superior canal and another through the axis of the modiolus, serve to demarcate the mastoid, perilabyrinthine, and petrous apex regions of pneumatization of the temporal bone. The perilabyrinthine region can be further subdivided into infralabyrinthine and supralabyrinthine areas; in the petrous apex, peritubal and apical areas are recognized.

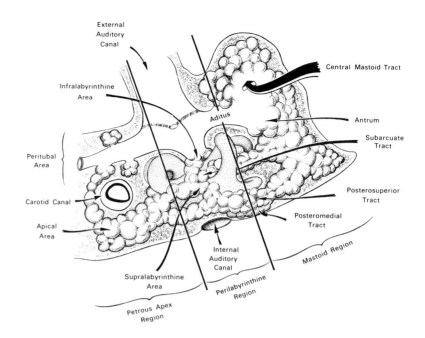

The Middle Ear Region

The middle ear region may be divided into five areas: 1) a mesotympanic area that lies medial to the pars tensa, 2) an epitympanic area that lies superior to a horizontal plane passing through the anterior and posterior tympanic striae, 3) a hypotympanic area located inferior to a horizontal plane passing through the most inferior level of the tympanic annulus, 4) a protympanic area, occupying that space anterior to a frontal plane passing through the anterior margin of the tympanic annulus, and 5) a posterior tympanic area located posterior to a frontal plane passing through the posterior margin of the tympanic annulus and including the sinus tympani and facial recess. For detailed anatomy see middle ear spaces (Chapter 3, p. 86).

The Mastoid Region

At birth the mastoid has a single cavity consisting of the antrum and small adjacent mastoid. It occupies a superficial position and is surrounded by diploic bone (Figs. 4.2 to 4.4).

In adult life the normal mastoid may be fully pneumatized, diploic, or sclerotic. In the diploic and sclerotic types, pneumatization is limited mainly to the antra and central mastoid tracts. The diploic type contains soft tissue in the form of bone marrow, whereas the sclerotic type consists predominantly of dense bone (Figs. 4.5 to 4.8). Even narrow mastoids may be well pneumatized (Figs. 4.9 and 4.10). Surgical access to the middle ear via the facial recess (posterior tympanotomy approach) is difficult or impossible in narrow mastoids such as those shown in Figures 4.5, 4.7, and 4.9.

In an examination of 250 adult human temporal bones, Zuckerkandl (1879) found 36.8% to be completely pneumatized, 43.2% to be partially pneumatized and partially diploic, and 20% to be completely diploic or sclerotic.

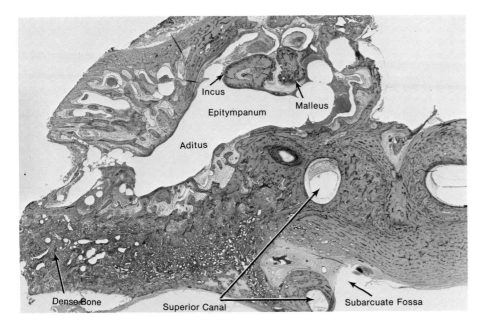

Labels on Fig. 4.2: Incus, Epitympanum, Malleus, Aditus, Dense Bone, Superior Canal, Subarcuate Fossa

FIG. 4.2: The following three photos are from the same temporal bone of a 41-day-old female infant. This view of a superior level shows the pneumatization of the epitympanum and aditus for this age. Occasionally mesenchyme will persist in the epitympanum and mastoid for some months after birth. The periantral cells have not yet appeared. The subarcuate fossa leads to the petromastoid canal, which in turn passes between the limbs of the superior canal.

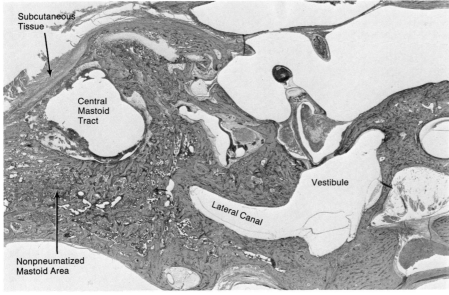

Labels on Fig. 4.3: Subcutaneous Tissue, Central Mastoid Tract, Nonpneumatized Mastoid Area, Lateral Canal, Vestibule

FIG. 4.3: At the level of the oval window there is pneumatization of the middle ear and central mastoid tract which is appropriate for this age (41 days). The cortical bone of the mastoid is normally thin.

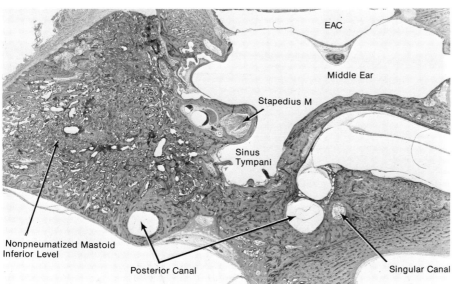

Labels on Fig. 4.4: EAC, Middle Ear, Stapedius M, Sinus Tympani, Nonpneumatized Mastoid Inferior Level, Posterior Canal, Singular Canal

FIG. 4.4: At a more inferior level the hypotympanum is seen to be fully pneumatized. The mastoid consists of solid bone. As the embryo nears term the resolution of mesenchyme proceeds from the hypotympanum and mesotympanum to the epitympanum and mastoid (female, age 41 days).

Pneumatization 113

Fig. 4.5: This section shows a lack of mastoid air cell development without evidence of inflammatory disease. The small mastoid is associated with an anterior and lateral location of the sigmoid sinus (male, age 79 years).

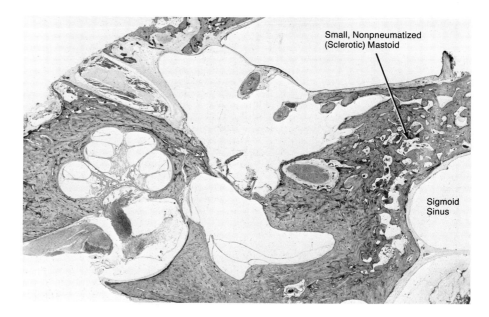

Fig. 4.6: The mastoid is markedly sclerotic in this specimen. Pathologic changes in the tympanic membrane document the previous occurrence of otitis media. The petrous apex contains bone marrow (female, age 65 years).

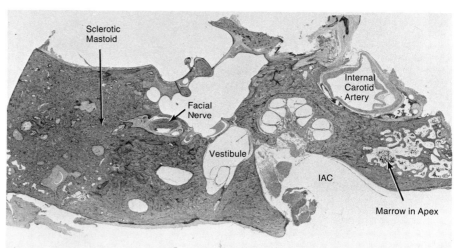

Fig. 4.7: A narrow mastoid is seen in association with a laterally situated sigmoid (lateral venous) sinus. The operculum overlying the endolymphatic sac is demonstrated. An otosclerotic focus is present anterior to the oval window. There is no evidence of previous otitis media (female, age 80 years).

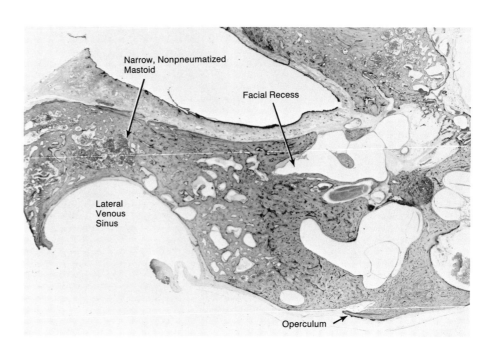

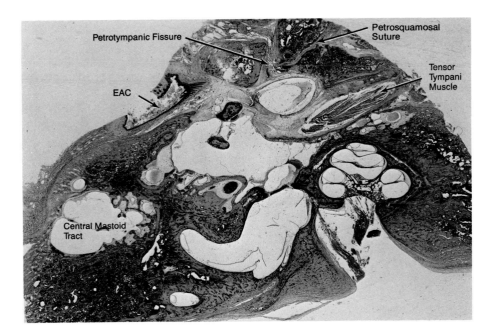

Labels on figure: Petrotympanic Fissure, Petrosquamosal Suture, EAC, Tensor Tympani Muscle, Central Mastoid Tract

FIG. 4.8: The middle ear and upper portion of the central mastoid tract are well pneumatized in this 9-week-old infant. Sclerotic bone surrounds the central mastoid tract. The bone of the mastoid cortex is normally thin.

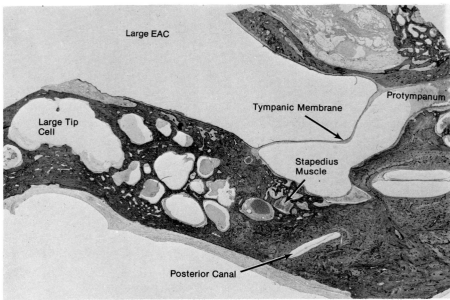

Labels on figure: Large EAC, Large Tip Cell, Tympanic Membrane, Protympanum, Stapedius Muscle, Posterior Canal

FIG. 4.9: In contrast to the large external auditory canal (EAC), the mastoid is narrow, although well pneumatized. The large tip cell abuts the bony external auditory canal (male, age 73 years).

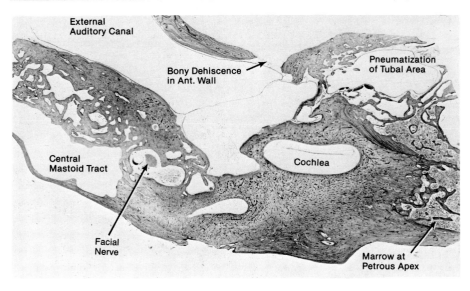

Labels on figure: External Auditory Canal, Bony Dehiscence in Ant. Wall, Pneumatization of Tubal Area, Central Mastoid Tract, Cochlea, Facial Nerve, Marrow at Petrous Apex

FIG. 4.10: This temporal bone shows a well-pneumatized narrow mastoid. The peritubal area is well pneumatized. The bony dehiscence of the anterior wall of the external auditory canal is an occasionally occurring anatomic variant (male, age 22 years).

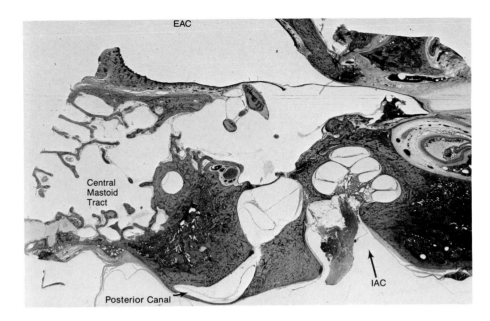

FIG. 4.11: The temporal bone of this 8-month-old infant shows advanced pneumatization of the mastoid but inhibited perilabyrinthine pneumatization; thus, the internal auditory canal (IAC) is short and wide and the posterior canal bulges into the posterior fossa. Anteriorly, the pars tensa has been artifactually separated from the tympanic annulus.

In temporal bones with inhibited pneumatization of the perilabyrinthine areas, the posterior canal may form a prominence on the posterior surface of the petrous bone (Fig. 4.11). The arcuate eminence, which marks the location of the superior canal in the floor of the middle cranial fossa, is also emphasized by inhibited pneumatization of this area of the temporal bone.

The anterolateral portion of the mastoid arises from the squamous part of the temporal bone; the posteromedial portion, including the mastoid tip, arises from the petrous part. The delineation of these areas is indicated on the outer surface by the petromastoid fissure, which is usually obliterated in early adult life. In most mastoids the plane of junction of these two parts is marked internally by an incomplete plate of bone, the petrosquamosal septum, also known as Koerner's septum (Møller, 1930). This bony partition is of variable thickness and descends to variable depths; in extensively pneumatized bones it may be missing altogether. Proctor (1964) proposes that Koerner's septum is the consequence of the "persistence and further development of the mucosal fold between saccus superior and saccus medius in the antrum and mastoid of the adult."

FIG. 4.12: The division of the mastoid into an anterolateral squamous portion and a posteromedial petrous portion by Koerner's septum is demonstrated in this photograph (female, age 65 years).

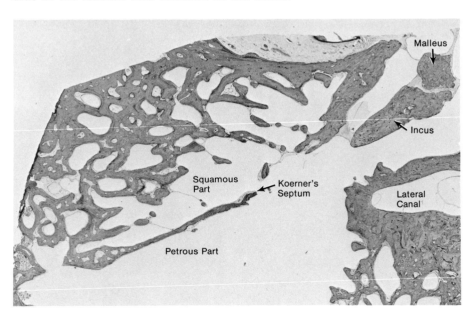

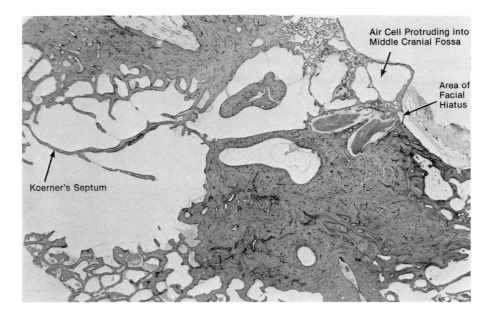

Air Cell Protruding into Middle Cranial Fossa

Area of Facial Hiatus

Koerner's Septum

FIG. 4.13: Koerner's septum delineates a normally smaller squamous part from the larger petrous part of the mastoid. In this specimen the anterior epitympanic recess protrudes into the middle cranial fossa (male, age 76 years).

When encountered during surgical procedures, Koerner's septum may be confused with the medial wall of the antrum (Figs. 4.12 to 4.14). The identity of Koerner's septum becomes obvious when it is realized that the usual anatomic landmarks such as the tegmen of the mastoid, the prominence of the lateral canal, the lateral venous sinus, and the antrum are not in view.

The mastoid region can be divided into three areas (Fig. 4.15): 1) The mastoid antrum area is a large superior central space which communicates with the epitympanic space of the middle ear via the aditus. The lateral wall is formed by the squamous part of the temporal bone. 2) The central mastoid tract area extends inferiorly from the mastoid antrum (Fig. 4.16). It may consist of a single space of varying size or of a series of cells and may be partly divided by the petrosquamosal (Koerner's) septum. 3) The peripheral mastoid area has five cell groups consisting of (a) the tegmental cells bordering the tegmen and lying superiorly in the mastoid bone, (b) the sinodural cells occupying the posterosuperior angle of the mastoid bone and bounded superiorly by the dural plate of bone as well as posteroinfer-

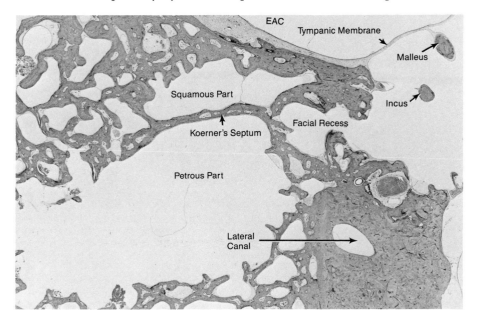

EAC

Tympanic Membrane

Malleus

Squamous Part

Incus

Facial Recess

Koerner's Septum

Petrous Part

Lateral Canal

FIG. 4.14: This more inferior view of the same ear shown in Figure 4.12 demonstrates the smaller size of the anterolateral squamous part when compared to the larger posteromedial part of the mastoid. Because of the differing origins of their pneumatization, the facial recess and mastoid are always separated by a bony partition (female, age 65 years).

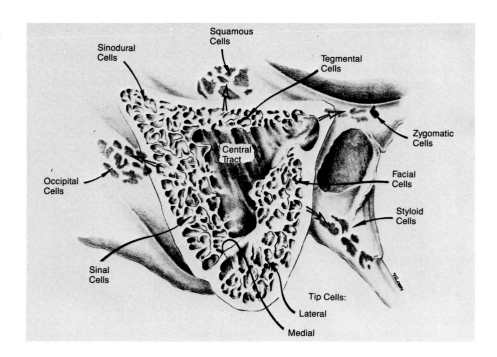

FIG. 4.15: This diagrammatic sketch illustrates the areas of pneumatization of the mastoid region and accessory regions of the temporal bone.

iorly by the sinus plate of bone, (c) the sinal cells lying lateral, medial, and posterior to the sigmoid sinus, (d) the facial cells lying in relation to the mastoid segment of the facial nerve, and (e) the tip cells occupying the inferior projection of the mastoid bone and divided by the digastric ridge into medial and lateral groups.

The Perilabyrinthine Region

The perilabyrinthine region is subdivided into: 1) the supralabyrinthine area (Fig. 4.24) and 2) the infralabyrinthine area (Fig. 4.17) which lie superior and inferior to the labyrinth, respectively.

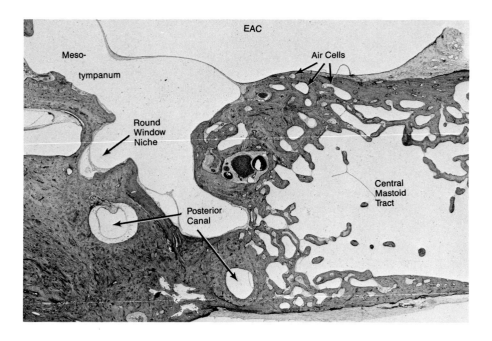

FIG. 4.16: The central mastoid tract extends inferiorly from the antrum and is surrounded by smaller air cells, some of which may extend into the cortex of the posterior wall of the external auditory canal (EAC) (female, age 58 years).

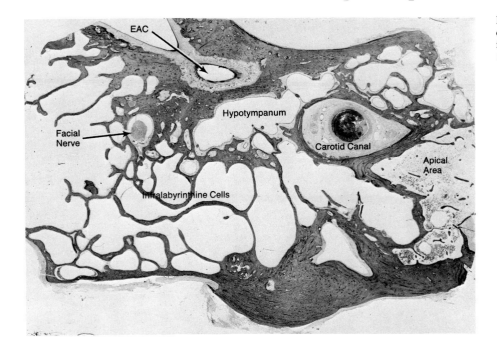

FIG. 4.17: This photomicrograph shows extensive pneumatization of the infralabyrinthine area (female, age 16 years).

The Petrous Apex Region

The petrous apex region is divided into: 1) the peritubal area (Figs. 4.18, 4.19) which surrounds the osseous portion of the eustachian tube and lies anterolateral to the carotid canal, and 2) the apical area (Figs. 4.20 to 4.24) which lies anteromedial to the carotid canal. Peritubal pneumatization is common; however, the apical area is not usually pneumatized (Fig. 4.25).

To the surgeon, the apical area is the most remote part of the temporal bone. It may be pneumatized by the peritubal, perilabyrinthine, posterosuperior, posteromedial, and subarcuate cell tracts. Surgical access for drainage of purulent accumulations (petrous apicitis) can usually be accomplished by following one of these routes (Jones, 1935; Mayer, 1937;

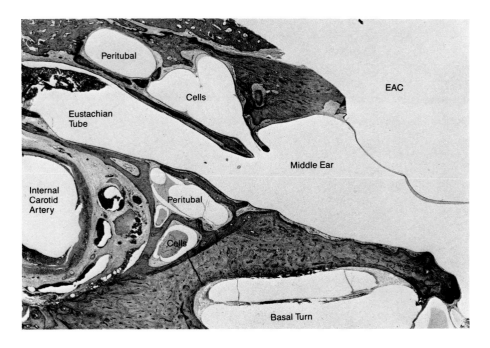

FIG. 4.18: In this ear peritubal air cells are located both medial and lateral to the eustachian tube. The internal carotid artery is separated from the bony part of the eustachian tube by a thin plate of bone (male, age 74 years).

FIG. 4.19: There is a dehiscence of the anterior wall of the external auditory canal. This anatomic variant is of significance in surgical procedures in this area (male, age 53 years).

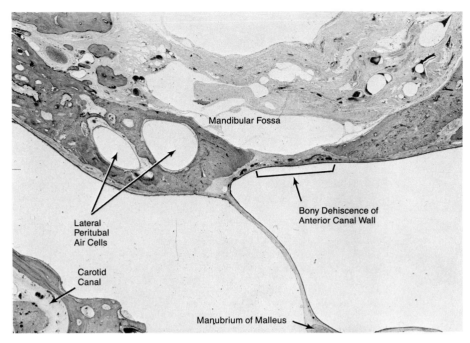

FIG. 4.20: This temporal bone shows extensive pneumatization of the peritubal and apical areas of the petrous apex region. Peritubal cells frequently serve as a route of pneumatization to the apical area (female, age 89 years).

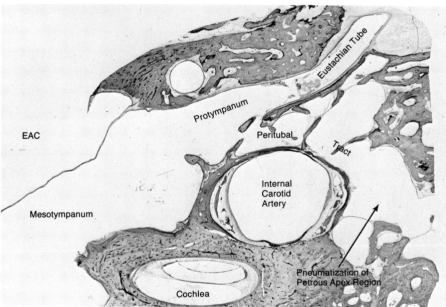

FIG. 4.21: The petrous apex is narrow but extensively pneumatized. The aditus is that constricted region posteromedial and superior to the body and short process of the incus leading from the epitympanum to the mastoid antrum (female, age 64 years).

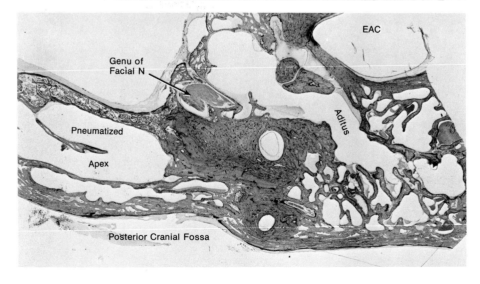

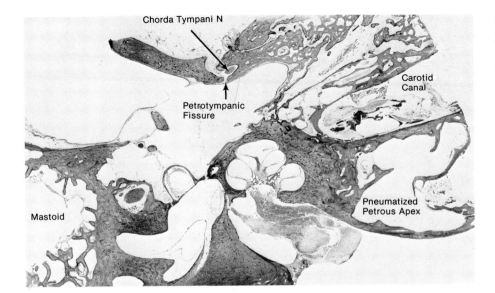

Figures labeled: Chorda Tympani N, Petrotympanic Fissure, Carotid Canal, Mastoid, Pneumatized Petrous Apex

FIG. 4.22: In this ear the petrous apex area is highly pneumatized. Serial sections show continuity with the peritubal and posterosuperior cell tracts (female, age 49 years).

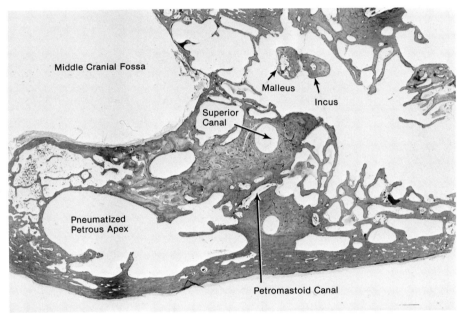

Figures labeled: Middle Cranial Fossa, Malleus, Incus, Superior Canal, Pneumatized Petrous Apex, Petromastoid Canal

FIG. 4.23: This temporal bone shows a single large apical air cell (male, age 40 years).

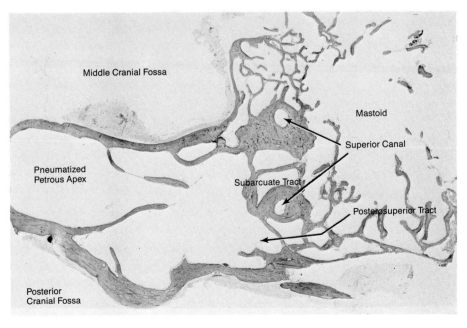

Figures labeled: Middle Cranial Fossa, Mastoid, Superior Canal, Pneumatized Petrous Apex, Subarcuate Tract, Posterosuperior Tract, Posterior Cranial Fossa

FIG. 4.24: Two common pathways to the petrous apex from the mastoid are the posterosuperior tract and the subarcuate tract (female, age 16 years).

FIG. 4.25: This temporal bone shows the usual state of nonpneumatization of the petrous apex. The carotid canal with its vascular and neural plexuses is also found in the petrous apex (male, age 60 years).

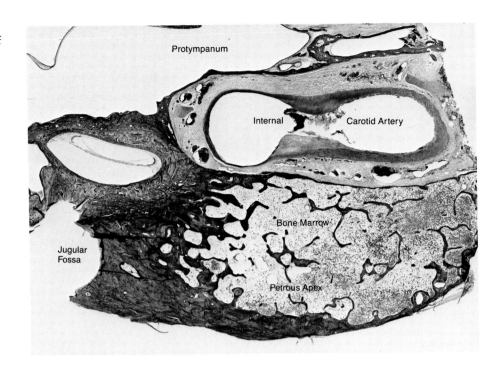

Lindsay, 1938, 1945). An alternative route, proposed by Ramadier (1933), is to drill through the bony labyrinth between the cochlea and carotid canal; most otologic surgeons, however, consider this approach to be too difficult to be practical. The limited space available between the cochlea posteriorly and the facial nerve and carotid artery anteriorly is demonstrated in Figures 4.20, 4.21, and 4.22. Infections of the petrous apex have become a rarity in most parts of the world.

The Accessory Regions

Occasionally, pneumatization extends beyond the middle ear, mastoid, perilabyrinthine, and petrous apex regions to involve adjacent portions of the temporal bone and even the adjacent cranial bones, thus forming the accessory cell areas (Fig. 4.15): 1) a zygomatic area that is an anterior extension from either the epitympanic or tegmental cell areas and occupies the root and sometimes the arch of the zygoma, 2) a squamous area which lies in the squamous portion of the temporal bone above the level of the infratemporal line as a superior extension from the tegmental cells, 3) an occipital area that lies within the occipital bone as a posterior extension from the sinal cells, and 4) a styloid area consisting of a rare accessory pneumatization occurring as an extension of the tip cells into the base of the styloid process.

The Tracts of Pneumatization

Pneumatization of the temporal bone is the result of a hollowing-out process in which mesenchyme is resolved to leave spaces. Each space becomes air-containing and is in free communication with all other pneumatized spaces. The tracts of pneumatization are well known to the otologic surgeon, for they serve as routes which can be followed to approach diseased areas of the temporal bone (Ziegelman, 1935; Diamant, 1940; Lindsay, 1940; Williams, 1966).

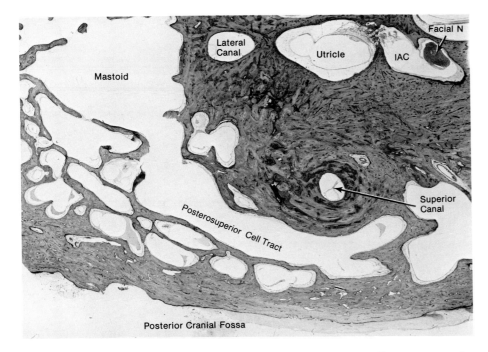

FIG. 4.26: This photomicrograph shows the posterosuperior cell tract as it extends anteromedially from the mastoid toward the internal auditory canal (IAC) in a course parallel to the posterior surface of the temporal bone. It lies in close anatomic relationship to the nonampullated limb of the superior canal (female, age 81 years).

These tracts are as follows: 1) The posterosuperior cell tract extends anteromedially from the superior part of the mastoid and lies in the angle between the dural plates of bone of the middle and posterior cranial fossae and the superior canal. This tract usually terminates near the internal auditory canal, but may pass superior to the internal auditory canal to reach the supralabyrinthine and apical areas (Figs. 4.26 and 4.27). 2) The posteromedial cell tract extends anteromedially from the mastoid along the posterior surface of the petrous bone at a level inferior to the posterosuperior cell tract (Figs. 4.28 and 4.29). On one side it is bordered by the endolymphatic duct and sac, and on the other by the bony wall of the posterior cranial fossa. It may lead to the supralabyrinthine and infralabyrinthine areas. 3) The subarcuate cell tract, occurring in 3% of temporal bones (Proctor, 1983), extends from the mastoid in an anteromedial direction

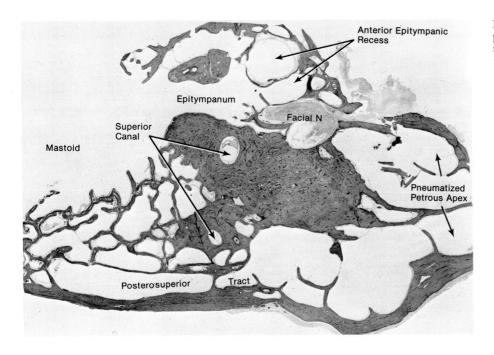

FIG. 4.27: In this case a large posterosuperior cell tract leads directly to a pneumatized apical area (female, age 16 years).

FIG. 4.28: This temporal bone has a well developed posteromedial cell tract (male, age 57 years). AICA—anterior inferior cerebellar artery, EAC—external auditory canal.

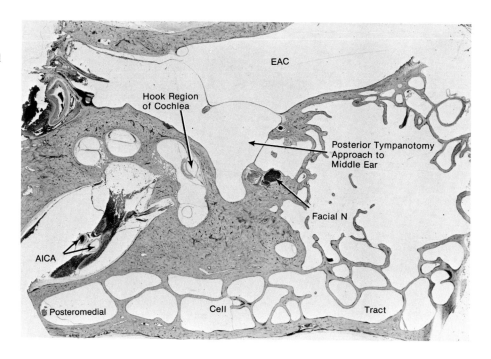

through the arc of the superior semicircular canal adjacent to the petromastoid canal. It may reach the apical area (Figs. 4.30 and 4.31). 4) The perilabyrinthine tracts extend from the epitympanic and hypotympanic areas of the middle ear into the supralabyrinthine and infralabyrinthine areas, respectively. 5) The peritubal tract arises from the protympanum or eustachian tube and takes a course anterior to the internal carotid artery to reach the apical area (Fig. 4.20).

FIG. 4.29: The posteromedial cell tract of this 79-year-old female is composed of large cells which bulge into the posterior cranial fossa.

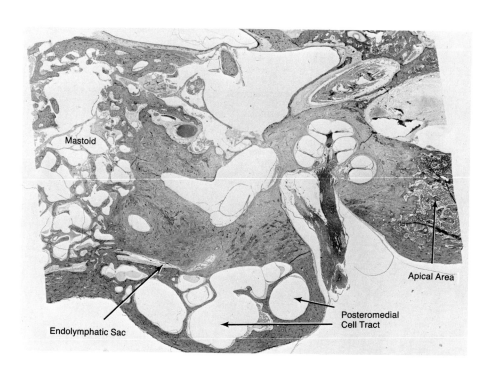

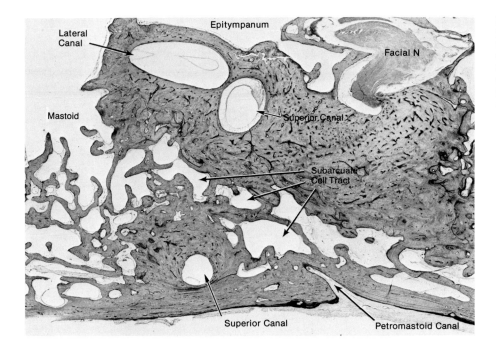

Lateral Canal

Epitympanum

Facial N

Mastoid

Superior Canal

Subarcuate Cell Tract

Superior Canal

Petromastoid Canal

FIG. 4.30: The subarcuate tract is seen passing between the ampullated and nonampullated limbs of the superior canal as it extends anteromedially from the mastoid. The petromastoid canal is also seen, passing posterolaterally from the posterior cranial fossa (male, age 44 years).

Pacchionian Bodies

Pacchionian bodies, also known as arachnoid granulations, are pseudo-podial projections of the pia-arachnoid which normally extend through the dura into venous sinuses or venous lacunae. There is a variability in the number and location of these bodies. The largest number can generally be found adjacent to the superior sagittal sinus, but they may also be found bordering the transverse, cavernous, and superior petrosal sinuses. With age, there is a tendency for the bodies to increase in size and number, and to undergo calcification. Each of these Pacchionian bodies is composed of several arachnoid villi; each of the villi consists of bundles of collagenous fibers interspersed with pia-arachnoid-like cells surrounded by a thin, outer membrane with small, oval epithelial cells on the surface. The space

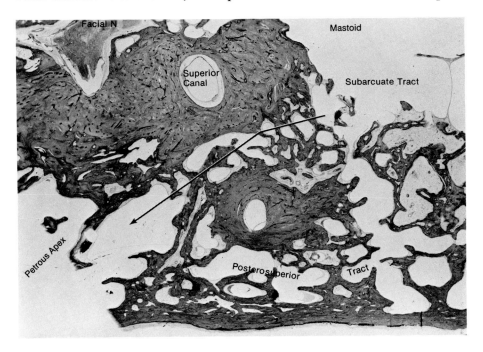

Facial N

Mastoid

Superior Canal

Subarcuate Tract

Petrous Apex

Posterosuperior Tract

FIG. 4.31: The subarcuate tract extends anteriorly through the arc of the superior canal. The posterosuperior tract parallels the posterior border of the temporal bone (male, age 80 years). The subarcuate tract is one of several surgical routes to the petrous apex. (See Fig. 1.45 and stereo reel II.)

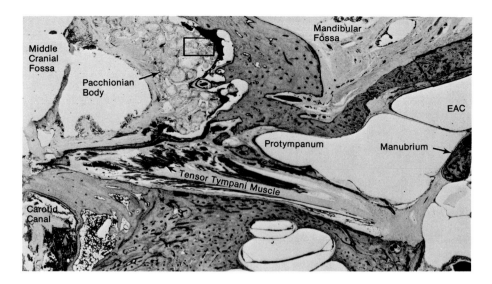

contained by the villi is a continuation of the subarachnoid space. The bodies are believed to serve principally as one-way, pressure dependent valves between the relatively high pressure cerebrospinal fluid system to the low pressure venous sinus system.

Pacchionian bodies are also found extending from the arachnoid of the middle cranial fossa (Figs. 4.32 and 4.33) and from the posterior fossa into the adjacent mastoid cells (Figs. 4.34 to 4.36). In these locations the bodies may be encountered by the surgeon, particularly in non-infected ears. Exposing them does not result in a cerebrospinal fluid leak. The function of these bodies in areas not related to venous channels is not known.

The Subarcuate Fossa and the Petromastoid Canal

In the adult, the subarcuate fossa is usually a small shallow depression on the posterior surface of the petrous pyramid, posterosuperior to the meatus of the internal auditory canal. In the fetus and the newborn the fossa is relatively larger than in the adult (Proctor, 1983) (Figs. 4.2 and

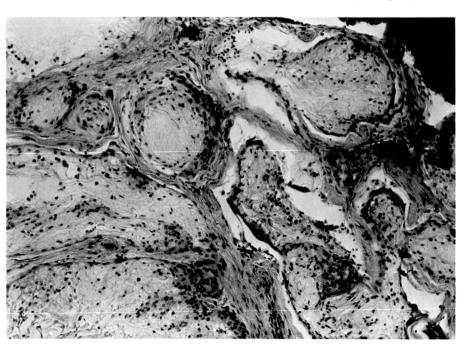

126 Anatomy of the Temporal Bone with Surgical Implications

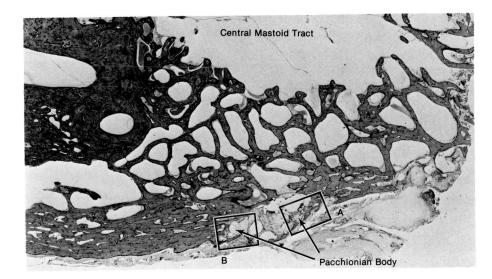

FIG. 4.34: In this case there is a large Pacchionian body arising from the meninges of the posterior cranial fossa. There is soft tissue continuity (osseous dehiscence) between the cranial cavity and the mastoid at the site of this body. It has not been demonstrated, however, that such sites provide pathways for bacterial spread or cerebrospinal fluid leak. Figures 4.35 and 4.36 are high-power views of areas A and B respectively (female, age 74 years).

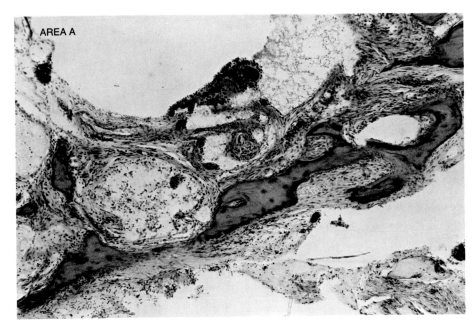

FIG. 4.35: Shown is a high-power view of area A in Figure 4.34 (female, age 74 years).

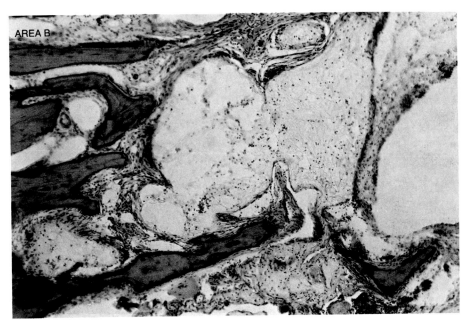

FIG. 4.36: Shown is a high-power view of area B in Figure 4.34 (female, age 74 years).

Pneumatization   127

FIG. 4.37: This ear demonstrates a persisting subarcuate fossa. If such an ear also had a well-pneumatized subarcuate tract, mastoidectomy could readily be complicated by a cerebrospinal fluid leak (male, age 1 year, 9 months).

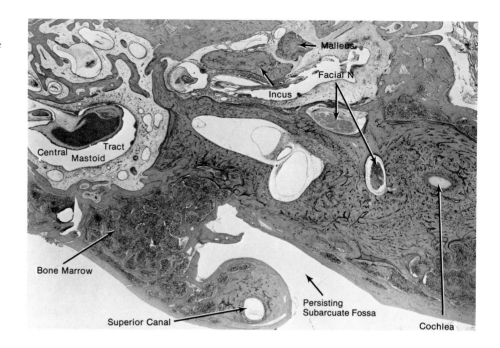

4.37). It leads into the petromastoid canal, a channel for the subarcuate artery and its accompanying vein as they course posteriorly through the arc of the superior canal (Figs. 4.23 and 4.30) (Mazzoni, 1970). The mastoid aperture of the petromastoid canal is usually found in a periantral cell anterior to the nonampullated end of the superior canal; however, in 5% of cases it opens directly into the antrum (Proctor, 1983).

5. The Inner Ear

The Bony Labyrinth

The bony labyrinth develops from the otic capsule. Its matrix is trilamellar, consisting of the internal periosteal (or endosteal) layer, the middle mixed layer of intrachondrial and enchondral bone, and the external periosteal layer. The internal and external periosteal layers are derived respectively from the embryonic internal and external perichondrium (see ossification, Chapter 9, p. 269). Scattered within the middle layer is intrachondrial bone (globuli interossei) (Figs. 5.1 and 5.2) which consists of islands of cartilage, the lacunae of which develop a thin layer of bone from invading osteoblasts. The amount of intrachondrial bone decreases with the age of the individual (Wolff et al., 1957). Following fracture, this middle layer of bone fails to heal by osteoid or callus formation. The endosteal (inner periosteal) layer also demonstrates poor reparative capability. Fractures of the temporal bone heal predominantly with fibrous tissue and some bone from the external periosteal layer.

The long axis of the bony labyrinth, measuring 20 mm in length (Anson & Donaldson, 1981), roughly parallels the posterior surface of the petrous pyramid. Its components are the vestibule, the semicircular canals, and the cochlea (Fig. 5.3).

THE VESTIBULE

The vestibule is the central chamber, measuring 4 mm in diameter; the irregular topography of its walls corresponds to the contained elements of the membranous labyrinth. At the posterosuperior aspect of its medial wall is a depression known as the elliptical recess which accommodates part of the utricular macula. The spherical recess is a similar depression for the saccular macula, located anteroinferiorly. The vestibular crest, an oblique elevation between these two recesses, bifurcates posteriorly into two wings which delimit the cochlear recess for the vestibular cecum (basal end) of the cochlear duct.

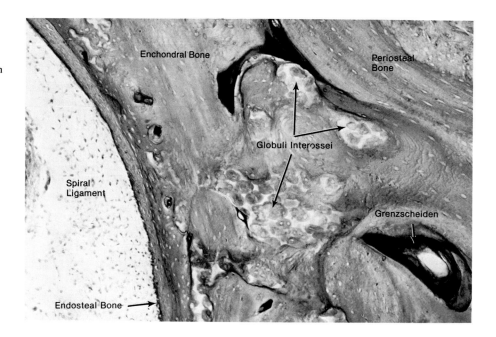

There are discrete openings in the bony walls of the vestibule. The opening for the cochlea lies anteriorly, while the openings for the semicircular canals are located posteriorly. The cribriform (or cribrose) areas are clustered tiny openings through which the vestibular and cochlear nerve bundles gain access to the inner ear. The oval window is an opening on the lateral wall, adjoining the tympanic cavity. The vestibular aqueduct with its contained endolymphatic duct opens into the posteroinferior aspect of the vestibule.

THE COCHLEA

The osseous cochlea (Figs. 5.4 to 5.6) derives its name from its resemblance to a snail shell; it consists of a 32-mm spiral canal which winds two and one-half turns about a central bony axis, the modiolus. The base

FIG. 5.2: Shown here are the three layers of the bony labyrinth of a newborn infant with osteogenesis imperfecta. The endosteal layer of bone is normal. The enchondral layer shows an increase in the fibrous tissue component. The delicate trabeculae of the enchondral layer are separated by moderately cellular fibrous tissue with some blood vessels. The periosteal bone is more dense than the enchondral layer, but also is composed of thin trabeculae separated by fibrous tissue.

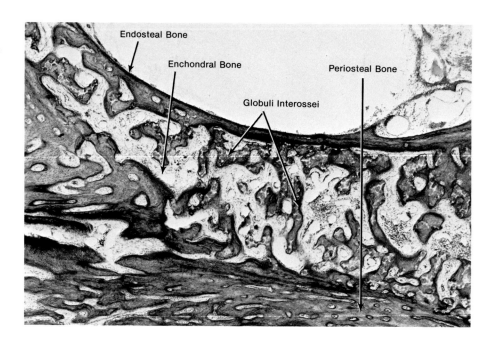

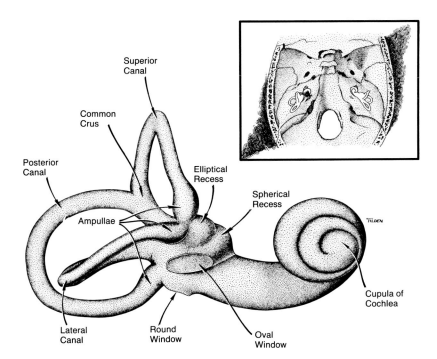

FIG. 5.3: This sketch of the bony laby-rinth in effect shows the configuration of the endosteal layer of bone. (After Sobotta, 1957.)

of the spiral is located at the anterolateral aspect of the internal auditory canal, corresponding to the cochlear cribrose area for the transmission of nerves supplying the cochlea; the apex points inferiorly, laterally, and ante-riorly. The height of the cochlea is 5 mm. The osseous spiral lamina is a slender bony projection which circles the modiolus to partially subdivide the cochlear canal into the scala vestibuli anteriorly and the scala tympani posteriorly; it terminates apically at the hamulus. The helicotrema is the apical communication of the two scalae. The secondary osseous spiral lam-ina is a thin, narrow, curved shelf of bone located on the external wall of the basal end of the cochlea, hugging the posterior surface of the spiral ligament. Defects in the interscalar septum between the middle and apical turns (scala communis) are common and of no functional significance (Fig. 5.7).

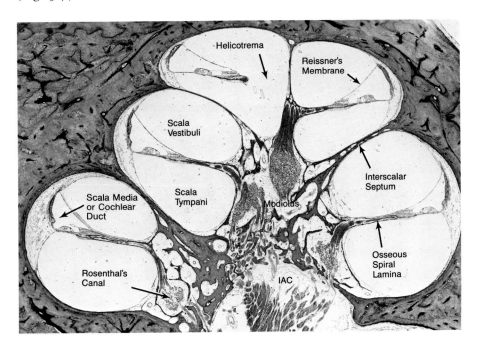

FIG. 5.4: This photograph shows the microscopic anatomy of a normal coch-lea. Note that from base to apex there is progressive narrowing of the spiral ligament and widening of the basilar membrane (female, age 63 years). Same ear as Figures 5.5 and 5.6.

FIG. 5.5: This view shows the normal cochlear duct. Compare with sketch in Figure 5.15. The areas of acellularity in the spiral ligament are normal for age. The protein precipitate is a normal consequence of histologic preparation (female, age 63 years). Same ear as Figures 5.4 and 5.6.

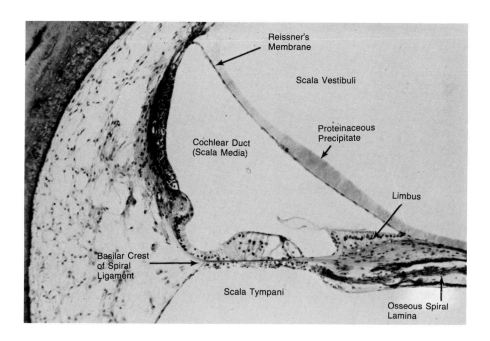

THE CANALS

The osseous semicircular canals (here referred to as the lateral, posterior, and superior canals) are situated posteriorly relative to the vestibule. Each canal is orthogonally related to the others, describing a 240° arc, and measuring 1 mm in diameter. Each canal expands to double its diameter at its osseous ampulla where it communicates with the vestibule. The nonampullated ends of the posterior and superior canals fuse, forming the common crus, while the nonampullated end of the lateral canal remains independent. Thus, the vestibule has five apertures for the semicircular canals.

MICROFISSURES

Microfissures, commonly occurring disruptions in the endosteal and enchondral layers of the bony labyrinth, are of no pathologic or functional significance. They contain a combination of fibrous tissue and an osteoid-like acellular matrix. Temporal bone fractures caused by trauma create

FIG. 5.6: This is a normal organ of Corti. Ciliary tufts are often visualized in well-preserved specimens. Note that the outer hair cell (OHC) nuclei and Deiters' cell nuclei are located in distinct rows (female, age 63 years). IHC—inner hair cell. Same ear as Figures 5.4 and 5.5. Compare with sketch in Figure 5.15.

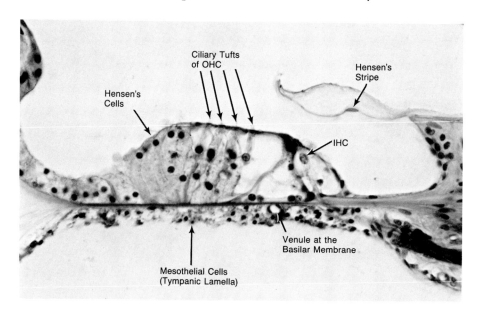

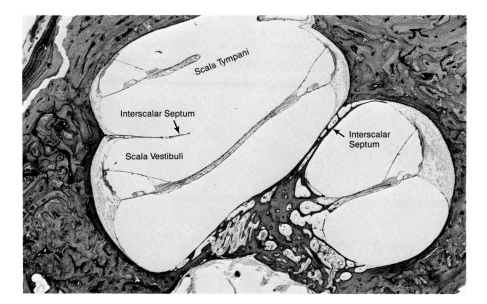

FIG. 5.7: A partially missing interscalar septum (scala communis) is a common developmental defect and is compatible with normal cochlear function (female, age 63 years).

wider, longer fissures which also involve the periosteal layer and may extend through the entire transverse dimension of the temporal bone. Increased numbers of microfissures may be seen in association with temporal bone fractures and in Paget's disease, in which case the more appropriate terminology would be microfractures. While the endosteal and enchondral layers of the bony labyrinth manifest minimal osseous reparative powers, the external periosteal layer is capable of osseous repair.

A constant microfissure is located between the round window niche and the ampulla of the posterior canal (Fig. 5.8) (Keleman, 1933; Harada et al., 1981). Okano, Harada and colleagues (Okano & Myers, 1976; Okano et al., 1977; Harada et al., 1981) related this microfissure to an embryologic communication between the round window niche and the ampulla of the posterior canal seen in 10- to 15-week fetuses. With further gestational age, mesenchymal tissue originally present in the channel is replaced by cartilage, so that no communication is discernible at term. After 1 year of age, the microfissure is observed with increasing incidence as a function of age. By the age of 6 years it is seen in all ears.

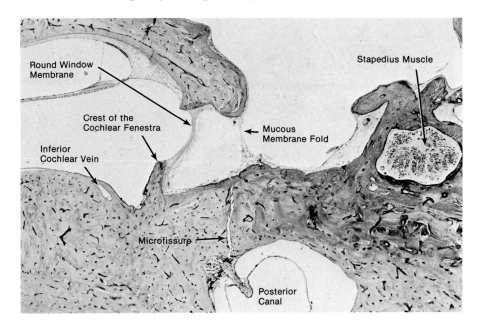

FIG. 5.8: The microfissure between the ampulla of the posterior canal and round window niche occurs in all adult temporal bones (Okano & Myers, 1976; Okano et al., 1977; Harada et al., 1981) (male, age 84 years). The crest of the cochlear fenestra (round window) is also known as the semilunar crest.

FIG. 5.9: The cochlea of this newborn infant shows the area of the tympanomeningeal (Hyrtl's) fissure. Rarely this fissure may persist into adulthood to become the site of cerebrospinal fluid otorrhea. Reichert's bar is seen as the cartilaginous precursor of the styloid process which ossifies only after birth.

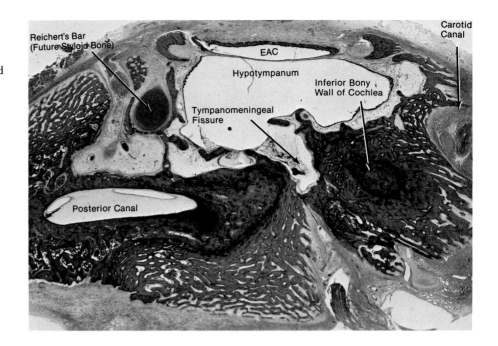

Mayer (1930, 1931) was the first to describe alternate sites of temporal bone microfissures. Harada et al. (1981) found microfissures in the oval window region in 25% of 331 temporal bone specimens, with an increased incidence after the age of 40. In two-thirds of the cases the microfissure extended in a vertical plane both superior and inferior to the oval window but it did not penetrate the footplate.

The etiology of these microfissures is unclear, but a popular hypothesis contends that they are stress fractures generated by ossification and remodeling processes occurring within the bony labyrinth (Mayer, 1930, 1931; Harada et al., 1981). Another proposal (Proops et al., 1984) suggests that they are caused by constant stresses transferred to the bony labyrinth by the act of mastication.

FIG. 5.10: The tympanomeningeal fissure runs parallel to the cochlear aqueduct (male, age 44 years).

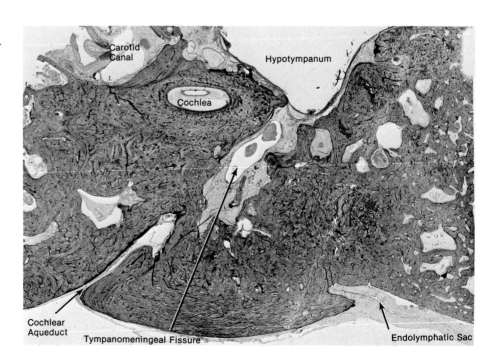

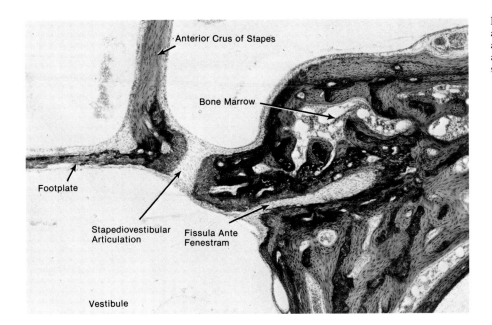

Labels on image: Anterior Crus of Stapes, Bone Marrow, Footplate, Stapediovestibular Articulation, Fissula Ante Fenestram, Vestibule

FIG. 5.11: This view shows the fissula ante fenestram and stapediovestibular articulation in a newborn infant. This area is the site of predilection for otosclerosis.

Because of firm fibrous healing and blockage of the fissure, it seems improbable that it could act as a conduit for the spread of middle ear inflammatory processes and ototoxic medications into the inner ear as suggested by Harada et al. (1981). The role that these microfissures may play as sites for spontaneous perilymph fistulae is a matter for speculation.

THE TYMPANOMENINGEAL FISSURE

The tympanomeningeal fissure, which apparently is open in early embryonic life, parallels the cochlear aqueduct extending from the area inferior to the round window to the meninges of the posterior fossa (Figs. 5.9 and 5.10). This fissure is a rare site for spontaneous cerebrospinal fluid otorrhea. It has been termed Hyrtl's fissure (Eggston & Wolff, 1947; Spector et al., 1980); search of the literature, however, has failed to reveal a description of this fissure by Hyrtl.

THE FISSURES OF THE VESTIBULE

The fissula ante fenestram is considered to be an appendage of the perilymphatic space (Fig. 5.11). It is a transcapsular channel formed by resorption of precartilage. In adult life it contains cartilage and/or fibrous tissue. It courses from the vestibule anterior to the oval window through an irregular slit-like space to the periosteum of the tympanic cavity near the cochleariform process (Anson & Donaldson, 1981).

The fossula post fenestram is an invagination of the periotic tissue into the otic capsule posterior to the oval window (Fig. 5.12) and extends about one-third of the way to the nonampullated end of the lateral canal. It occurs inconsistently, contains fibrous tissue (Anson & Donaldson, 1981), and when present is likely to communicate only with the vestibule.

The Membranous Labyrinth

The membranous labyrinth is encased within the bony labyrinth and is surrounded by the perilymphatic space with its fluid, blood vessels, and

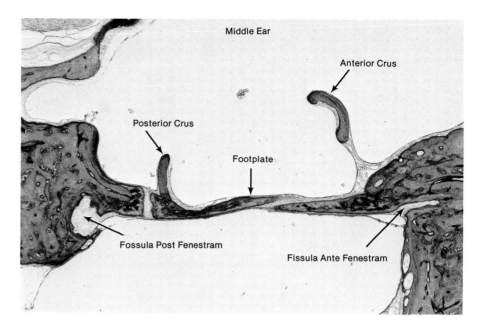

FIG. 5.12: The normal histologic appearance of the fossula and fissula is demonstrated. The apparent overlapping of the footplate onto the anterosuperior margin of the oval window is the normal consequence of the angle of sectioning (female, age 34 years).

supporting connective tissue. The constituents of the membranous labyrinth are the cochlear duct, the three semicircular ducts and their ampullae, the otolithic organs (the utricle and saccule), and the endolymphatic (otic) duct and sac (Fig. 5.13). This system of epithelially lined channels and spaces is filled with endolymph (Scarpa's fluid); the utricular duct, the saccular duct, and the ductus reuniens interconnect the major structures.

Vesiculations which may be seen in the walls of the membranous canals were described by Rüdinger approximately a century ago. Lempert et al. (1952) theorized that these vesiculations were the result of viral infection of the labyrinth and that their rupture was responsible for the symptoms of Ménière's disease. Today they are considered to be of no pathologic significance; it is not known whether they are premortem alterations of aging, postmortem changes, or artifacts of preparation (Altmann, 1968).

FIG. 5.13: This sketch shows the membranous labyrinth as viewed from medially. Note the "Y" configuration of the utricular and saccular ducts as they join to form the sinus of the endolymphatic duct. The endolymphatic duct parallels the common crus and posterior semicircular duct on its way to the posterior surface of the temporal bone. (After Anson & Donaldson, 1981.)

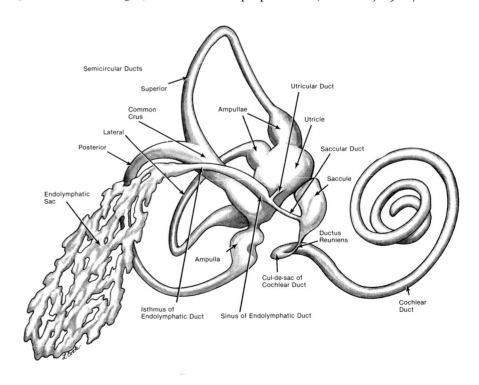

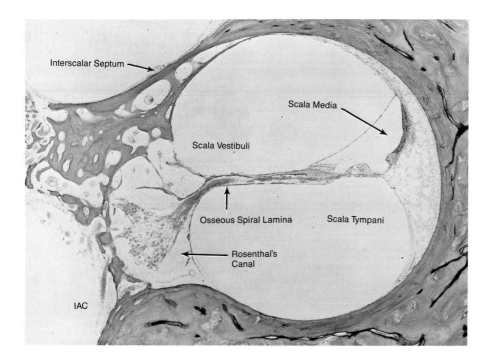

FIG. 5.14: This photomicrograph shows a cross-sectional view of the basal turn (male, age 28 years).

THE COCHLEAR DUCT

The cochlear duct (scala media) is the spiral epithelial duct coursing between the osseous spiral lamina internally and the bony wall of the cochlea externally (Fig. 5.14). It begins in the vestibule (vestibular cecum) as a blind pouch connected to the saccule via the ductus reuniens (Fig. 5.13). Mimicking the bony cochlea, the cochlear duct forms a 32-mm spiral around two and one-half turns (a basal, middle, and an incomplete apical turn) to end immediately distal to the hamulus of the osseous spiral lamina in another cul-de-sac, the cupular cecum. With the osseous spiral lamina, this duct completes the subdivision of the bony cochlear canal into the scala vestibuli and scala tympani.

In a shallow sulcus in the outer wall of the bony cochlear canal lies a specialized layer of thickened periosteum, the spiral ligament (Fig. 5.15).

FIG. 5.15: This sketch shows most of the structures of the cochlear duct. (After Davis, 1962.)

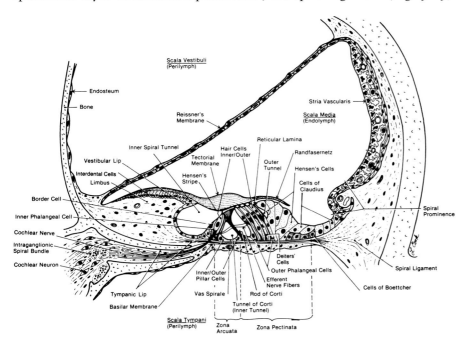

This ligament is an intricate arrangement of connective tissue cells (fibrocytes), intercellular substance, and blood vessels. On its inner surface it is lined by the stria vascularis, the spiral prominence, the basilar crest, and the external sulcus cells. The spiral prominence consists of a single layer of small cuboidal cells interposed between the external sulcus cells and the stria vascularis (vascular stripe). The outer sulcus cells lie posterior to the spiral prominence, and are external to and distinct from the cells of Claudius. Duvall (1969), in an electron microscopic study of guinea pig cochleae, confirmed Shambaugh's (1908) finding that these external sulcus cells are arranged as a "continuous band" for the entire length of the cochlear duct. He noted that they form peg-like projections into the spiral ligament external to the stria vascularis and are surrounded by the capillary network of the stria vascularis and the spiral prominence. In the basal and middle turns, these external sulcus cells are beneath both the Claudius' cells and the cells of the spiral prominence, but in the apical turn, they insinuate themselves between these two cell types and border the endolymphatic surface.

The stria vascularis is a band of specialized tissue which lies on the spiral ligament between the spiral prominence and the attachment of Reissner's membrane. It is composed of three cell types (Fig. 5.16): 1) marginal cells located on the endolymphatic surface, 2) intermediate cells, and 3) basal cells which border the spiral ligament (Smith, 1957). A rich capillary network lies within the stria vascularis. The floor (posterior wall) of the cochlear duct is composed of the thickened periosteum of the osseous spiral lamina and a fibrous tissue continuation, the basilar membrane, which stretches from the tympanic lip of the osseous spiral lamina to the basilar crest of the spiral ligament. Reissner's membrane forms the roof (anterior wall) of the cochlear duct. It bridges from its site of attachment at the spiral ligament (the vestibular crest) to the spiral limbus, and consists of an epithelial layer at its endolymphatic surface and a mesothelial layer at its perilymphatic surface. The limbus is a specialized mound of thickened periosteum of the osseous spiral lamina; its surface can be divided into three zones: 1) facing the scala media, 2) facing the inner spiral sulcus, and 3) facing the scala vestibuli.

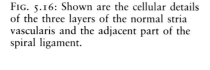

FIG. 5.16: Shown are the cellular details of the three layers of the normal stria vascularis and the adjacent part of the spiral ligament.

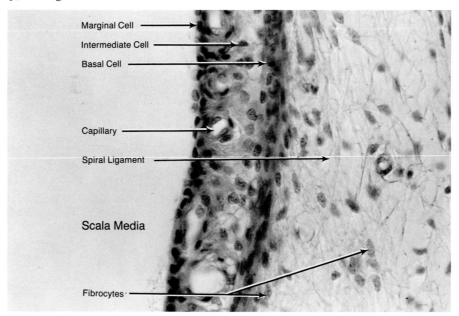

Marginal Cell

Intermediate Cell

Basal Cell

Capillary

Spiral Ligament

Scala Media

Fibrocytes

The epithelium of the floor of the cochlear duct is highly specialized and is dominated by the organ of Corti (the spiral organ). Huschke (1824a, 1824b) termed this organ the basilar papilla. Corti (1851) was the first to provide a detailed description of the cytoarchitecture of this structure, subsequently known as the organ of Corti. The light microscopic details have since been further described by Boettcher (1869), Retzius (1884), Held (1926), and Kolmer (1927). Transmission electron microscopy (Smith, 1957; Engström & Wersäll, 1958a, 1958b; Friedmann, 1959; Flock, 1965; Kimura, 1966; Spoendlin, 1966; Iurato, 1967; Duvall, 1969) and scanning electron microscopy (Lim, 1969; Bredberg et al., 1970) have revealed a whole order of magnitude of greater detail.

The basilar membrane which supports the organ of Corti consists of connective tissue layers and extracellular matrix (Iurato, 1967). In man it is about 32 mm in length and measures 104μ in width at its basal end and 504μ at the apical end (Retzius, 1884). The basilar membrane is divided into two portions (Fig. 5.15): 1) the zona arcuata which is located under the tunnel of Corti and extends to the outer pillars, and 2) the zona pectinata which extends from the outer pillars to the basilar crest of the spiral ligament. This membrane separates the bases of the supporting cells, which rest on a thin basement membrane, from the perilymph of the scala tympani. It consists of three main elements: a fibrous portion, a homogeneous ground substance, and mesothelial cells (Cabezudo, 1978). The tympanic border cells (mesothelial cells) form a layer on the posterior surface of the basilar membrane; there is a general increase in their number proceeding apically (Cabezudo, 1978). The basilar membrane permits nearly unimpeded passage of small particles (horseradish peroxidase, thorium dioxide) to the extracellular fluid of the organ of Corti; hence that fluid should very closely approximate perilymph (Angelborg & Engström, 1973). Engström (1960) believes that this fluid is a separate entity and calls it "cortilymph".

The primary cytologic elements of the organ of Corti are Deiters' cells, Hensen's cells, hair cells, internal and external sulcus cells, and pillar cells. According to Retzius (1884), there are 3,500 inner hair cells and 12,000 outer hair cells in the human cochlea. The term "hair cells" stems from the tufts of stereocilia which protrude from their apices. The outer hair cells, cylindrical in shape, are supported by the reticular membrane apically and by concavities of Deiters' cells basally. The inner hair cells are flask-shaped and are completely surrounded, except apically, by internal pillar cells, inner phalangeal cells, and border cells. The inner and outer hair cells are the primary auditory receptors; their cell bodies are partially enveloped by the synaptic terminations of the cochlear nerve fibers.

Several types of supporting cells are associated with the inner and outer hair cells (Fig. 5.15). Proceeding radially outward from the inner sulcus cells they are: the inner border cells, inner phalangeal cells, inner and outer pillar cells, Deiters' cells (outer phalangeal cells), Hensen's cells, and Claudius' cells. Save for the pillar cells, all of the supporting cells possess numerous microvilli at their free surfaces, hypothesized to function either in endolymph ion exchange or in attachment to the tectorial membrane.

The inner border cells stretch from the basilar membrane to the surface, forming a thin band of cells internal to the inner hair cells; they are rich in mitochondria and microvilli and are believed to act in a nutritional role for the inner hair cells (Angelborg & Engström, 1973).

The inner phalangeal cells are arranged in a single row with a single phalanx stretching between two inner hair cells. They are tall, slender cells, extending from the basilar membrane to the surface; it is unclear whether they possess fibrils as do Deiters' cells and the outer phalangeal cells.

There are 5,600 inner pillar cells and 3,850 outer pillar cells (or rods) (Angelborg & Engström, 1973). These cells also rest on the basilar membrane. By electron microscopy it has been shown that they contain an abundance of fibrillar structures; hence, their function is presumed to be supportive. Along with Deiters' cells, they form the reticular membrane, which supports and surrounds the apices of all the hair cells.

Deiters' cells (outer phalangeal cells) reach from the basilar membrane to the bases of the outer hair cells for which they provide supporting cups. These large, filament-containing cells also provide slender processes which extend to, and are integrated into, the reticular membrane.

Hensen's cells are tall, columnar cells. The extent of their contact with the tectorial membrane has been a matter of some dispute and it is felt that after birth this contact is very tenuous, consisting only of small strands (Angelborg & Engström, 1973).

Claudius' cells are shorter than Hensen's cells and have no intracellular filaments (Iurato, 1967).

The inner sulcus cells, along with Hensen's cells, are the least differentiated of the epithelial cells of the organ of Corti. They lie internal to the inner border cells. Boettcher's (Böttcher's) cells form a layer between the basilar membrane and Claudius' cells.

The organ of Corti contains constant intercellular spaces including the tunnel of Corti, the spaces of Nuel (the outer tunnel), and the spaces between the outer hair cells. All of these spaces communicate with each other. Iurato (1967) describes the "lacuna of Corti" which is bounded superiorly by the reticular lamina, inferiorly by the upper surface of Deiters' cells, radially outwards by Hensen's cells, and radially inwards by the inner pillar cells.

The tectorial membrane is a gelatinous leaf which stretches out from its attachment at the vestibular lip of the limbus and ends in the border net (Randfasernetz). It is divided into three zones (Iurato, 1960; Lim, 1972): 1) the inner limbal zone, which inserts into the interdental cells, 2) the middle zone which overlies the organ of Corti, and 3) the outer marginal zone or border net (Held, 1926; Kolmer, 1927; de Vries, 1949; Lawrence, 1981) which overlies Hensen's cells. Hardesty's membrane is that part of the marginal zone in which the cilia of the outer hair cells are embedded (Lim, 1972). Hensen's stripe marks the area at which the tectorial membrane is attached to the inner phalangeal and border cells.

THE UTRICLE

The utricle (Fig. 5.17) is an irregular, elliptical tube, the superior part of which occupies the elliptical recess of the posterosuperior aspect of the medial wall of the vestibule; here it is held in place by filaments of the utricular nerve and strands of fibrous tissue. The utricular sense organ (the macula) is an ovoid, thickened area which lies predominantly in the horizontal plane at the dilated anterior portion of the utricle (the utricular recess). The maculae of both the utricle and the saccule are divided into two regions by the striola, a narrow curvilinear area extending through their middle regions. The maculae contain the sensory hair cells of the otolithic organs with their retinue of supporting cells (see also semicircular ducts, p. 143). The otolithic membrane is the gelatinous blanket into which the stereocilia of the macular hair cells project. This membrane is studded

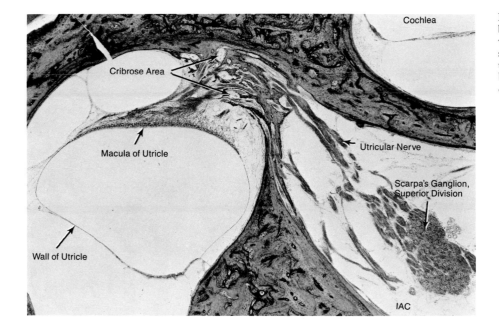

FIG. 5.17: The utricular nerve is a branch of the superior division of the vestibular nerve. All nerve fibers to the sense organs of the inner ear pass through tiny channels in the wall of the bony labyrinth known as the cribrose or cribriform areas (male, age 24 years).

with otoconia, which are calcium carbonate concretions in calcite crystalline structure with a specific gravity of approximately 2.71. Extending from the inferior aspect of the utricle is the utricular duct, skirting the utricular wall to open into the sinus of the endolymphatic duct. The utriculo-endolymphatic valve is a thickening found at the utricular aspect of the cleft-shaped opening into the endolymphatic duct (Retzius, 1884; Werner, 1940) (Figs. 5.18 and 5.19). The semicircular ducts open into the utricle via its posterior wall, while the anteriorly located utricular and saccular ducts provide a route of communication with the saccule.

THE SACCULE

The saccule is an elliptical, flattened sac, the macula of which is located in the spherical recess of the medial and anterior wall of the vestibule, inferior to the utricle; it is held in position by connective tissue fibers and

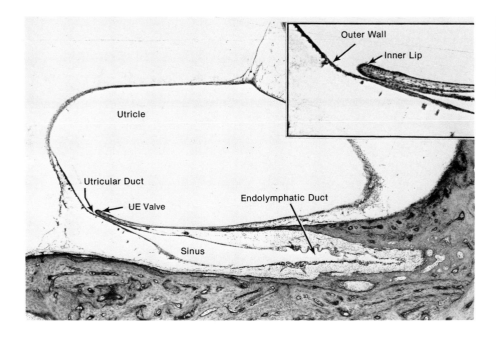

FIG. 5.18: This photomicrograph illustrates the utriculo-endolymphatic (UE) valve. The outer wall is formed by the utricular wall. The inset shows the composition of the inner lip which consists of a connective tissue core and a lining surface epithelium (infant, age 41 days).

The Inner Ear **141**

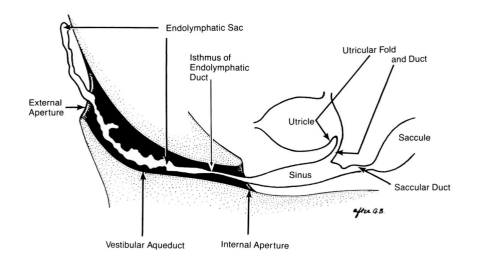

FIG. 5.19: This diagram illustrates the interrelationships of the endolymphatic sinus, duct, and sac. Illustrated, but not labeled, are the intraosseous and intradural segments of the endolymphatic sac. (After Anson & Donaldson, 1981.)

filaments of the saccular nerve. The hook-like macula of the saccule is oriented primarily in the vertical plane. The reinforced area is a discrete thickening of the saccular wall located at its anterolateral part where it is adjacent to the vestibular wall (Perlman, 1940). Superiorly, the wall of the saccule abuts and adheres to the membranous wall of the utricle; however, the only communication with the utricle is indirectly through the saccular and utricular ducts. Inferiorly, the saccule narrows into the ductus reuniens through which communication with the cochlear duct is maintained. Occasionally the saccule and utricle are widely confluent (Fig. 5.20).

MACULAR ORIENTATION

The otolithic surface of the macula of the utricle faces posteromedially, while the otolithic surface of the macula of the saccule faces posterolaterally (Fig. 5.21). Thus, when the utricle is viewed through an open oval window, the dull white surface of the utricular nerve will be seen; in con-

FIG. 5.20: In both ears of this subject, the utricle and saccule are widely confluent and communicate directly with the endolymphatic sinus. The condition may represent a phylogenetically based failure of development of the utriculo-endolymphatic valve (see Chapter 9, p. 255). The clinical history revealed no evidence of auditory or vestibular dysfunction (male, age 55 years).

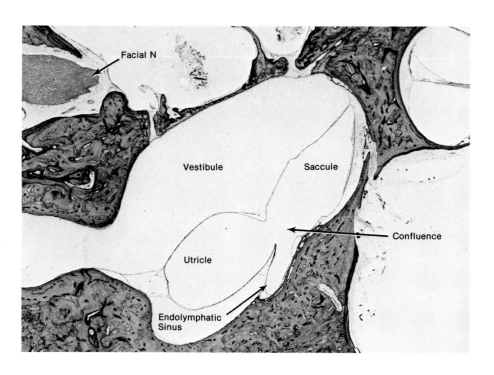

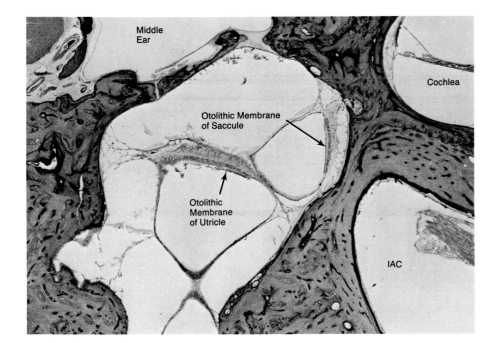

Middle Ear

Cochlea

Otolithic Membrane of Saccule

Otolithic Membrane of Utricle

IAC

FIG. 5.21: When viewed through the oval window during surgical procedures, the utricular macula has a dull, white appearance due to its neural presenting surface. In contrast, the saccular macula has a slightly granular, more brilliant, whitish appearance because its presenting surface is its otolithic membrane viewed through the almost transparent saccular wall (female, age 68 years).

trast, the saccule will present a more glistening, slightly granular surface because of the reflective properties of the otoconia.

THE SEMICIRCULAR DUCTS

The three semicircular membranous ducts course along the external walls of the bony semicircular canals (Figs. 5.22 and 5.23). Like their bony channels, each of the ducts is orthogonally related to the other. The lateral canal in man forms a 30° angle with respect to the horizontal plane. Near its utricular orifice, each duct enlarges to form the membranous ampulla, which is attached to bone at its base. The walls of the semicircular ducts are trilaminar. A loose connective tissue layer lies adjacent to the perilymphatic space and contains blood vessels and pigment cells. The internal

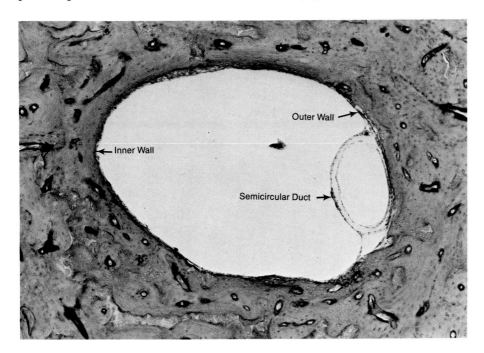

Inner Wall

Outer Wall

Semicircular Duct

FIG. 5.22: The semicircular ducts invariably pass along the outer walls of their bony canals, as seen in the nonampullated end of this posterior canal (female, age 77 years).

The Inner Ear   **143**

FIG. 5.23: The bony wall of the posterior canal shows a scalloped appearance. This is an unusual but not pathologic finding in the semicircular canals (female, age 22 years).

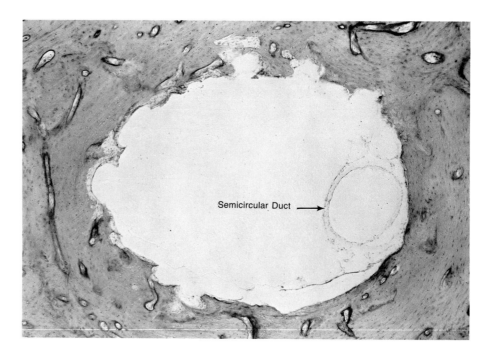

Semicircular Duct →

lining is a simple low epithelium. Interposed between these layers is a basement membrane. The cristae are mound-like elevations which cross the bases of the ampullae; they are representative of a thickening of the three layers of the membranous wall and consist of connective tissue, blood vessels, nerve fibers, and sensory neuroepithelium, all capped by a gelatinous cupula. The cupula extends diametrically from the neuroepithelium to the opposing wall of the ampulla. The semilunar planes are half-moon shaped zones of cuboidal or cylindrical cells which are located on the ampullary walls at either end of each crista. Transitional epithelium occupies a zone along the sides of the crista; adjacent to it is a zone of dark cells (Kimura, 1969; Mira & dal Negro, 1969). The dark cells are thought to have a secretory capacity (Kimura, 1969). The sensory epithelium of the maculae of the otolithic organs has the same general morphological structure as the cristae (Smith, 1956).

Like the organ of Corti, the maculae of the otolithic organs and the cristae of the semicircular ducts contain two types of ciliated hair cells, type I and type II (Wersäll, 1956). The type I hair cell is analogous to the inner hair cell of the organ of Corti, with a flask-like configuration and a surrounding chalice of vestibular nerve endings. The type II hair cell is the vestibular counterpart of the outer hair cell and has a cylindrical shape. Like the cochlear hair cells, the vestibular hair cells are studded with stereocilia at their free surface; however, the vestibular hair cells are distinguished by the presence of a true kinocilium (Hamilton, 1969) in addition to the stereocilia. The stereocilia of the cristae are embedded in a gelatinous cupula, while those of the maculae project into the gelatinous otolithic membrane.

THE CRISTA NEGLECTA

The crista neglecta is a small vestigial endorgan located in the vestibular labyrinth. Its prevalence in man has been reported as 7.6% by Okano et al. (1978) and 0.9% by Montandon et al. (1970). In the former study, every section of the serial set was stained and studied; therefore it probably represents the more accurate figure. The crista neglecta is found on the antero-lateral wall of the ampulla of the posterior canal (Okano et al., 1978). It possesses all the morphologic attributes of a true crista ampullaris, including a cupula, types I and II sensory cells, and transitional epithelium, as well as efferent and afferent nerve fibers (Montandon et al., 1970; Okano et al., 1978) (Fig. 5.24). Its size averages 70.3μ in height, 17.5μ in width, and 228.2μ in length in the 17 cases studied by Okano et al. (1978); however, there was a large range of values for each of these parameters. The nerve supply is derived from the posterior ampullary nerve, either by the main trunk or by a discrete branch which runs in its own bony canal. Although the clinical significance of the crista neglecta is not established, it is closely related to the posterior canal crista and, perhaps, as suggested by Montandon et al. (1970), is normally incorporated into the posterior canal crista in man.

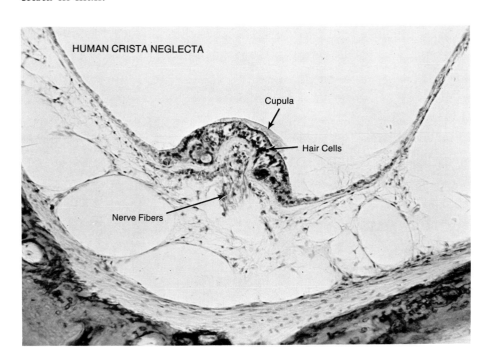

HUMAN CRISTA NEGLECTA

Cupula

Hair Cells

Nerve Fibers

FIG. 5.24: The crista neglecta is a small accessory crista, occurring regularly in felines and certain other species and occasionally in man. It has an ampulla, sensory epithelium, cupula, and nerve fibers, and is located in the anterior wall of the ampullated end of the posterior canal (female, age 77 years).

The Endolymphatic Duct and Sac

THE UTRICULO-ENDOLYMPHATIC VALVE

In the anteroinferior wall of the utricle at the orifice of the utricular duct is a slit-shaped opening (Fig. 5.18) known as the utriculo-endolymphatic valve. This structure was first described by Bast (1928) and more recently has been evaluated regarding its functional significance in man (Schuknecht & Belal, 1975). The utricular wall, in continuity with the utricular duct, forms its outer wall. The inner lip is specially constructed to function as a valve. It has a central core of loosely knit fibrocytes and capillaries and a surface layer of large cuboidal cells. As endolymphatic pressure increases in the utricle, the outer membranous wall is displaced from the more rigid inner lip, permitting the escape of endolymph into the utricular duct (Fig. 5.25). As the utricular endolymphatic pressure is lowered, the valve again closes to prevent excess loss of endolymphatic fluid. In view of the absence of any neural or muscular components in its structure, the action of this valve probably is entirely passive. Phylogenetically,

FIG. 5.25: Sketch to demonstrate the probable mechanical action of the utriculo-endolymphatic valve. Its apparent purpose is to maintain the fluid volume and preserve the membranous contours of the pars superior (utricle and canals). (Schuknecht & Belal, 1975.)

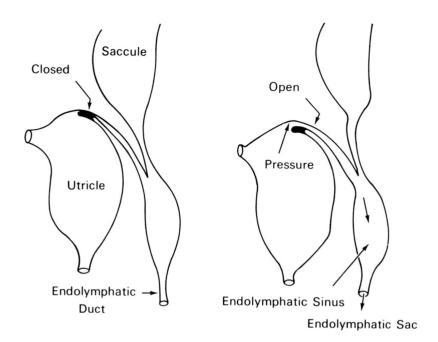

this valve develops coincidentally with the appearance of the auditory pars inferior (cochlea and saccule). Its purpose may be to prevent collapse of the walls of the pars superior (utricle and semicircular ducts) in the event of a rupture of the pars inferior. Absence of the utriculo-endolymphatic valve may occur as an anatomical variant (Fig. 5.26).

THE ENDOLYMPHATIC DUCT

The sinus of the endolymphatic duct is located in a groove on the posterolateral wall of the vestibule (Fig. 5.20) and terminates at the mouth of the vestibular aqueduct. The vestibular aqueduct is a bony channel coursing posteriorly and then laterally; it houses the intermediate segment of the endolymphatic duct as it passes from the vestibule to the posterior surface

FIG. 5.26: In this ear the utriculo-endolymphatic (UE) valve is missing. The medical records of this patient made no mention of a vestibular disorder (male, age 3-1/2 months). E—endolymphatic.

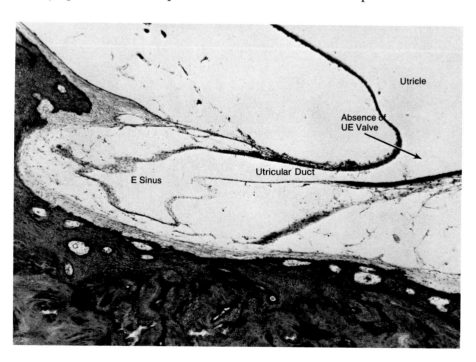

of the petrous pyramid (Figs. 5.19 and 5.27). In embryologic development, the vestibular aqueduct initially pursues a straight course paralleling the common crus to reach the endolymphatic sac in the posterior cranial fossa. While the otic capsule has attained its final adult dimensions by 20 weeks of gestation, the posterior cranial fossa continues to grow. This distal part of the endolymphatic system is pulled inferiorly by the migrating sigmoid sinus and dura of the posterior cranial fossa (Fig. 5.19). Thus, in the adult configuration the vestibular aqueduct, and consequently the endolymphatic duct, are curved laterally and inferiorly. From such developmental considerations, one can expect the anatomic relationships of the first part of the vestibular aqueduct to be quite constant and the course of the second portion to be highly variable.

The isthmus (narrowest part) of the endolymphatic duct is about 1 mm from the vestibular orifice and averages 0.3 mm in diameter (Valvassori & Clemis, 1978). The total length of the vestibular aqueduct is determined by the degree of perilabyrinthine and infralabyrinthine pneumatization (Arenberg et al., 1977).

The dimensions of the vestibular aqueduct render visualization of this structure by radiologic methods technically feasible. In Ménière's disease there is an increased incidence of nonvisualization of the vestibular aqueduct (Clemis & Valvassori, 1968; Stahle & Wilbrand, 1974a). Arenberg et al. (1977) believe that such nonvisualization is not caused by anatomic obliteration of the vestibular aqueduct, but by technical or morphologic factors. They found that ears with Ménière's disease showed reduced periaqueductal pneumatization and a higher incidence of a shortened vestibular aqueduct, which ran straighter and closer to the posterior canal than in ears without Ménière's disease. In association with the reduced periaqueductal pneumatization, they also noted an increased incidence of an anteriorly located sigmoid sinus and a superiorly located jugular bulb. The surgeon performing drainage procedures on the endolymphatic sac should keep in mind that it may be more inferiorly located in ears with Ménière's disease than in normal ears.

The lining epithelium of the endolymphatic duct, as well as that of the saccular and utricular ducts, is either simple squamous or low cuboidal;

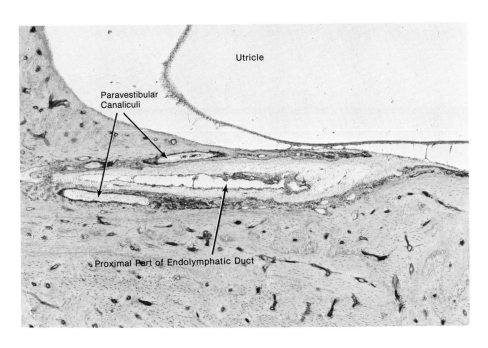

FIG. 5.27: Between the endolymphatic duct and the bony walls of the vestibular aqueduct is a layer of loose fibrous tissue. The epithelial lining varies from simple squamous to low columnar. The paravestibular canaliculi carry blood vessels which supply the endolymphatic duct and sac (female, age 40 years).

subepithelially there is a continuous basement membrane and loose connective tissue with sparse capillaries. From recent electron microscopic observations (Rask-Andersen et al., 1981) in both the guinea pig and man, the morphologic characteristics of the cells lining the endolymphatic duct suggest a functional role in water and solute absorption from endolymph.

THE ENDOLYMPHATIC SAC

Externally, approximately 10 mm posterolateral to the porus of the internal auditory canal and 10 mm inferior to the superior petrosal sulcus, the vestibular aqueduct expands to accommodate the terminal enlargement of the endolymphatic duct, the endolymphatic sac. The sac lies on the posterior surface of the petrous pyramid in a slight depression termed the foveate impression (Anson & Donaldson, 1967) or the endolymphatic fossette (Portmann, 1927); here it is partially covered by a scale of bone, the operculum. It is not simply an epithelially lined pocket, but a network of interconnected ducts and sacs (Fig. 5.28). It is closely related to the lateral venous sinus and the posteromedial cell tract. In an electron microscopic study, Lundquist (1965) divided the endolymphatic sac into three parts: 1) a proximal part located within the vestibular aqueduct and lined by cuboidal epithelium on a loose connective tissue with numerous capillaries, 2) an intermediate or rugose part located partially within the vestibular aqueduct and partially between layers of dura mater outside the vestibular aqueduct, and 3) a distal part adjacent to the sigmoid sinus, resting completely within layers of dura mater (Figs. 5.29 to 5.34).

FIG. 5.28: A graphic reconstruction of the endolymphatic sac shows it to consist of a series of interconnected saccules and channels. (Courtesy of Anson et al., 1968.)

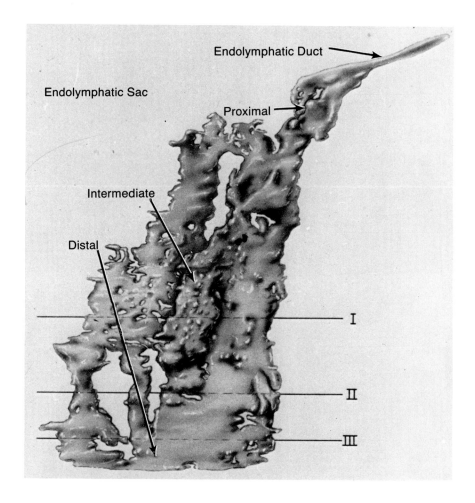

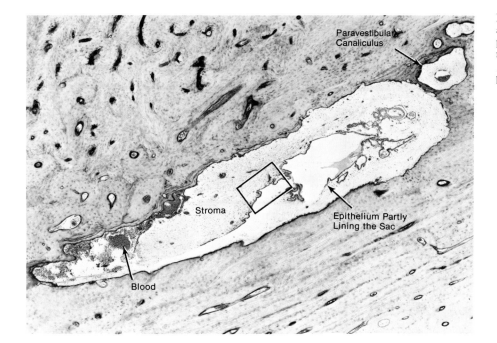

FIG. 5.29: Shown here is the intermediate part of the endolymphatic sac. The paravestibular canaliculus carries its nutrient vascular supply (male, age 50 years). Figure 5.30 shows a high power view of the outlined area.

The intermediate portion of the endolymphatic sac has a highly differentiated epithelium consisting of tall cylindrical cells irregularly dispersed into papillae and crypts, which uniformly possess microvilli and pinocytotic vesicles; it seems to be primarily engaged in pinocytotic activity (Lundquist et al., 1964; Adlington, 1967). The subepithelial connective tissue is areolar with a rich capillary supply; deep to the epithelium the connective tissue assumes a more fibrous character as it merges with the endosteum of the surrounding bone or with the dura. In the distal portion the epithelial cell height decreases, so that at its distal extreme only ductlike cuboidal cells are found, and the walls are approximated. In this area the subepithelial connective tissue has an extensive capillary meshwork, and as the sigmoid sinus is approached, the connective tissue gradually merges with that surrounding the sinus.

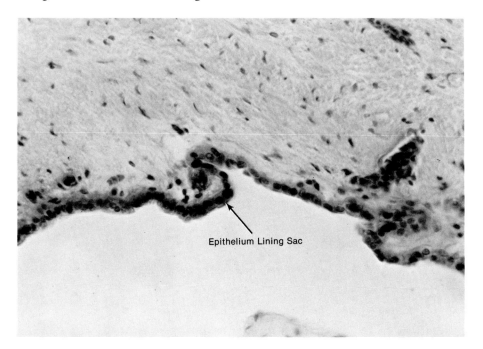

FIG. 5.30: This high power view of the outlined area in Figure 5.29 shows the cuboidal, epithelial lining of the intermediate part of the endolymphatic sac (male, age 50 years).

FIG. 5.31: In the rugose portion of the endolymphatic sac the lining epithelium is irregularly folded into papillae and crypts, which probably reflects an increased metabolic activity of this region (male, age 50 years). See Figure 5.32 for a high power view of the outlined area.

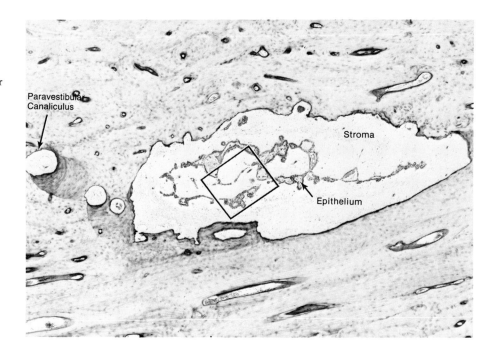

Anson and Donaldson (1981) divide the sac into a proximal portion (segments 1 and 2 of Lundquist) and a distal portion.

The portion of the sac that extends beyond the operculum is variable and is determined by the degree of pneumatization of the petrous bone. A long subosteal and a short intradural apportionment is associated with rich pneumatization, and conversely (Stahle & Wilbrand, 1974a).

The lumen of the endolymphatic sac normally contains a mixture of cellular debris, free-floating macrophages, and a variety of blood cells, predominantly leukocytes. Thus one function of the sac appears to be phagocytosis, acting as an arm of local immunodefense (Rask-Andersen et al., 1981).

FIG. 5.32: This high power view of the outlined area in Figure 5.31 shows the convoluted architecture of the lining epithelium of the rugose portion of the endolymphatic sac (male, age 50 years).

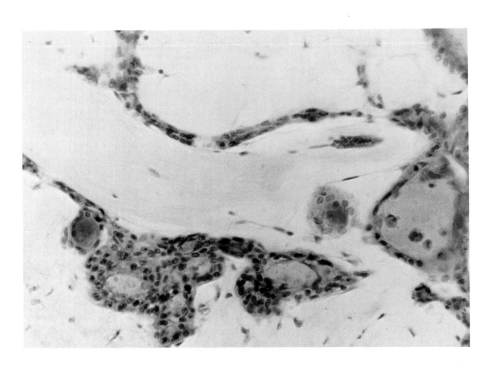

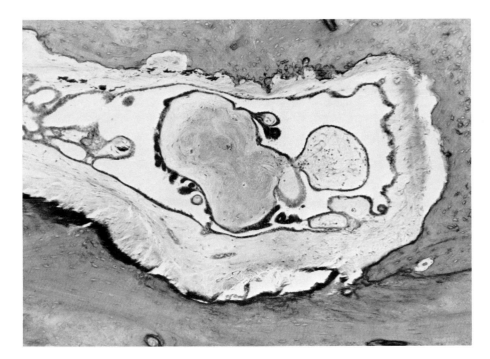

FIG. 5.33: The lining epithelium of the rugose portion of the endolymphatic sac. Its papillary projections result in islands of epithelium surrounding connective tissue cores (female, age 50 years).

The arterial supply of the vestibular aqueduct and its contents is from a branch of the posterior meningeal artery and a branch of the internal auditory artery. Venous drainage is supplied by the vein of the vestibular aqueduct (see p. 152). Lymphatics in the perisaccular connective tissue were first described by Arnvig (1951). Rask-Andersen et al. (1981) also identified lymphatic channels in association with the endolymphatic duct, and they believed that these vessels, which seemed to drain directly into the vein of the vestibular aqueduct, played a role in the resorptive function of the endolymphatic duct.

THE PARAVESTIBULAR CANALICULI (AQUEDUCTS)

The vestibular aqueduct is accompanied by the paravestibular canaliculi (Fig. 5.35), of which there are usually two. The main channel, first described by Cotunnius (Cotugno) in 1761, originates in the vestibule su-

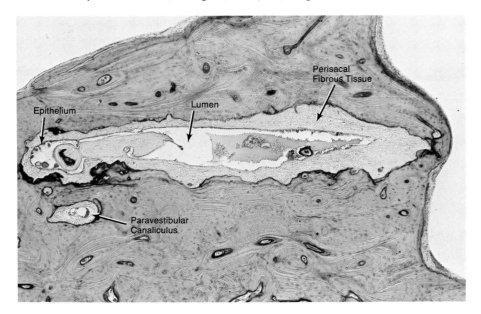

Perisacal Fibrous Tissue

Lumen

Epithelium

Paravestibular Canaliculus

FIG. 5.34: The irregular contour of the rugose portion of the endolymphatic sac is seen in this photomicrograph (female, age 16 years).

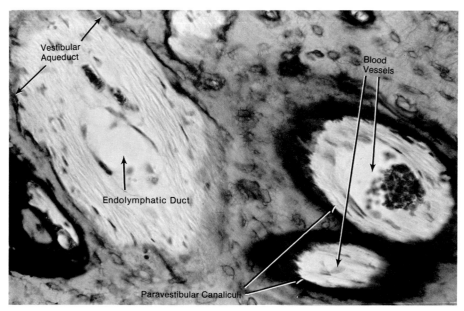

perior and medial to the aperture of the vestibular aqueduct; it houses an important vein as well as a small artery and loose connective tissue. In its intracranial appearance the vein of the vestibular aqueduct is found adjacent to the inferior aspect of the cranial orifice of the vestibular aqueduct. In this position it is well removed from the site of surgical procedures on the endolymphatic sac and internal auditory canal.

According to Mazzoni (1979), the course of this vein, which drains much of the vestibular labyrinth and part of the basal turn of the cochlea, may be divided into three segments: 1) The first segment begins as the vein enters the bony paravestibular canaliculus to travel dorsally. In this segment it parallels the vestibule and is cranial to the vestibular aqueduct. 2) The second segment sweeps dorsally and inferiorly, leaving the labyrinthine capsule and coursing through the retrolabyrinthine cell tract, first superior, then inferomedial, and finally anteromedial to the aqueduct. 3) The third segment lies within the dura mater, where it ramifies in proximity to the endolymphatic sac and terminates either in the inferior petrosal sinus or in the jugular bulb. The canaliculus enlarges as it runs from the vestibular aperture to the posterior cranial fossa, with average diameters increasing from 0.095 mm (Sando et al., 1980) to 0.3 mm (Ogura & Clemis, 1971) as it receives tributaries from the bone, dura, and the endolymphatic sac (Mazzoni, 1979). There is some controversy as to the course of this paravestibular aqueduct. Sando et al. (1980) found that in 80% of the temporal bones there were two vestibular orifices instead of one as reported by Mazzoni (1979). Ogura and Clemis (1971) and Stahle and Wilbrand (1974b) found that in 70% of cases the paravestibular canaliculus merged with the vestibular aqueduct before reaching the posterior cranial fossa.

The Perilymphatic System

THE PERILYMPHATIC LABYRINTH

The perilymphatic labyrinth consists of fluid-filled spaces interposed between the membranous labyrinth and the bony labyrinth. Its components include the vestibule (periotic cistern), the scalae tympani and vestibuli, the perilymphatic spaces of the semicircular canals, the periotic duct contained within the cochlear aqueduct, the cul-de-sac of the scala tympani, and the space around the proximal portion of the endolymphatic sinus and duct.

The remnants of the primordial reticulum are represented by scattered strands of fine connective tissue which traverse the perilymphatic spaces to the membranous walls of the utricle, saccule, semicircular ducts, and to a lesser extent the cochlear duct, often in association with small blood vessels.

The scala vestibuli is an extension of the vestibule along the anterior surface of the cochlear duct (Fig. 5.36). It is bordered by a mesenchymal epithelium which, with the epithelium of the anterior wall of the cochlear duct, forms Reissner's membrane. The scala vestibuli communicates with the scala tympani at the helicotrema.

The scala tympani is identical to the scala vestibuli in structure, but rests on the posterior side of the cochlear duct and osseous spiral lamina. From its union with the scala vestibuli at the helicotrema, it coils basalward to the round window. The anterior wall of the scala tympani contributes to the formation of the basilar membrane. The perilymph of the scala tympani communicates directly with the fluid surrounding the organ of Corti through small openings in the osseous spiral lamina known as canaliculae perforantes (Schuknecht, 1974).

At the opening of the vestibular aqueduct the contained endolymphatic duct is sheathed by a short extension of the periotic labyrinth.

THE COCHLEAR AQUEDUCT AND PERIOTIC DUCT

The cochlear aqueduct (or canaliculus) traverses the petrous pyramid from the scala tympani of the basal turn of the cochlea, close to the round window membrane (Figs. 5.37 and 5.38), to an external, funnel-shaped aperture on the inferior surface of the petrous pyramid at the anterior division of the jugular foramen. Specialized, loose connective tissue and fluid, constituting the periotic duct, fill the aqueduct and connect the scala

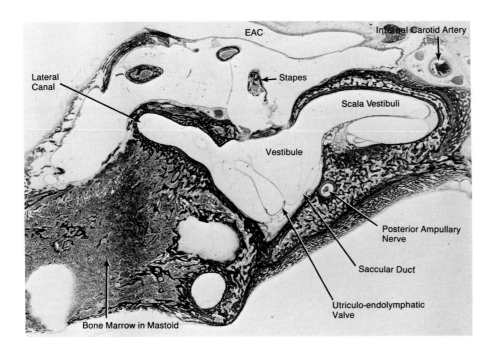

EAC

Internal Carotid Artery

Lateral Canal

Stapes

Scala Vestibuli

Vestibule

Posterior Ampullary Nerve

Saccular Duct

Utriculo-endolymphatic Valve

Bone Marrow in Mastoid

FIG. 5.36: This view demonstrates the normal relationship of the vestibule with the scala vestibuli of the basal turn (male, age 3 days).

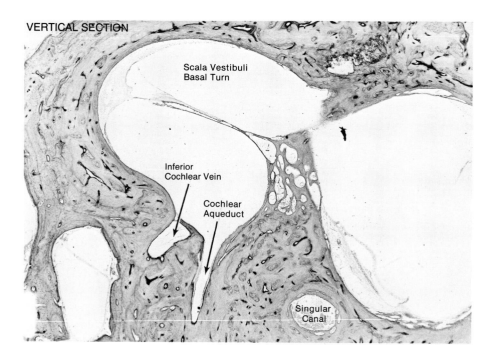

VERTICAL SECTION

Scala Vestibuli
Basal Turn

Inferior
Cochlear Vein

Cochlear
Aqueduct

Singular
Canal

tympani with the subarachnoid space. The length of the aqueduct varies
considerably, ranging from 6.2 to 12.9 mm in different studies, mainly
because of variance in choice of measurement points (Meurman, 1930;
Anson et al., 1965; Ritter & Lawrence, 1965; Palva & Dammert, 1969;
Rask-Andersen et al., 1977). Its narrowest point, or isthmus, generally is
located in the otic capsule.

The tissue of the periotic duct, as studied in the guinea pig by transmission electron microscopy, consists of two primary types of cells (Duckert,
1974): 1) The lining cells are spindle-shaped and extend from the tympanic
ostium to the external infundibulum as a continuous layer up to three
strata in thickness. 2) The reticular cells form a loose, cellular network
throughout the entirety of the ductal lumen, and possess numerous pores
as well as interdigitating cytoplasmic processes which increase their surface

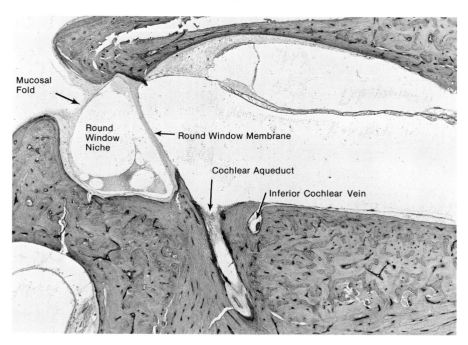

Mucosal
Fold

Round
Window
Niche

Round Window Membrane

Cochlear Aqueduct

Inferior Cochlear Vein

area and equip them for a fluid exchange function. Macrophages and erythrocytes are found among the reticular cells. The cellular elements are supported in a meshwork of connective tissue fibers. At the tympanic ostium the reticular cells of the aqueduct extend to the round window membrane, while the lining cells merge imperceptibly with the endosteum of the scala tympani.

Waltner (1948) described a "barrier membrane" occluding the cochlear opening of the aqueduct, but subsequent studies (Schuknecht & Seifi, 1963; Anson et al., 1964; Palva & Dammert, 1969; Palva, 1970) have refuted this claim. The lumen of the aqueduct is irregular, with bony excrescences (Keleman et al., 1979) as well as corpora amylacea. These latter structures were first described by Waltner (1947), who felt that they presented an impedance to cerebrospinal fluid flow. Later studies (Palva & Dammert, 1969; Keleman et al., 1979) documented that corpora amylacea could be found throughout the lumen of the cochlear aqueduct, especially at its cranial end. Palva and Dammert in 1969 demonstrated that the preponderance of corpora amylacea were composed of degenerated and contracted arachnoid cells and fibers impregnated with calcium salts and precipitates. There was no evidence, however, to indicate that these structures impeded fluid exchange between perilymph and cerebrospinal fluid.

The cranial aperture of the cochlear aqueduct is a flattened funnel that is anatomically adjacent to the trunk of the glossopharyngeal nerve. Extending into the aperture are dura and arachnoid membranes contiguous with the cranial meninges.

The patency and the function of the cochlear aqueduct have been the focus of multiple investigations (Figs. 5.39 and 5.40). Palva and Dammert (1969), in a histologic study of human temporal bones, concluded that it serves as a channel for exchange of fluids between the perilymphatic and subarachnoid spaces. The adaptation of the reticular cells for fluid exchange would facilitate such a flow. Moreover, the meshwork of the lumen could also serve to dampen sudden pressure variations between the cerebrospinal fluid and perilymph. Foreign particle transport studies (Schuknecht & Seifi, 1963), in conjunction with the microscopic visualiza-

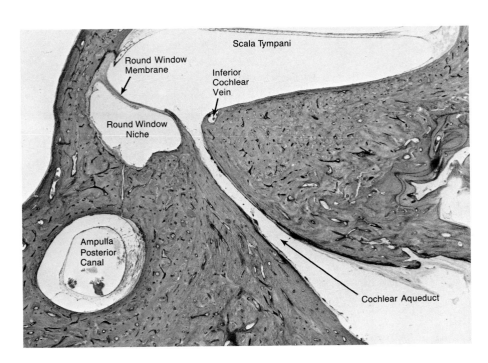

FIG. 5.39: A large patent cochlear aqueduct, as the one shown here, is unusual (male, age 67 years). The condition is probably responsible for the outflow of perilymphatic fluid (and cerebrospinal fluid) which occasionally occurs upon fenestrating the footplate of the stapes during surgical procedures. The clinical vernacular is "perilymph oozer."

Scala Tympani

Round Window Membrane

Inferior Cochlear Vein

Round Window Niche

Ampulla Posterior Canal

Cochlear Aqueduct

FIG. 5.40: The cranial end of the cochlear aqueduct may show a flared enlargement (male, age 69 years).

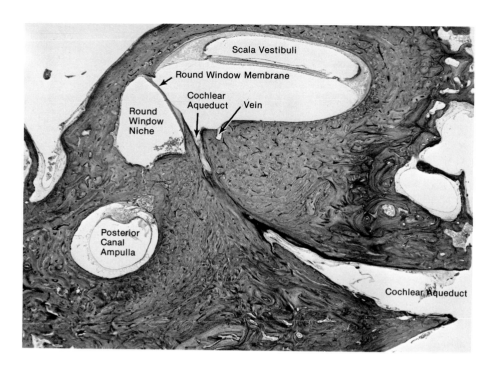

tion of macrophages and erythrocytes within the connective tissue meshwork, support the concept that the duct passes particulate matter as well as
fluid between the perilymph and cerebrospinal fluid.

It has been conjectured by surgeons that the outflow of cerebrospinal
fluid that occasionally occurs when the oval window is opened, particularly in ears with congenital hearing losses, is the result of large patent
cochlear aqueducts. This explanation seems reasonable for mild outflows,
commonly referred to as "perilymph oozers." It is doubtful, however, that
voluminous outflows, known as "perilymph gushers," could be accounted
for on this basis. Defects in the modiolus have been suspected as the basis
for this phenomenon (Schuknecht, 1980) and such defects have now been
demonstrated (Shi, 1985) (Fig. 5.41).

There are two accessory canals (Siebenmann, 1890) which course in
close association with the cochlear aqueduct. The first accessory canal shel-
ters the inferior cochlear vein and exits the scala tympani adjacent to the
cochlear aqueduct. The vein empties into either the inferior petrosal sinus
or the jugular bulb. This bony canal is eponymically referred to as the
"canal of Cotugno" (or Cotunnio), named for the Neapolitan anatomist
who originally described it in 1761. Less constant is the second accessory
canal which transmits a vein from the tympanic cavity and eventually joins
the canal of Cotugno (Palva, 1970).

The Internal Auditory Canal

The internal auditory canal is a bony, neurovascular channel providing
a tunnel for the facial, cochlear and vestibular nerves, the nervus intermedius, and the labyrinthine artery and vein from the posterior cranial fossa
into the petrous bone. It has three distinguishable regions: 1) the porus
(meatus) or inlet, located on the posterior surface of the temporal bone,
2) the canal proper, and 3) the fundus, abutting upon the medial aspect of
the labyrinth. The dura and arachnoid membranes of the internal auditory
canal extend to the lamina cribrosa which marks the lateral boundary of

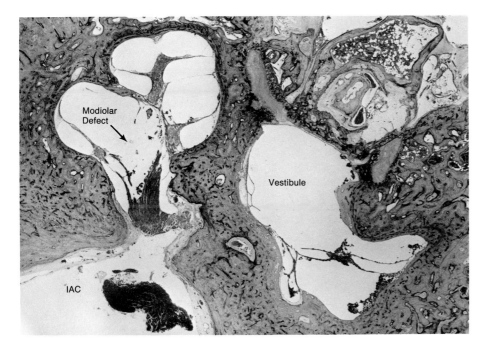

FIG. 5.41: The cochlea of this 2-1/2-year-old child with congenital conductive hearing loss shows a developmental defect in the modiolus of the basal turn resulting in a wide confluence between the subarachnoid space of the internal auditory canal (IAC) and the scala vestibuli of the basal turn. The stapes is fixed. In such cases, fenestrating the footplate of the stapes during surgical procedures results in a voluminous outpouring of perilymph and cerebrospinal fluid. The clinical vernacular is "perilymph gusher."

the fundus. The falciform (transverse) crest, a transverse ridge of bone, divides the lamina cribrosa into upper and lower compartments and provides an attachment site for the dura. The upper compartment is further divided into anterior (containing the facial nerve and nervus intermedius) and posterior (containing the superior vestibular nerve) quadrants by the vertical crest. In the lower compartment, the cochlear nerve courses in the anterior quadrant while the inferior vestibular nerve occupies the posterior quadrant (Fig. 5.42).

The term "semilunar lip" is used clinically to denote the combined inferior, superior, and posterior margins of the porus. Neoplasms arising within the internal auditory canal often erode this lip, thus widening the porus and canal as well as shortening the length of the floor, roof, and posterior wall.

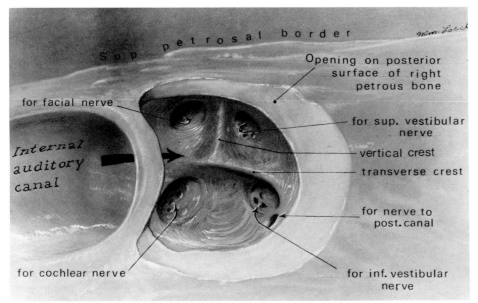

FIG. 5.42: The fundus of the internal auditory canal is compartmentalized by the vertical and transverse crests. (After Anson & Donaldson, 1981.)

Embryologically, the ossification of the fundus and the adjacent walls of the internal auditory canal are intimately related with that of the otic capsule; this establishes the constant relationship of structures of the inner ear to the internal auditory canal.

Variations in size and degree of pneumatization of the encasing petrous bone have an impact upon the size, shape, and orientation of the internal auditory canal. X-ray studies by Carnelis, as cited by Portmann et al. (1975), show that the axis of the internal auditory canal makes an 80° to 90° angle with the sagittal plane in 58% of ears, and 91° to 100° in 37% of ears. There is great variability in both the vertical and horizontal diameters of the internal auditory canal. A recent study by Pérez Olivares and Schuknecht (1979) showed horizontal diameter measurements ranging from 2.5 to 5.26 mm, with a mean of 3.68 mm, and vertical diameter measurements of 2.0 to 5.8 mm, with an average of 3.72 mm. The average length of the internal auditory canal is 8 mm (Portmann et al., 1975), but large variations occur (Fig. 5.43). In each individual, there is relative constancy in the diameter of the paired internal auditory canals; differences of more than 2 mm are considered to be abnormal. However, there may be interaural differences in internal auditory canal length of some 6 mm. Portmann et al. (1975) believe that this relative constancy of the diameter of the canal reflects the constancy of the volume of the contained neurovascular bundle for a particular individual. The variable length of the internal auditory canal is in great part determined by the degree of pneumatization of the temporal bone. The internal auditory canal is usually uniformly cylindrical, although variations of 1 to 2 mm in the horizontal and vertical dimensions can occur. Thus, one may see funnel-shaped canals with a smaller diameter at either the medial or lateral aspects of the canal, or canals presenting a central hourglass-like narrowing.

A common anatomic variant is a localized area of widening (cupping) in the anterior wall of the canal (Figs. 5.44 and 5.45).

The exposure of the internal auditory canal and its contents by way of a middle cranial fossa approach, popularized by House (1961), has been

FIG. 5.43: The internal auditory canal (IAC) in this ear measures 12 mm in length (normal: 8 mm) which is considered to be a normal anatomic variant (female, age 90 years).

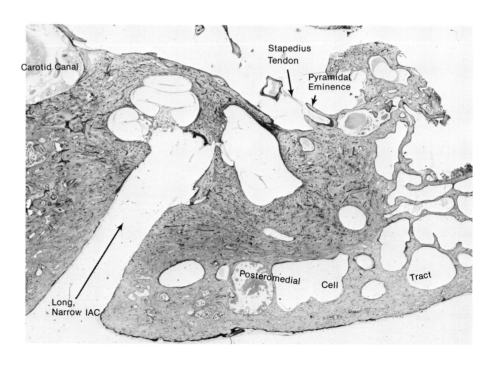

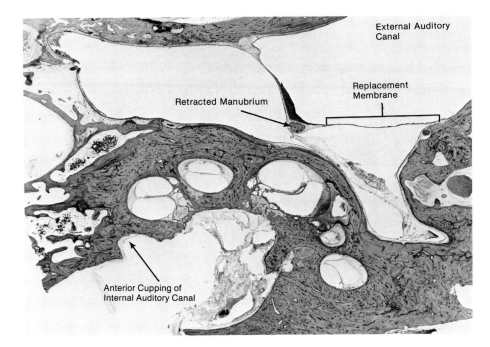

External Auditory Canal

Replacement Membrane

Retracted Manubrium

Anterior Cupping of Internal Auditory Canal

FIG. 5.44: The internal auditory canal (IAC) measures 7.5 mm in length which is considered to be normal. The cupping at its anterior aspect is an occasional occurrence that may create a diagnostic dilemma on imaging studies. The pathologically thin replacement membrane is the result of a healed perforation. As a result, the manubrium is medially displaced because of lessened opposition to the traction of the tensor tympani muscle (male, age 46 years).

successfully used for removal of small vestibular schwannomata, for vestibular and/or cochlear nerve section, and for facial nerve decompression. This approach to the internal auditory canal demands a thorough knowledge of the normal anatomy as well as of the typical variations one may encounter. In the House (1961) approach, once the squamosal craniotomy has been performed, the middle meningeal artery entering the cranium via the foramen spinosum is the first intracranial landmark to be identified; it forms the anterior limit of dissection. Further dural elevation is carried out to expose the arcuate eminence posteriorly and the superior petrosal sinus medially. The greater superficial petrosal nerve, a crucial landmark in the localization of the internal auditory canal, is next identified and dural elevation proceeds posteriorly, parallel to its course. The geniculate ganglion serves as a reference point for further dissection. The facial nerve is medial

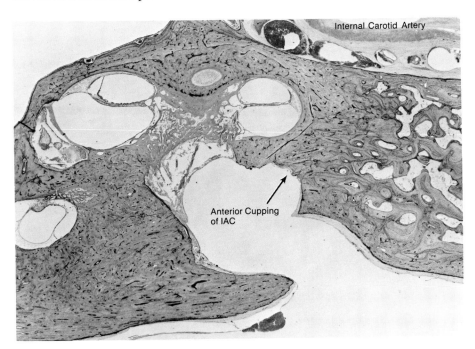

Internal Carotid Artery

Anterior Cupping of IAC

FIG. 5.45: The temporal bone of a 66-year-old man shows anterior cupping of the middle portion of the internal auditory canal (IAC) occurring as an anatomic variant.

to the geniculate ganglion, while the superior canal is posteromedial to it. The exposure of the internal auditory canal is achieved by drilling in the area between the superior canal and the basal turn of the cochlea just medial to the geniculate ganglion. Medial dissection follows the facial nerve up to the ridge of the superior petrosal sinus corresponding to the superior lip of the porus acousticus. This dissection is facilitated by the anteromedial divergence of the internal auditory canal from the superior canal, which widens the surgical field.

Suggestions have appeared in the literature that a narrow internal auditory canal may cause sensorineural hearing loss and vertigo, and that surgical decompression of the canal is an appropriate therapy (House & Brackmann, 1977). Pérez Olivares and Schuknecht (1979) studied 144 temporal bone specimens from subjects with a history of slowly progressive sensorineural hearing loss and found a distribution of canal dimensions similar to that of normals; they also reported the absence of any soft tissue lesions which could have caused a canal narrowing. Hence they believe that radiologic documentation of a small internal auditory canal is merely coincidental to, and not causative of, cochlear and/or vestibular peripheral symptomatology.

Parisier (1977) conducted a temporal bone study, utilizing both dissected and serially sectioned specimens, to examine the variations in anatomic landmarks used in the middle cranial fossa approach. He found that those structures which were of otic placode derivation and encased in enchondral bone (for instance, the cochlea, superior canal, and facial nerve at the area nervi facialis) demonstrated relatively little variability in anatomic relationships. In contrast, neural and vascular structures showed a considerable degree of variability, both with respect to each other as well as to inner ear landmarks.

Fisch (1970) has modified the House (1961) approach to the internal auditory canal, using the arcuate eminence as his primary reference point; however, as noted by Parisier (1977), the prominence as well as its relationship to the superior canal is quite variable, depending upon the pattern and degree of temporal bone pneumatization. According to Fisch, the superior canal forms a 60° angle with respect to the superior vestibular nerve; he uses this fact to locate the posterior margin of the internal auditory canal. Parisier noted considerable variability in this relationship.

6. Neuroanatomy

The Facial Nerve

THE FUNCTIONAL COMPONENTS

The facial nerve is the nerve of the second branchial arch, and as such innervates structures derived from Reichert's cartilage (see embryology, Chapter 9). Five populations of fibers contribute to the facial nerve trunk (Gray, 1959; Carpenter, 1972): 1) *special visceral efferent fibers,* which supply the striated muscles of facial expression, the stapedius muscle, the stylohyoid muscle, and the posterior belly of the digastric muscle; 2) *general visceral efferent fibers* (preganglionic secretory fibers) which are distributed to the lacrimal and seromucinous glands of the nasal cavity via the greater superficial petrosal nerve (see also nervus intermedius, p. 176) and to the submaxillary and sublingual glands through the chorda tympani nerve; 3) *special sensory fibers* for taste from the anterior two-thirds of the tongue through the chorda tympani nerve and from the tonsillar fossae and palate via the greater superficial petrosal nerve; 4) *somatic sensory fibers* supplying the external auditory canal and adjacent conchal region, as well as conveying proprioceptive information from the facial muscles; and 5) *visceral afferent fibers* serving the mucosa of the nose, pharynx, and palate. Three nuclei supply the fibers to the facial nerve: 1) The *motor nucleus* is located in the caudal aspect of the pons. Its superior part, which supplies the frontal and orbicularis oculi muscles, receives both crossed and uncrossed fibers from the precentral gyrus (motor cortex). The inferior part of the facial motor nucleus receives only homolateral, uncrossed cortical information to innervate the remainder of the facial musculature, save for the levator palpebrae superioris. The blink reflex and stapedius reflex are mediated through internuclear connections in the medulla oblongata (Miehlke, 1964). 2) The *superior salivatory nucleus* is situated dorsal to the motor nucleus and carries parasympathetic secretory stimuli to the submaxillary, sublingual, lacrimal, nasal, and palatine glands. 3) The *nucleus of the solitary tract* which is located in the medulla oblongata receives the taste, proprioceptive, and cutaneous sensory fibers of the facial nerve.

The origins of the motor roots and sensory roots (nervus intermedius) are located at the inferior border of the pons; there, in a recess between the inferior cerebellar penduncle and the olive, the motor root lies medially with respect to the nervus intermedius and the acoustic nerve lies laterally. A schema of the distribution of the motor, taste, and parasympathetic fibers is seen in Figure 6.1.

THE NORMAL COURSE IN THE TEMPORAL BONE

The combined sensory and autonomic components of the facial nerve are separated from the motor component distally as far as the geniculate ganglion into the nervus intermedius (see p. 176) and motor trunk. Distal to the geniculate ganglion, the sensory component is segregated into a discrete bundle within the trunks of the facial nerve. The question as to whether there is a topographical organization in the facial nerve has been argued positively (May, 1973; Crumley, 1980; Kempe, 1980) and negatively (Harris, 1968; Thomander et al., 1981), but the issue appears finally to have been resolved by Gacek and Radpour (1982). Using an anterograde degeneration technique in combination with selective lesions of the facial nerve in cats, they could find no topographic segregation of the motor fibers.

The course of the facial nerve may be divided anatomically into five segments: 1) The first or *intracranial segment* of the facial nerve spans the 23 to 24 mm between its origin at the pons and the internal auditory canal, cradled in a groove on the superior surface of the cochlear nerve. The nervus intermedius parallels the facial nerve and joins it in a spiraling fashion in the fundus of the internal auditory canal (Guerrier, 1977).

2) The second or *internal auditory canal segment* is 7 to 8 mm in length. The facial nerve maintains its superior position relative to the cochlear nerve and passes above the transverse (falciform) crest to enter the fallopian canal at the area nervi facialis.

3) The third, *labyrinthine* (intratemporal) *segment* (Fig. 6.2), is the shortest at only 3 to 4 mm. It begins at the area nervi facialis and heads

FIG. 6.1: Schematic diagram of the facial nerve illustrating the distribution of motor ⊞, taste ▬, and parasympathetic = fibers. (Schuknecht & Shinozaki, unpublished data.)

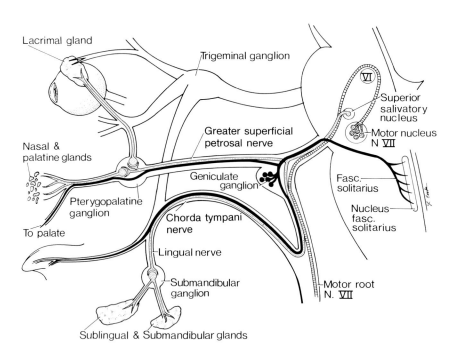

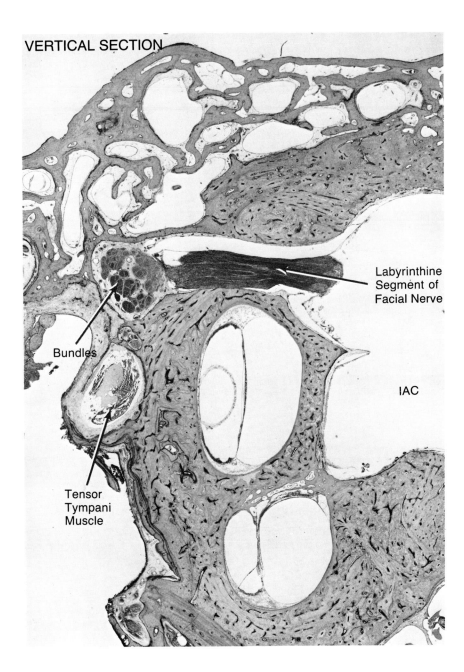

VERTICAL SECTION

Labyrinthine Segment of Facial Nerve

Bundles

Tensor Tympani Muscle

IAC

FIG. 6.2: This vertical section shows the labyrinthine segment of the facial nerve. In this region the nerve is susceptible to injury by transverse fractures of the temporal bone (male, age 71 years).

anteriorly and laterally, running superior to the cochlea and vestibule and nearly perpendicular to the petrous pyramid, until it reaches the geniculate ganglion. The geniculate ganglion houses the cell bodies serving both the sensory (taste) fibers of the chorda tympani nerve and the greater superficial petrosal nerve, and the preganglionic secretory fibers for the sphenopalatine ganglion. Ganglion cells serving pain reception are also believed to be within the geniculate ganglion (Kuré & Sano, 1936) and are held responsible for the pain of petrosal neuralgia. In a topographic study, Dobozi (1975) consistently found that the geniculate ganglion, which appears triangular in the horizontal plane of sectioning, averaged 1.09 mm in length, 0.76 mm in width, and 0.6 to 0.8 mm in height, showing little variability among the specimens examined. Ultrastructural studies of the guinea pig geniculate ganglion (Kitamura et al., 1982) have demonstrated two types of ganglion cells, light cells and smaller dark cells. However, the exact functional significance of these two types of cells remains obscure. The anterior limit of the geniculate ganglion lies in close relation to the middle cranial fossa, from which it is usually separated by a bony plate; however, it may lie free in a bony dehiscence in the floor of the middle cranial fossa (see facial hiatus, p. 172). Distal to the geniculate ganglion, the facial nerve turns abruptly posteriorly, forming the first genu of the facial nerve (Figs. 6.3 to 6.5). The bony fallopian canal, dubbed with a misnomer of "aqueductus" by Gabriele Falloppio (cited by Politzer, 1907) because it reminded him of a water pipe, courses about 30 mm from the area nervi facialis to the stylomastoid foramen. Not only is this bony canal riddled with multiple deficiencies in its walls (see dehiscences of the facial nerve, p. 168), but also it can act as a strangulating tunnel in the presence of facial nerve edema and facial palsy.

4) The fourth or *tympanic segment* parallels the longitudinal axis of the petrous pyramid, running posteriorly and laterally on the medial wall of the tympanic cavity between the lateral canal superiorly and the oval window inferiorly for 12 to 13 mm. At the sinus tympani the nerve turns inferiorly. This second genu marks the beginning of the mastoid segment.

5) The fifth or *mastoid segment* carries the nerve vertically downward in the posterior wall of the tympanic cavity and the anterior wall of the mastoid, a distance of 15 to 20 mm, to the nerve's egress from the skull at the stylomastoid foramen.

Ogawa and Sando (1982) studied the relative cross-sectional area of the facial nerve with respect to its canal in histologic preparations of 18 normal temporal bone specimens. They found that in its labyrinthine and tympanic segments the nerve occupied, on the average, somewhat more than 45% of the canal, whereas in the mastoid segment the figure was 32%.

ABNORMAL COURSES IN THE TEMPORAL BONE

The otologic surgeon must be aware of the various anomalous courses of the facial nerve. Working in bone with a high-speed cutting bur, the surgeon must develop a technique which will allow for an unexpected encounter with the nerve without injury to it.

FIG. 6.3: In approximately 5% of cases (House & Crabtree, 1965), the genu of the facial nerve lies dehiscent in the middle cranial fossa (female, age 16 years).

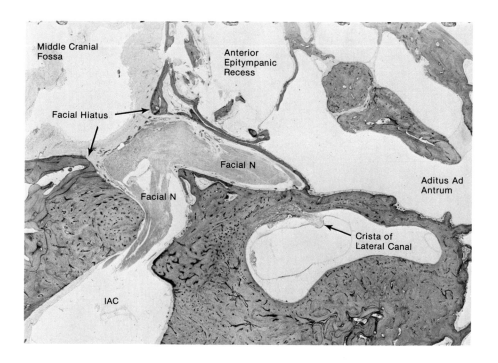

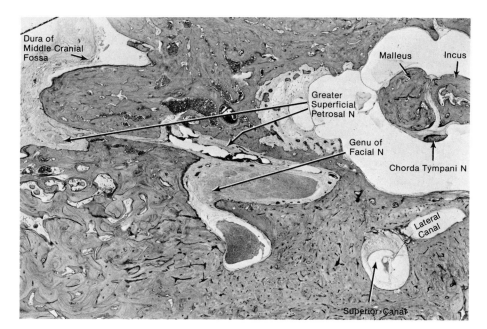

FIG. 6.4: In this ear the genu of the facial nerve lies deeply buried in the petrous bone far from the dura of the middle cranial fossa. The greater superficial petrosal nerve channels anteriorly through bone to emerge from a small facial hiatus (female, age 53 years).

There are numerous examples of cases in which the facial nerve pursues an anomalous course through the petrous bone (Basek, 1962; Miehlke, 1964, 1965; Durcan et al., 1967; Shambaugh, 1967; Wright et al., 1967; Greisen, 1975; Gerhardt & Otto, 1981; Proctor & Nager, 1982a, 1982b). The most common example is that in which the main nerve trunk runs anterior and inferior to the oval window (Hough, 1958, 1977). Rarely, the nerve pursues a course anterior to both the oval window and the round window (Fowler, 1961; Dickinson et al., 1968).

The infant lacks a true mastoid process and possesses only a rudimentary tympanic ring, leaving the facial nerve vulnerable to injury at the stylomastoid foramen. In subsequent development, the nerve becomes more secluded by the medial migration of the stylomastoid foramen dictated by the growth of the tympanic ring and mastoid.

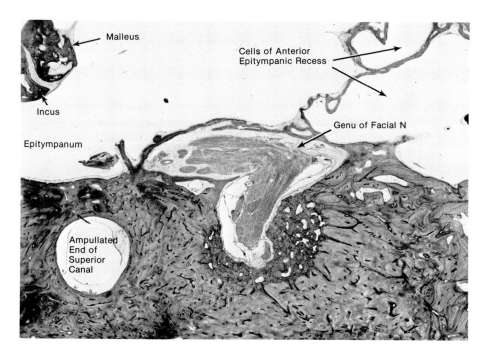

FIG. 6.5: The genu of the facial nerve normally lies in the medial wall of the epitympanum and is protected by a bony covering. There is an otosclerotic focus partly surrounding the labyrinthine segment of the nerve (male, age 62 years).

Neuroanatomy **165**

FIG. 6.6: The sketch shows the second genu of the facial nerve more posteriorly located than usual. (After Miehlke, 1973.)

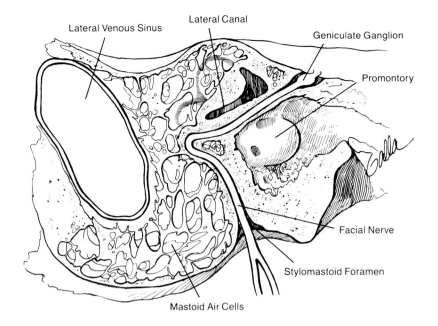

Lateral Venous Sinus

Lateral Canal

Geniculate Ganglion

Promontory

Facial Nerve

Stylomastoid Foramen

Mastoid Air Cells

Dehiscences in the bony canal also render the facial nerve potentially vulnerable to surgical injury. The mastoid segment of the nerve may be displaced several millimeters posteriorly and/or laterally (Fig. 6.6). There are cases of bi- or even tri-partition of the nerve in which the individual branches course to their separate points of exit from the skull, each in its own canal (Figs. 6.7 to 6.9). The nerve may pass anterosuperiorly to the cochlea rather than posterosuperiorly as it normally does (Figs. 6.10 and 6.11). In its mastoid segment it may swerve more posteriorly than normal (Fig. 6.12).

Other anomalous courses are more generally associated with aural malformations, such as an hypoplastic facial nerve passing through the obturator foramen of the stapes (Altmann, 1951).

FIG. 6.7: The mastoid segment of the facial nerve in this ear has divided into three separate bundles, each of which exits separately from the temporal bone (female, age 61 years).

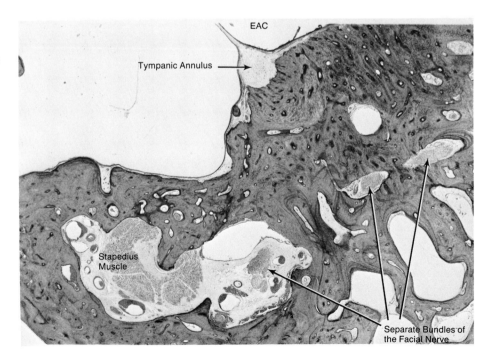

EAC

Tympanic Annulus

Stapedius Muscle

Separate Bundles of the Facial Nerve

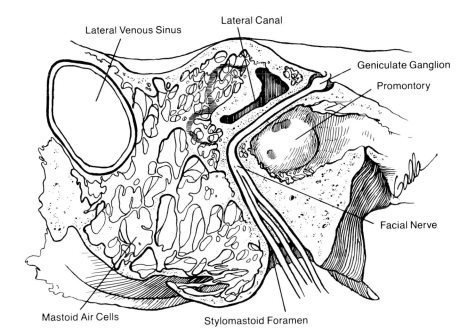

Labels for top figure:
Lateral Venous Sinus
Lateral Canal
Geniculate Ganglion
Promontory
Facial Nerve
Mastoid Air Cells
Stylomastoid Foramen

FIG. 6.8: The sketch demonstrates tripartition of the facial nerve distal to the second genu. Compare to Figure 6.7. (After Miehlke, 1973.)

Litton et al. (1969) studied the anatomic relationship of the facial nerve in adults with respect to the tympanic annulus and noted great variability in the course of the facial nerve through its tympanic and mastoid segments. It is to be remembered that the tympanic annulus in the adult is not in the sagittal plane, but rather is directed anteriorly and inferiorly. The usual location of the facial nerve is 1.4 mm posterior and 2.3 mm medial to the posterosuperior part of the tympanic annulus. The descending segment of the facial nerve is consistently located posterior to the posteroinferior margin of the tympanic annulus. The facial canal, as it heads laterally and inferiorly, crosses the plane of the tympanic annulus in its lower one-half.

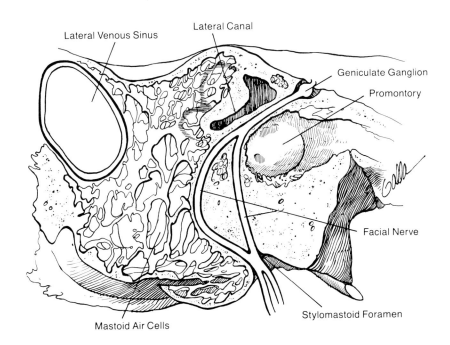

Labels for bottom figure:
Lateral Venous Sinus
Lateral Canal
Geniculate Ganglion
Promontory
Facial Nerve
Mastoid Air Cells
Stylomastoid Foramen

FIG. 6.9: The sketch demonstrates bifurcation of the facial nerve. (After Miehlke, 1973.)

FIG. 6.10: The facial nerve may pass anterior to the cochlea as shown here. The nerve may also course between the oval and round windows or over the promontory just anterior to both windows. (After Miehlke, 1973.)

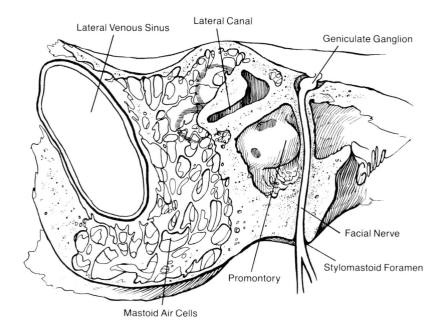

Lateral Venous Sinus Lateral Canal Geniculate Ganglion Facial Nerve Stylomastoid Foramen Promontory Mastoid Air Cells

DEHISCENCES OF THE FACIAL NERVE

The facial nerve passes through the temporal bone, protected throughout most of its course by the bony sheath of the fallopian canal. Politzer (1894) described "congenital gaps in the facial canal." As documented by Baxter (1971), it is not unusual for gaps to exist in the continuity of this bony sheath; he found dehiscences of the fallopian canal, defined as non-pathologic gaps of 0.4 mm or greater in diameter, in either the tympanic or mastoid segments of the facial nerve in 55% of the temporal bones studied. Moreover, more than one dehiscence was found in 22% of the ears examined. The most common site of dehiscence of the bony canal involved the tympanic segment adjacent to the oval window (Figs. 6.13 to 6.15), where the facial nerve normally overhangs the oval window niche. The average width of the dehiscences was 0.92 mm in the oval window region and

FIG. 6.11: In this ear the facial nerve in its labyrinthine segment takes an aberrant course anterosuperior to the cochlea (male, age 56 years).

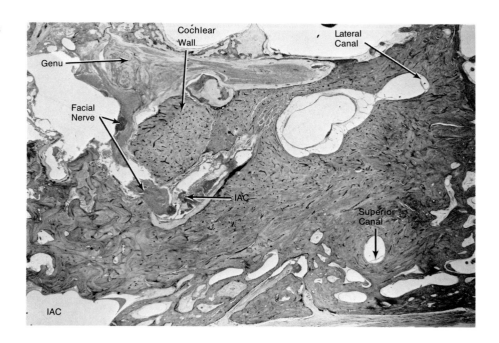

Cochlear Wall Lateral Canal Genu Facial Nerve IAC Superior Canal IAC

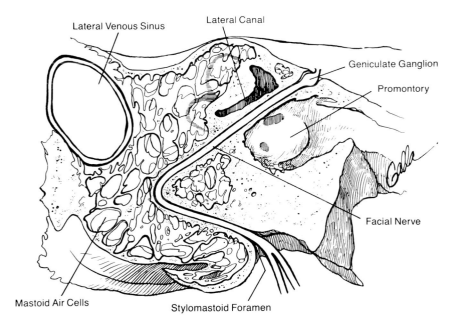

Lateral Venous Sinus
Lateral Canal
Geniculate Ganglion
Promontory
Facial Nerve
Mastoid Air Cells
Stylomastoid Foramen

FIG. 6.12: The sketch demonstrates the facial nerve coursing in the mastoid far posterior to its normal location. (After Miehlke, 1973.)

0.73 mm in the mastoid segment. Other histologic studies of the temporal bone (Kikuchi, 1907; Iida, 1951) and other observations (Fowler, 1947; Guild, 1949; Hough, 1958; Kaplan, 1960; Beddard & Saunders, 1962) also confirm that the oval window area of the canal is the most common site for dehiscence. Dehiscences of the facial nerve may also be found adjacent to the tensor tympani tendon, in the facial recess (Fig. 6.16), and in the medial wall of the anterior epitympanic recess (Figs. 6.17 and 6.18).

Dehiscences in the bony covering of the facial nerve provide areas of vulnerability to surgical injury. This risk is increased when the nerve bulges out of the dehiscence, as sometimes occurs in the oval window area (Figs. 6.19 and 6.20) (Johnsson & Kingsley, 1970). It is possible that dehiscences predispose the facial nerve to inflammatory disease of the middle ear. Facial palsy may occur as a complication of acute otitis media.

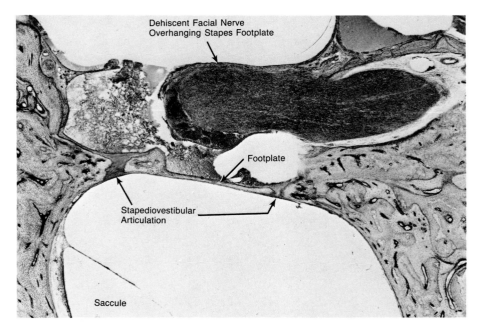

Dehiscent Facial Nerve
Overhanging Stapes Footplate
Footplate
Stapediovestibular
Articulation
Saccule

FIG. 6.13: The most common area for dehiscence of the facial nerve is in the region of the oval window. In this case, the facial nerve protrudes from the fallopian canal and overlies part of the stapes footplate (male, age 51 years).

FIG. 6.14: The facial nerve in its tympanic segment is seen protruding from its canal and encroaching on the oval window. This ear also shows the pathologic condition of endolymphatic hydrops (female, age 68 years).

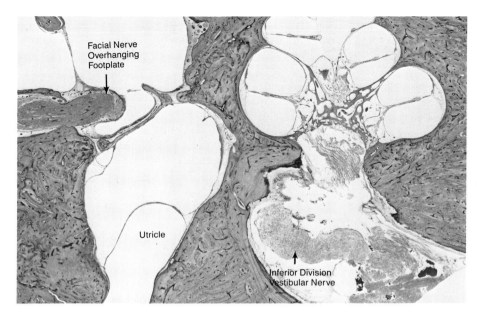

FIG. 6.15: The facial nerve protrudes from its canal to overlie the footplate partially and nearly abut a posteriorly located cochleariform process (male, age 82 years).

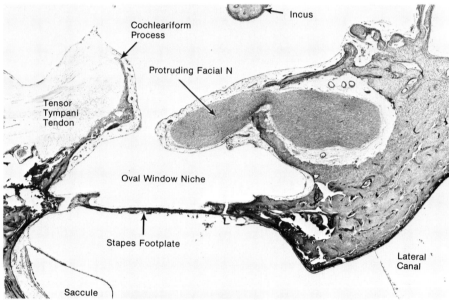

FIG. 6.16: In this ear there is a bony dehiscence of the fallopian canal in the medial wall of the facial recess (female, age 50 years).

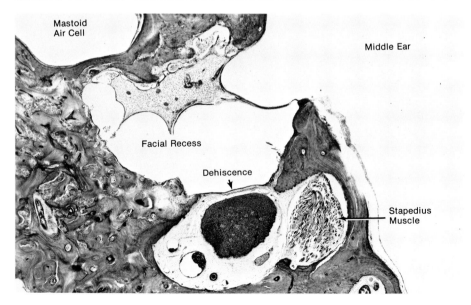

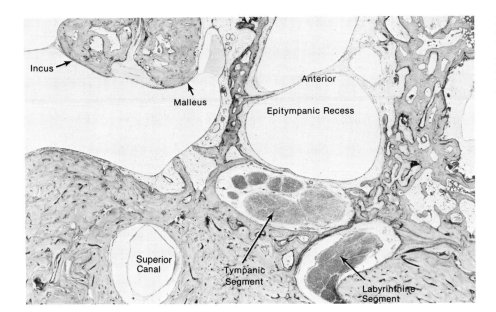

Fig. 6.17: The anterior epitympanic recess appears as a single large cell with the facial nerve dehiscent of bone in its medial wall. In many cases, as shown here, the facial nerve trunk in both its tympanic and labyrinthine segments is composed of several bundles (female, age 65 years).

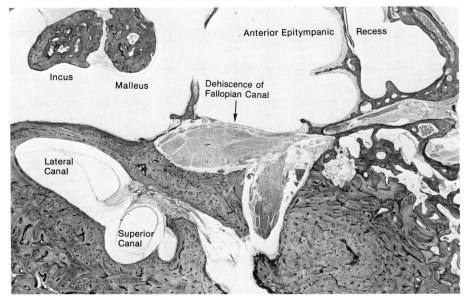

Fig. 6.18: There is a bony dehiscence of the facial nerve canal in the medial wall of the anterior epitympanic recess. The nerve bulges slightly into the recess (female, age 72 years).

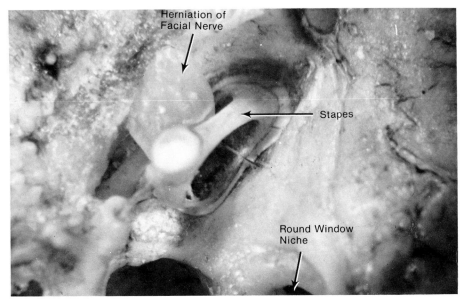

Fig. 6.19: This photograph of a partially dissected temporal bone shows a tumor-like herniation of the facial nerve from the fallopian canal just superior to the oval window (see Fig. 6.20). (Courtesy of Johnsson & Kingsley, 1970.)

FIG. 6.20: Same specimen as Figure 6.19, showing a histologic cross section of the nerve after it has been removed from the facial canal. The entire nerve trunk takes an omega-shaped course out of its canal. (Courtesy of Johnsson & Kingsley, 1970.)

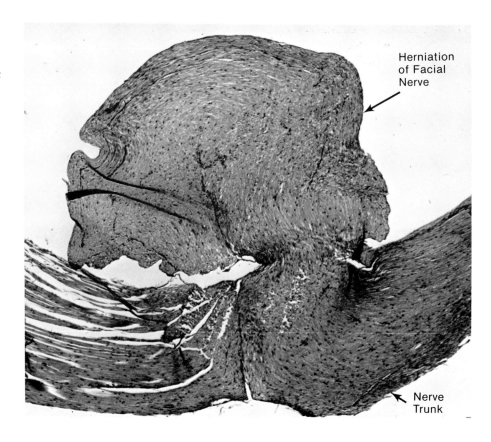

Herniation of Facial Nerve

Nerve Trunk

THE FACIAL HIATUS

The facial hiatus (hiatus canalis nervi petrosi majoris) is a dehiscence of variable size present in the petrous part of the temporal bone in the floor of the middle cranial fossa; it marks the entrance of the greater superficial petrosal nerve into the middle cranial fossa. This nerve originates from the geniculate ganglion, located on the anterior aspect of the genu of the facial nerve. Usually the geniculate ganglion lies deep to the hiatus, in which case the greater superficial petrosal nerve passes through a bony canal to reach the hiatus. In some cases the geniculate ganglion lies under the dura (Fig. 6.21) within the hiatus (Hall et al., 1969). According to Ge and Spector (1981), at 15 weeks' gestation the geniculate ganglion lies in a dural condensation superior to the anterior part of the epitympanum, and the "primitive facial hiatus" provides a route of communication between the middle cranial fossa and the middle ear cavity. As the squamous part of the temporal bone develops, it separates the geniculate ganglion from the epitympanic space. The superior surface of the geniculate ganglion, however, is still dehiscent in the 35-week-old embryo, and its perineural tissues are directly attached to the dura and middle cranial fossa. This dehiscence may persist to a variable extent even into adulthood. House and Crabtree (1965) found that the geniculate ganglion was exposed to the middle cranial fossa without a bony covering in 5% of cases. Hall et al. (1969) found a 15% incidence of partial or total exposure of the geniculate ganglion to the middle cranial fossa in a study of 100 adult temporal bones. Saito et al. (1970) reviewed 400 temporal bones in the collection of the Massachusetts Eye and Ear Infirmary and found that in 9% of the cases the facial hiatus measured more than 1.5 mm in its greatest dimension, leaving the geniculate ganglion open to the middle cranial fossa.

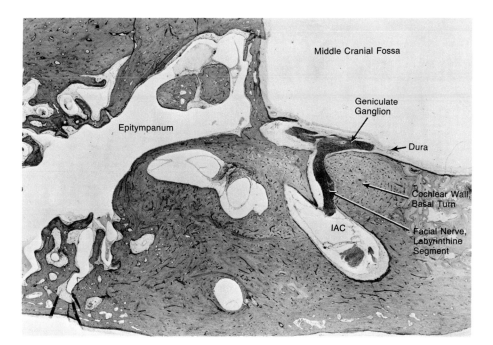

Middle Cranial Fossa

Geniculate
Ganglion

Epitympanum

Dura

Cochlear Wall,
Basal Turn

IAC

Facial Nerve,
Labyrinthine
Segment

FIG. 6.21: The genu of the facial nerve lies under the dura of the middle cranial fossa. This ear does not have an anterior epitympanic recess (female, age 79 years).

Variations in the anatomy of the facial hiatus are of significance for two reasons: 1) when the geniculate ganglion and facial nerve lie within the hiatus, they are vulnerable to injury during neurosurgical procedures involving the floor of the middle cranial fossa, and 2) the facial hiatus is used as an anatomic landmark in the middle fossa approach to the internal auditory canal.

BRANCHES OF THE FACIAL NERVE

The facial nerve gives off three major branches in its course through the temporal bone: 1) The first is the *greater superficial petrosal nerve* (Fig. 6.4), which originates from the anterior aspect of the geniculate ganglion. It surfaces at the facial hiatus and enters the middle cranial fossa, from which this mixed nerve of parasympathetic and sensory fibers courses anteriorly towards the foramen lacerum. It unites with the sympathetic fibers of the deep petrosal nerve to form the vidian nerve (nerve of the pterygoid canal). Leaving its canal anteriorly, the vidian nerve passes through the pterygopalatine fossa to enter the sphenopalatine ganglion. 2) The second branch is the *nerve to the stapedius muscle*. It arises from the mastoid segment of the facial nerve in the region of the pyramidal eminence. 3) The fibers of the third branch, the *chorda tympani nerve*, are located in the sensory bundle of the facial nerve trunk which occupies approximately 10% of its total cross-sectional area (Fig. 6.22) (Saito et al., 1970). The sensory bundle (chorda tympani fibers) occupies an anterolateral position in the tympanic segment and posterolateral position in the mastoid segment of the facial nerve before separating from the facial nerve trunk. The nerve usually arises about 4 mm superior to the stylomastoid foramen, although it may arise distal to the stylomastoid foramen. The nerve follows a course which is phylogenetically determined; it is the pretrematic branch of the second branchial arch, and connects the Vth cranial nerve (the nerve of the first branchial arch) with the nerve of the second branchial arch (the facial nerve). Thus it runs with the facial nerve in the area derived from the second branchial arch and with the trigeminal nerve (mandibular division) in the region derived from the first arch.

FIG. 6.22: In the mastoid segment the sensory component of the facial nerve is located in the posterolateral part of the nerve trunk (male, age 62 years).

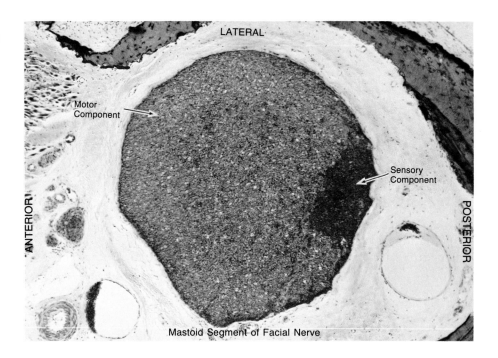

It follows a recurrent route superiorly in its own canal (the canaliculus chordae tympani), and enters the tympanic cavity through an opening in the posterior wall, the iter chordae posterius, at the horizontal level of the round window and the cochlear aqueduct. Here it is accompanied by the posterior tympanic artery. The iter chordae posterius generally lies between the pyramidal eminence and the tympanic annulus in the vertical plane. In its transtympanic course the chorda tympani nerve is housed in a fibrous sheath and shrouded in a layer of mucous membrane. As it heads anteriorly, it lies medial to the posterior malleal ligament (Fig. 6.23) and then passes lateral to the long process of the incus and medial to the neck of the malleus, suspended between these two ossicles. The chorda tympani

FIG. 6.23: This photomicrograph illustrates the pretympanic spine and its relationship to the chorda tympani nerve. The posterior malleal ligament is the thickened inferior margin of the posterior malleal (mucosal) fold. The posterior pouch of von Tröltsch is located between the posterior tympanic stria and the posterior malleal ligament (female, age 72 years).

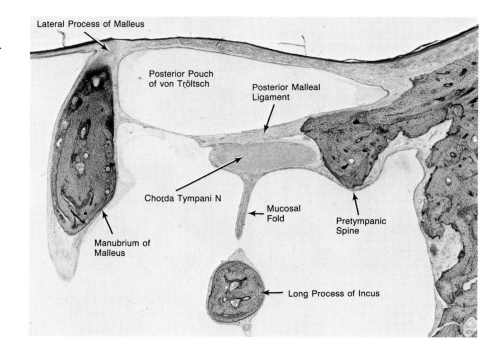

nerve passes from the neck of the malleus, in which it may occupy a groove (Fig. 6.24), thus paralleling the anterior process of the malleus. The chorda tympani nerve takes a direct route from the iter posterius to the iter anterius; stretching of this nerve by disease processes or surgical manipulation causes temporary loss of secretion of the submandibular gland and loss of taste on the ipsilateral anterior two-thirds of the tongue (Bull, 1965; Chilla et al., 1982). The iter chordae anterius (canal of Huguier) marks the exit of the chorda tympani nerve from the tympanic cavity as it enters the petrotympanic (Glaserian) fissure; here the nerve is accompanied by the anterior tympanic artery. The nerve then exits the skull at the medial surface of the spina angularis of the sphenoid bone; occasionally it occupies a groove in this spine—the groove of Lucas—as it travels anteriorly to join the lingual nerve.

Variations in the anatomy of the chorda tympani nerve may also occur. The chorda of the infant normally separates from the facial nerve beyond the skull which it re-enters by its own canal, anterior to the stylomastoid foramen. This separate canal may persist into adulthood (Gray, 1959). At the other extreme, the chorda tympani nerve may exit from the facial nerve at the level of the lateral canal (Haynes, 1955). The chorda tympani nerve varies in size and, like the facial nerve, it may be bipartite (Hough, 1958; Durcan et al., 1967). The chorda tympani nerve's point of entry into the middle ear cavity may be as much as 1 to 2 mm lateral to the rim of the external auditory canal, and the nerve may pass laterally, instead of medially, to the neck of the malleus (Hough, 1958; Durcan et al., 1967).

Variations in the location of the chorda tympani nerve are of significance in transcanal surgery. In these procedures the posterior part of the tympanic membrane is elevated and the adjacent bony tympanic annulus is removed to expose the posterior mesotympanum. Section of the chorda tympani nerve in some patients may cause symptoms of partial ageusia or dysgeusia and dry mouth. Stretching of the nerve may also cause these symptoms with partial recovery after some months (Chilla et al., 1982).

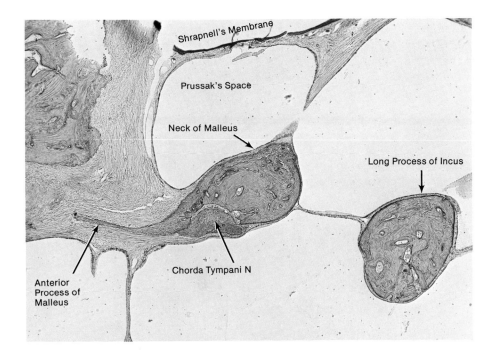

FIG. 6.24: The chorda tympani nerve frequently passes in a sulcus on the medial surface of the neck of the malleus at the base of the anterior process. Prussak's space is located medial to Shrapnell's membrane (female, age 55 years).

The sensory component of the facial nerve, known variously as the nervus intermedius, the nerve of Wrisberg, or the glossopalatine nerve (Gray, 1959), contains visceral afferent (taste) fibers and general visceral efferent (secretory) fibers (Figs. 6.1 and 6.25).

Its efferent neurons lie in the superior salivatory nucleus, located dorsomedial to the motor nucleus of the facial nerve. The chorda tympani nerve and the greater superficial petrosal nerve, both branches of the nervus intermedius, carry these secretory fibers to the submaxillary and sphenopalatine ganglia, respectively. The fibers from the submaxillary ganglion innervate the submaxillary and sublingual glands, while those fibers from the sphenopalatine ganglion supply the lacrimal gland and mucosal glands of the nose and palate.

The neurons serving the sensory function of taste lie in the geniculate ganglion; their fibers, which travel with the fibers of the tractus solitarius, end in the nucleus of this tract. These fibers from the ipsilateral palatal and pharyngeal mucosa travel in the greater superficial petrosal nerve, while those from the ipsilateral anterior two-thirds of the tongue travel in the chorda tympani nerve.

There also appears to be a somatic sensory component, serving the skin of the external auditory canal by fibers which travel with the auricular branch of the vagus (Arnold's nerve); the facial nerve is linked to Arnold's nerve via branches which pass between the two nerves just before the facial nerve leaves the stylomastoid foramen. The cell bodies are located in the geniculate ganglion, and centrally their fibers end in the spinal tract of the Vth cranial nerve (Gray, 1959).

Through histologic study of the temporal bones of two patients with facial nerve lesions, Saito et al. (1970) traced the course and the position of the sensory nerve bundle within the facial nerve trunk. In the internal auditory canal the nervus intermedius courses between the superior division of the vestibular nerve and the facial nerve (Fig. 6.25). In the tympanic segment of the facial nerve the sensory bundle is located dorsally, while in the

FIG. 6.25: The nervus intermedius is seen in the posterior portion of the facial nerve trunk in the internal auditory canal. Part of this nerve continues beyond the genu as the sensory bundle where it assumes a lateral position within the tympanic segment of the nerve trunk (female, age 5 years).

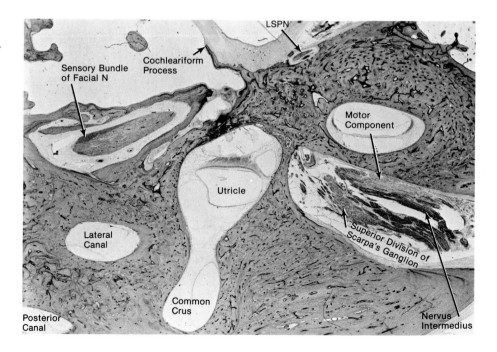

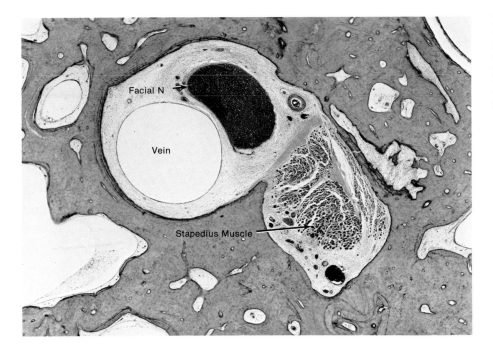

FIG. 6.26: Occasionally a large vein accompanies the facial nerve in the fallopian canal. This vein may cause troublesome bleeding during surgical procedures on the facial nerve. A fibrous partition separates the fallopian canal from the compartment for the stapedius muscle (male, age 40 years).

vertical segment it assumes a more lateral and posterior position. It finally exits anteriorly as the chorda tympani nerve.

THE VASCULAR SUPPLY OF THE FACIAL NERVE

The arterial supply of the facial nerve is derived from a variety of vessels as it courses from the pons to the stylomastoid foramen. In its intracranial segment it is supplied by the anterior inferior cerebellar artery and in its internal auditory canal segment by the labyrinthine artery. The geniculate ganglion is richly supplied by the superficial petrosal artery, a branch of the middle meningeal artery. For the remainder of its course in the fallopian canal, the nerve is supplied by the anastomosing branches of the superficial petrosal and stylomastoid arteries (Groves, 1976).

The vascular supply of the facial nerve is not uniform throughout the course of the nerve, nor does it occupy a constant proportion of the fallopian canal. Ogawa and Sando (1982) found that in the labyrinthine segment of the facial nerve canal the vascular channels occupied 12% of the cross-sectional area, while in the tympanic segment the figure was 63% and in the mastoid segment 54%. A large vein is frequently present in the fallopian canal (Fig. 6.26).

The Sensory Nerves of the Middle Ear

Jacobson's nerve is the eponymic name for the inferior tympanic nerve; it arises from the inferior ganglion of the IXth nerve which is located in the petrosal fossula at the caroticotympanic spine. Referred pain in the ear caused by pharyngeal disorders is mediated by this nerve. Like the chorda tympani nerve, this is a pretrematic nerve, and serves to interconnect the VIIth (facial) and IXth (glossopharyngeal) nerves of the second and third branchial arches, respectively. Having gained access into the middle ear via

FIG. 6.27: Jacobson's nerve (the inferior tympanic nerve) emerges from the inferior tympanic canaliculus and then ascends the promontory in a groove or tunnel to exit into the superior tympanic canaliculus in the region of the cochleariform process (male, age 83 years). (See Fig. 6.28.)

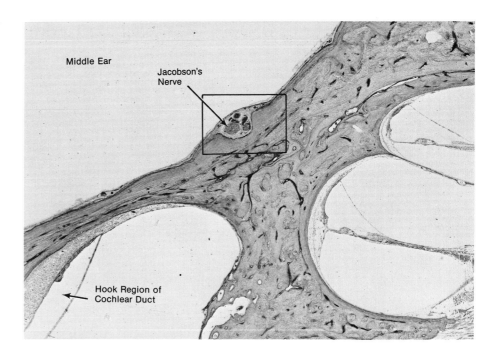

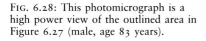

the inferior tympanic canaliculus, the tympanic nerve scales the medial wall of the tympanic cavity and the promontory partly in a bony canal and partly in a groove (Figs. 6.27 and 6.28). It innervates the eustachian tube as well as the middle ear mucosa. At the level of the round window, the tympanic nerve is joined by the caroticotympanic nerves (usually two) from the pericarotid sympathetic plexus (Arnold, 1831; Mitchell, 1953). This union forms the lesser superficial petrosal nerve (Arnold, 1831; Rosen, 1950) which enters the superior tympanic canaliculus beneath the cochleariform process; as it courses toward the middle cranial fossa, it runs parallel to, and sometimes within, the semicanal for the tensor tympani muscle (Figs. 6.29 and 6.30) (Wolff et al., 1957).

Immediately after its union with the caroticotympanic nerve, the tympanic nerve may send a twig to a more superior level of the carotid canal

FIG. 6.28: This photomicrograph is a high power view of the outlined area in Figure 6.27 (male, age 83 years).

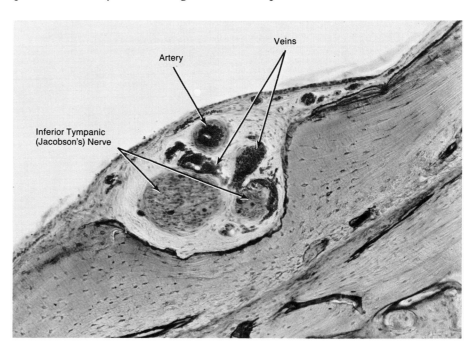

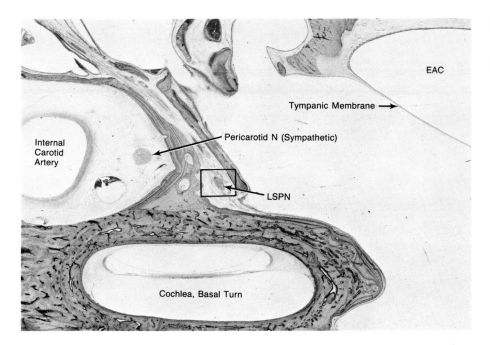

Internal
Carotid
Artery

Pericarotid N (Sympathetic)

Tympanic Membrane →

EAC

LSPN

Cochlea, Basal Turn

FIG. 6.29: The internal carotid artery is accompanied by both veins and sympathetic nerves. Also seen is the lesser superficial petrosal nerve (LSPN) (male, age 5 years). (See Fig. 6.30.)

(Fig. 6.31). According to Montandon (personal communication), this branch is synonymous with the lesser deeper petrosal nerve of Arnold (1831) and the superior caroticotympanic nerve (Portmann, 1955a, 1955b).

As the lesser superficial petrosal nerve passes by the geniculate ganglion, it is joined by a small twig from the facial nerve (Vidić & Young, 1967) and sends branches to the greater superficial petrosal nerve. The lesser superficial petrosal nerve leaves the middle cranial fossa either through the foramen ovale or through a channel of its own. It carries preganglionic parasympathetic and postganglionic sympathetic fibers to the otic ganglion, where it terminates.

The auricular branch of the vagus nerve is also known as Arnold's nerve. It is a composite of a large branch from the superior ganglion of the vagus nerve and a small branch from the inferior ganglion of the glosso-

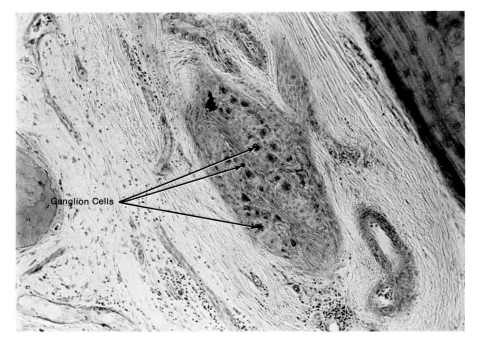

Ganglion Cells

FIG. 6.30: This photomicrograph is a high power view of the outlined area of Figure 6.29 showing a cluster of ganglion cells in association with the lesser superficial petrosal nerve (male, age 5 years).

FIG. 6.31: This sketch shows the nerves that are anatomically related to the middle ear: 1) vestibular nerve, 2) vestibular (Scarpa's) ganglion, 3) facial nerve, 4) vestibulofacial anastomosis, 5) extension of the geniculate ganglion within the labyrinthine segment of the facial nerve, 6) geniculate ganglion and genu of the facial nerve, 7) greater superficial petrosal nerve, 8) branch from the facial nerve to the lesser superficial petrosal nerve, 9) tympanic segment of the facial nerve, 10) area of the second genu and beginning of the mastoid segment of the facial nerve, 11) nerve to the stapedius muscle, 12) cutaneous branch from the facial nerve, 13) chorda tympani nerve, 14) inferior ganglion of the glossopharyngeal nerve in the jugular foramen, 15) tympanic (Jacobson's) nerve, 15b) junction of caroticotympanic and tympanic (Jacobson's) nerve, 16) branch of the tympanic nerve to the eustachian tube, 17) caroticotympanic nerve, 18) external branch of the internal carotid nerve, 19) lesser superficial petrosal nerve, 20) branch of the lesser superficial petrosal nerve to the facial canal, 21a) tympanic ganglia, 21b) ganglion associated with the lesser superficial nerve, 21c) ganglion with sensory fibers of the facial canal, 22) branch of the tympanic plexus, 23) variably present twig of the tympanic nerve to a superior level of the carotid canal (also known as the superior caroticotympanic nerve or the lesser deeper petrosal nerve), 24) superior ganglion (nodosa) of the vagus (Xth cranial) nerve, 25) large vagus twig to Arnold's nerve, 26) small glossopharyngeal twig to Arnold's nerve, 27) auricular branch of the vagus (Arnold's) nerve, 28) inferior branch of Arnold's nerve for cutaneous innervation of the external auditory canal, 29) superior branch of Arnold's nerve, 30) fibers from the superior branch of Arnold's nerve entering the facial nerve trunk, 31) fibers from the superior branch of Arnold's nerve ending in the sheath of the facial nerve, 32) nerve twig arising in the facial nerve and ending in the facial canal, 33) twig of Arnold's nerve ending in the facial recess of the middle ear. (Montandon, unpublished data.)

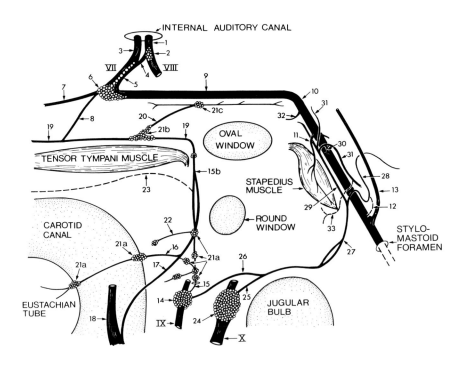

pharyngeal nerve (Fig. 6.31) (Arnold, 1831). From its origin in the jugular foramen it passes over the dome of the jugular bulb to the fallopian canal by way of either the mastoid canaliculus or a groove in the inferior aspect of the temporal bone (Guild, 1953); in this passage the nerve divides into two branches. Its superior branch emits multiple twigs which course superiorly and inferiorly in the facial nerve sheath in which they appear to terminate. The inferior branch of Arnold's nerve receives a small slip from the facial nerve (the cutaneous branch) and traverses the tympanomastoid fissure to distribute its somatic afferent fibers to the posterior surface of the external auditory canal and adjacent conchal area (Foley & Dubois, 1943). These fibers provide the pathway for the herpetic involvement of the skin of the external auditory canal in herpes zoster oticus (Hunt, 1915). Also, the tickling sensation in the throat and the coughing that is sometimes elicited by touching the skin of the ear canal is mediated by Arnold's nerve (the Alderman's nerve).

Clusters of ganglion cells, as opposed to a distinct ganglion, may be found scattered along the course of many of the nerves of the middle ear. Ganglion cells in small groups of 2 to 10 cells are also frequently seen within the trunk of the facial nerve central to the geniculate ganglion (Orzalesi & Pellegrini, 1933; Montandon, personal communication).

The ganglion cells which are located along the course of the tympanic nerve on the promontory are collectively referred to as the tympanic plexus (Portmann, 1955a, 1955b). The role of these ganglion cells is not known. The area of the tympanic plexus, particularly anterior to the oval window, is highly sensitive and painful to surgical manipulation.

There are also scattered ganglion cells along the course of the lesser superficial petrosal nerve, a clustering of which forms a distinct ganglion at the site of departure of the branch that courses to the facial nerve (Bötner & Ancetti, 1956) (Figs. 6.29 to 6.31). At the point where this branch joins the facial nerve (horizontal segment) there is another cluster of ganglion cells. Goycoolea et al. (1980) reported finding ganglion cells not only in the medial portion of the tensor tympani muscle, but also immediately proximal and lateral to the muscle fibers.

The Vestibular Nerves

There are three major interneural connections worthy of emphasis: 1) Voit's anastomosis is a small branch which leaves the superior vestibular nerve to supply the superior part of the macula of the saccule. 2) The vestibulofacial anastomosis is a bundle of fibers uniting the superior division of the vestibular nerve and facial nerve (Fig. 6.32) (Orzalesi & Pellegrini, 1933). It has been suggested that these fibers may be motor fibers of the facial nerve which have traveled with the vestibular nerve for some distance and are returning to the facial nerve trunk. This anastomosis may also transmit unmyelinated sympathetic fibers to the vestibular ganglion from the periphery (Spoendlin & Lichtensteiger, 1967). 3) Oort's anastomosis (the vestibulocochlear anastomosis) is composed of efferent fibers (Rasmussen, 1946) reaching from the saccular branch of the inferior division of the vestibular nerve to the cochlear nerve.

The innervation of the superior canal crista and the lateral canal crista is derived, respectively, from the superior and lateral ampullary nerves, which are branches of the superior division of the vestibular nerve. The posterior ampullary nerve is a branch from the inferior division of the vestibular nerve. It passes through the singular canal and may itself be subdivided (Fig. 6.33).

Gacek (1961) described a small accessory branch of the posterior ampullary nerve located posterosuperior to the main nerve trunk which innervates only the most posterior aspect of the crista of the posterior canal. Subsequent reports (Montandon et al., 1970; Bergstrom, 1973) have confirmed this finding. Okano et al. (1980) reviewed 223 human temporal bones for the purpose of mapping the intratemporal path of this accessory branch of the posterior ampullary nerve. In 87% of specimens examined, this accessory branch was present. While it usually joins the main posterior ampullary nerve after a short distance, in 5.8% of the cases it pursued a solitary course all the way to the ampulla of the posterior canal. Montandon et al. (1970) proposed that this accessory branch innervates the crista neglecta when that organ is present (0.9% of human ears). When the

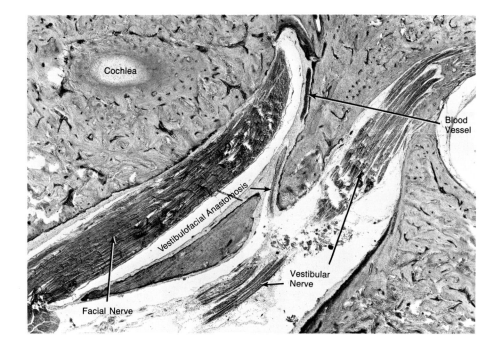

FIG. 6.32: This view shows the vestibulofacial anastomosis (male, age 70 years).

FIG. 6.33: In this case the posterior ampullary nerve is comprised of three discrete bundles. The pattern of division can be quite variable (female, age 5 years).

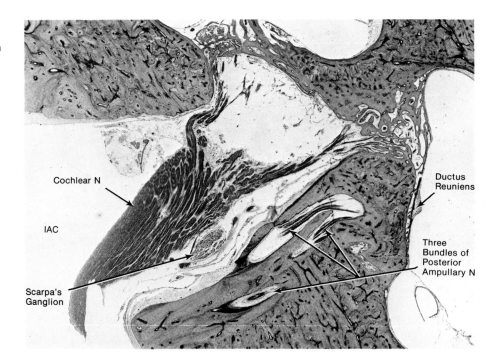

crista neglecta is not present, the accessory nerve innervates the crista of the posterior canal which has incorporated the crista neglecta into its structure. Surgical attempts to achieve total denervation of the crista of the posterior canal by sectioning the posterior ampullary nerve in the singular canal, as proposed by Gacek (1974) for the treatment of benign paroxysmal positional vertigo, would not be successful in cases where the accessory nerve pursued a solitary course all the way to the crista.

The macula of the utricle is innervated by the utricular branch of the superior division of the vestibular nerve. The innervation of the macula of the saccule is of dual origin. The superior division of the vestibular nerve gives off a small branch to the macula of the saccule (the anastomosis of Voit); the majority of the macula of the saccule is innervated by the main branch of the inferior division of the vestibular nerve.

The Cochlear Nerve

Only those aspects of cochlear and vestibular neuroanatomy which are of practical consequence to the surgeon will be discussed in this section. For details of light and electron microscopic neuroanatomy see *Pathology of the Ear* (Schuknecht, 1974).

The afferent cochlear nerve fibers all arise about the receptor hair cells as unmyelinated nerve fibers which then pass through the osseous spiral lamina to the modiolus where they acquire a myelin sheath and attain their originating cell body located in the spiral ganglion. The ganglion cells of the spiral ganglion are bipolar neurons, the central processes of which, having aggregated at the fundus of the internal auditory canal, traverse the internal auditory canal in close relationship to the vestibular and facial nerves. The VIIIth cranial nerve enters the brain stem caudal (approximately 5 mm) to the Vth cranial nerve (Guerrier, 1977) and cephalad to the IXth, Xth, XIth root entry zone. The efferent or descending cochlear pathways parallel those of the afferent.

The anatomic interrelationships of the cochlear nerve with the vestibular nerve as they gradually merge, and with the facial nerve as the VIIth/VIIIth nerve complex undergoes a 90° rotation in its journey through the internal auditory canal, have attained new significance in the light of the popularization of the retrolabyrinthine approach to these nerves. At the fundus of the internal auditory canal (Fig. 5.42) the superior vestibular and facial nerves occupy the superior hemisphere, separated by the vertical crest; the cochlear nerve and inferior vestibular nerve are located in the inferior hemisphere as discrete entities. The superior vestibular and inferior vestibular nerves fuse just proximal to the transverse crest (Silverstein, 1984). As one traces the VIIth/VIIIth nerve complex medially in the internal auditory canal, the cochlear nerve migrates posteriorly (as viewed from the postauricular approach) and unites with the superior vestibular/inferior vestibular nerve trunk; conversely, the facial nerve migrates anteriorly (Fig. 6.34). By the time the nerves have reached the porus of the internal auditory canal, they have completed a 90° rotation; the cochlear nerve, however, always remains in a relatively inferior location with respect to the facial and vestibular nerves (Silverstein, 1984).

In addition to the previously described rotation, the cochlear and vestibular nerves, which exist as multiple discrete bundles at the fundus of the internal auditory canal, gradually merge to form two major branches (the cochlear and vestibular nerve trunks) which are separated by a septum at the porus of the internal auditory canal. Histologic examination of this merger (Rasmussen, 1940; Silverstein, 1984) shows great variability in the completeness of this divisional septum, with some 20% of the cases lacking a discrete septal cleavage plane (Silverstein, 1984). In such cases selective vestibular nerve section would seem to be precluded; however, other features may be used to determine the cochlear-vestibular nerve trunk inter-

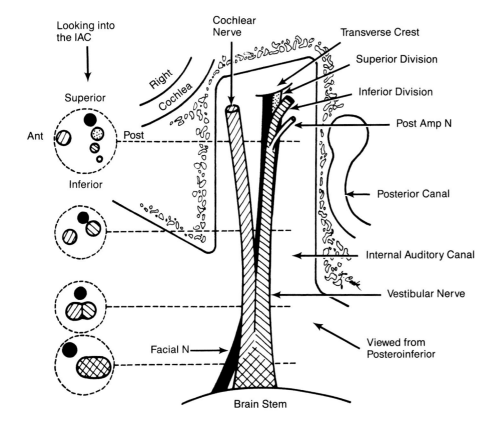

FIG. 6.34: This highly diagrammatic sketch shows the most common relationships of the nerve trunks in the right cerebellopontine angle and the internal auditory canal (IAC) as viewed from posteroinferiorly. The cleavage plane between the cochlear and vestibular nerve trunks is evident at the porus of the IAC in about 70% of dissected specimens. At the brain stem the facial nerve lies anterior to the cochlear and vestibular nerves, but as it passes peripherally it becomes intimately related to the superior division of the vestibular nerve. The close anatomic relationship of the posterior canal and the cochlea limits surgical access to the internal auditory canal. (After Silverstein, 1984.)

face. Firstly, the vestibular nerve trunk appears gray when compared to the cochlear, due to differing amounts of myelin in the two trunks; secondly, a small vessel which courses longitudinally along the lateral aspect of the cochlear-vestibular nerve trunk interface may be useful in selective sectioning (House et al., 1984; Silverstein, 1984). In some specimens (Brackmann, cited by Silverstein, 1984), a cleavage plane may be more readily detected at the medial, rather than the lateral, aspect of the nerve trunks; additionally, the nervus intermedius frequently can be found coursing adjacent to the cochlear-vestibular cleavage plane at its medial aspect. The facial nerve, at the point where selective vestibular nerve section is carried out, is located anteriorly and often is separated from the cochleovestibular nerve by the lateral branch of the anterior inferior cerebellar artery; hence, selective preservation of the facial nerve is readily accomplished.

7. Vascular Anatomy

The Vascular Supply of the External Auditory Canal and Pinna

The blood supply to the auricle derives from branches of the external carotid artery: the posterior auricular artery from the external carotid artery, the anterior auricular artery from the superficial temporal artery, and the mastoid branch from the occipital artery. The supply of the external auditory canal comes from the posterior auricular artery, the internal maxillary artery, and the superficial temporal artery. The veins accompany the corresponding arteries.

The Major Arteries

There are several major vessels which are intimately related to the temporal bone and consequently of significance in otologic surgery. Prime among these is the internal carotid artery. This vessel gains access to the petrous bone through the carotid canal which is located medial to the styloid process. It courses upward anterior to the middle ear and cochlea and then turns abruptly forward and medially (the "knee" segment) (Moniz, 1927) to pass beneath the eustachian tube (Figs. 7.1 and 7.2). It then again ascends, leaving its canal to enter the cranial cavity between the lingula and the petrosal process of the sphenoid.

Throughout its petrous course, the internal carotid artery is housed in a bony canal, the wall of which often measures less than 0.5 mm in thickness (Goldman et al., 1971), and which in approximately 1% of the cases (Myerson et al., 1934) shows dehiscent areas. The artery is surrounded in its canal by a venous plexus and by the pericarotid sympathetic plexus derived from the ascending branch of the superior cervical ganglion of the sympathetic trunk. As with major arteries elsewhere, it may undergo atherosclerotic changes with consequent weakening of its arterial wall (Fig. 7.3).

FIG. 7.1: The relationship between the internal carotid artery, eustachian tube, and peritubal cells is shown. The carotid canal bulges slightly into the protympanum (female, age 89 years).

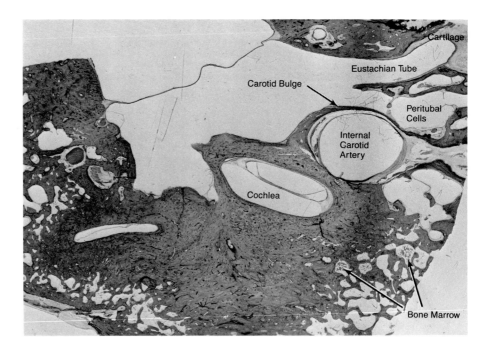

Atherosclerotic change of the internal carotid artery with dilation and thinning of the wall is a common occurrence in aged subjects. In some cases, the arterial wall appears to be totally atrophied and its function replaced by the bony wall of the carotid canal (Figs. 7.4 and 7.5). The surgical importance of this observation is clear: opening the carotid canal of an aged patient could lead to rupture of the artery.

Major anomalies of the petrous segment of the internal carotid artery are rare. Absence or hypoplasia may occur infrequently (Steffen, 1968). Lapayowker et al. (1971) reported aberrant positioning of an otherwise normal artery; in his cases, as well as those reported by Goodman and Cohen (1981), Glasscock et al. (1980), and Glasgold and Horrigan (1972), the anomalous internal carotid artery was located lateral and posterior to the "vestibular line" (on anteroposterior radiographic projection, a vertical

FIG. 7.2: The transition from bony to cartilaginous eustachian tube is seen here. In this case the carotid canal bulges into the protympanum (female, age 48 years).

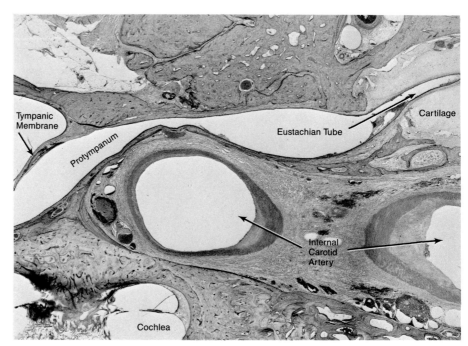

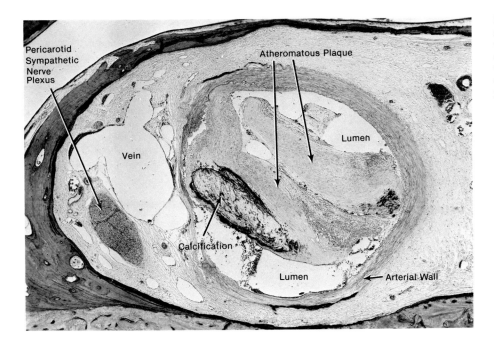

Labels on image: Pericarotid Sympathetic Nerve Plexus; Atheromatous Plaque; Vein; Lumen; Calcification; Lumen; Arterial Wall

FIG. 7.3: This internal carotid artery shows severe atheromatous degeneration with partial luminal occlusion. The pericarotid sympathetic nerve plexus and venous system travel in the carotid canal with the artery (female, age 70 years).

line passing through the lateral aspect of the vestibule). The carotid normally is found medial to this line.

An anomalous location of the internal carotid artery or an aneurysm of the artery may appear clinically as a pulsating mass behind the anterior part of the tympanic membrane. A common symptom is pulsatile tinnitus. The obvious clinical implication is that the mass should not be biopsied. The diagnosis is readily made by angiography.

Aneurysms of congenital origin are believed to arise in areas where the tunica media is occasionally deficient, such as at the site of obliterated embryonic arteries or at points of bifurcation (Steffen, 1968).

The middle meningeal and the accessory meningeal arteries which arise from the internal maxillary branch of the external carotid artery are occasionally seen in temporal bone specimens. They lie lateral to the facial hiatus and the petrous apex (Fig. 7.6).

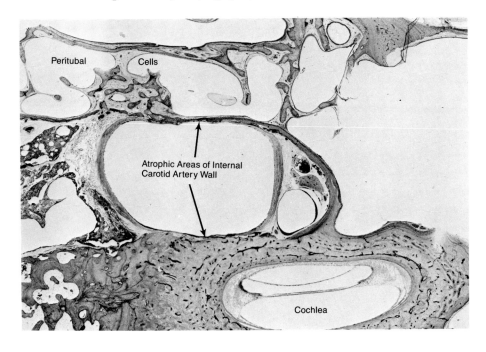

Labels on image: Peritubal Cells; Atrophic Areas of Internal Carotid Artery Wall; Cochlea

FIG. 7.4: A common finding in older subjects is stretching and dilation of the internal carotid artery, bringing the arterial wall into contact with the bone of the carotid canal. In the areas of contact there is severe atrophy of the arterial wall (female, age 72 years). (See Fig. 7.5.)

FIG. 7.5: A higher magnification of Figure 7.4 shows the atrophic changes in the wall of the internal carotid artery (female, age 72 years).

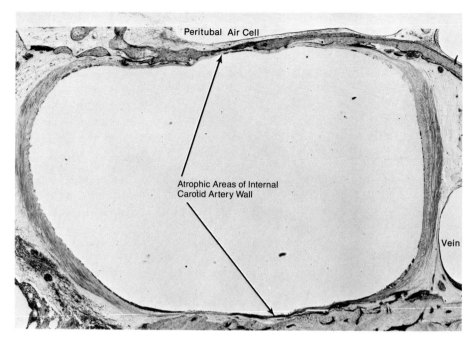

The anterior inferior cerebellar artery is frequently encountered in temporal bone sections. Mazzoni (1969) found that there was often an arterial loop within or near the internal auditory canal. In his review of 100 human temporal bone specimens, this arterial loop was either the main trunk or a branch of the anterior inferior cerebellar artery in 80%, the accessory anterior cerebellar artery in 17%, and a branch of the posterior inferior cerebellar artery in 3%. In 40% the loop was located within the internal auditory canal, in 27% it was at the meatus, and in 33% in the cerebellopontine angle (Figs. 7.7 to 7.11).

Blockage of the anterior inferior cerebellar artery causes necrosis of labyrinthine and brain stem structures, but is rarely fatal. Disruption of the anterior inferior cerebellar artery during surgical procedures in the internal auditory canal or cerebellopontine angle may result in uncontrollable bleeding.

FIG. 7.6: An accessory meningeal artery may occasionally be seen in horizontal temporal bone sections. It occupies a bony canal lateral to the facial hiatus (female, age 49 years).

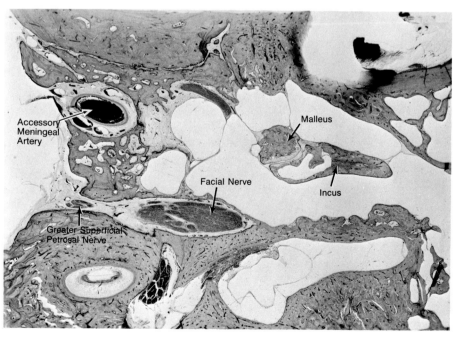

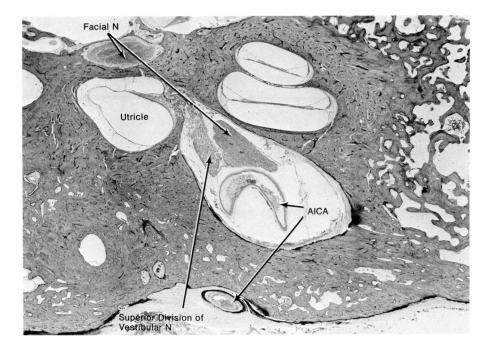

Figure labels: Facial N, Utricle, AICA, Superior Division of Vestibular N

FIG. 7.7: The anterior inferior cerebellar artery (AICA) frequently loops deeply into the internal auditory canal as shown here (male, age 87 years).

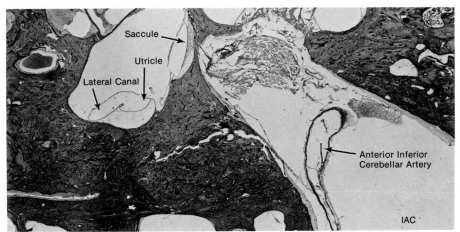

Figure labels: Saccule, Utricle, Lateral Canal, Anterior Inferior Cerebellar Artery, IAC

FIG. 7.8: The anterior inferior cerebellar artery is seen in the internal auditory canal (IAC) (female, age 96 years).

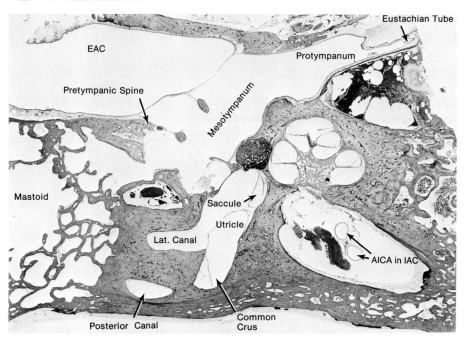

Figure labels: Eustachian Tube, EAC, Protympanum, Pretympanic Spine, Mesotympanum, Mastoid, Saccule, Utricle, Lat. Canal, AICA in IAC, Posterior Canal, Common Crus

FIG. 7.9: Here is another example of the anterior inferior cerebellar artery (AICA) looping deeply into the internal auditory canal (IAC). An incidental feature is an otosclerotic focus at the anterior margin of the oval window (female, age 75 years).

FIG. 7.10: In this case the anterior inferior cerebellar artery lies in a groove on the posterior wall of the petrous bone and enters the internal auditory canal (IAC) to form a tortuous loop (male, age unknown).

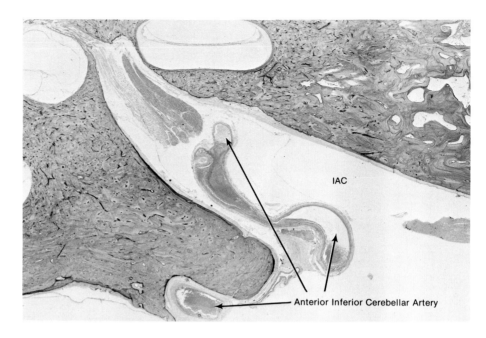

IAC

Anterior Inferior Cerebellar Artery

The Major Veins

The venous sinuses of the dura mater are low-pressure, valveless venous channels which drain the temporal bone, orbit, and brain. They are located between the two layers of the dura mater and are lined with an endothelium which is a continuation of that which lines the tributary veins. Of special relevance to temporal bone anatomy are the lateral sinus, the superior petrosal sinus, and the inferior petrosal sinus.

The lateral sinuses provide the major venous drainage from the head to the neck and are appropriately the largest of the sinuses. They begin at the internal occipital protuberance as continuations of either the superior sagittal sinus (usually on the right side) or of the straight sinus, and then course in the attached margin of the tentorium cerebelli to the bases of the petrous bones. Each lateral sinus heads medially and inferiorly in an S-

FIG. 7.11: The anterior inferior cerebellar artery extends deeply into the internal auditory canal (IAC) (male, age 83 years).

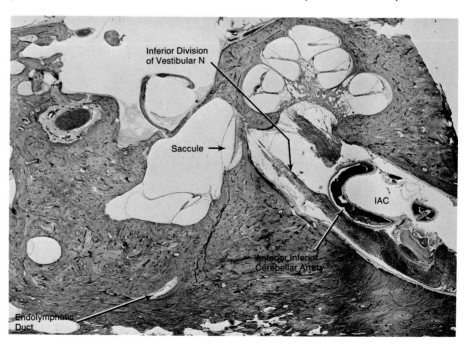

Inferior Division of Vestibular N

Saccule

IAC

Anterior Inferior Cerebellar Artery

Endolymphatic Duct

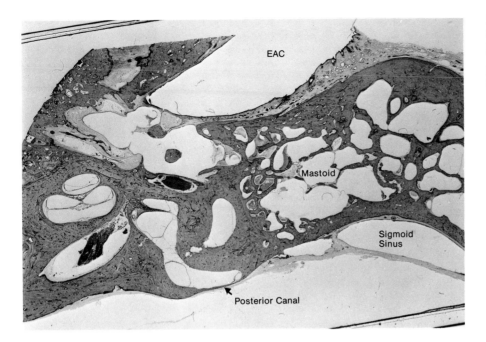

Fig. 7.12: The relationship of the sigmoid part of the lateral venous sinus to the mastoid air cell system is shown. The posterior canal produces a slight prominence on the posterior wall of the petrous bone (male, age 72 years).

shaped sulcus in the mastoid bone (the sigmoid sulcus) to end in the internal jugular vein (Fig. 7.12). The sigmoid part of the lateral venous sinus may bulge anteriorly into the mastoid air cell system where it is vulnerable to surgical injury (Fig. 7.13). The intimate relationship of the lateral venous sinus to the mastoid also makes it susceptible to thrombosis in severe mastoid infections. The position of the sigmoid sinus in relation to the labyrinth is variable (Figs. 7.14 to 7.18) and, according to Montgomery (1971), anterior positioning of the sinus usually indicates underdevelopment of the mastoid air cell system.

The superior petrosal sinus occupies the superior petrosal sulcus which runs along the petrous ridge enveloped in the attached margin of the tentorium cerebelli. It links the cavernous sinus with the lateral sinus; among its tributaries are veins from the tympanic cavity, cerebellar veins, and inferior cerebral veins.

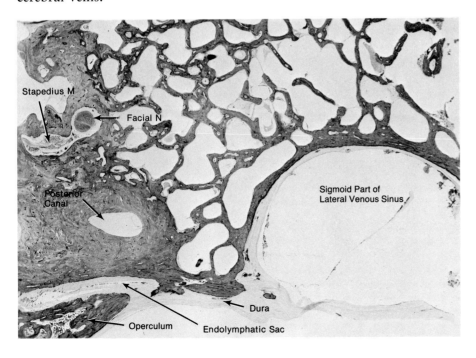

Fig. 7.13: The sigmoid sinus is that portion of the lateral venous sinus which occupies the sigmoid sulcus. It may protrude deeply into the posterior part of the mastoid air cell system. The operculum overlies the endolymphatic sac (female, age 75 years).

FIG. 7.14: In this case the lateral venous sinus heads toward the jugular bulb without forming a sigmoid segment. It forms a membranous party wall with the posterior canal (male, age 54 years). (See Fig. 7.15.)

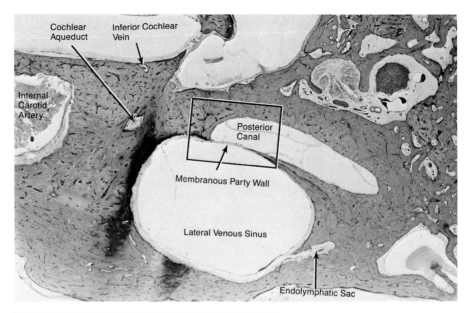

FIG. 7.15: High power view from Figure 7.14 showing the membranous party wall between the lateral venous sinus and the posterior canal (male, age 54 years).

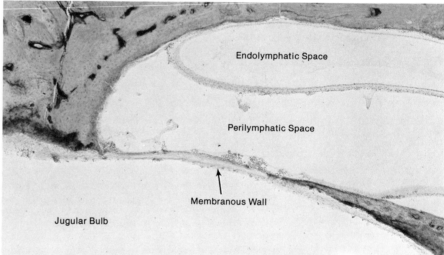

FIG. 7.16: In this case the lateral sinus passes directly to the jugular bulb without forming a sigmoid segment. The endolymphatic sac lies in close proximity to the sinus (male, age 56 years).

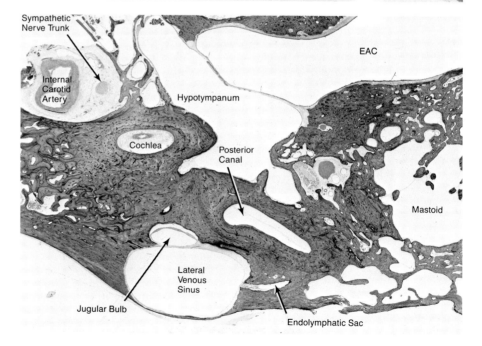

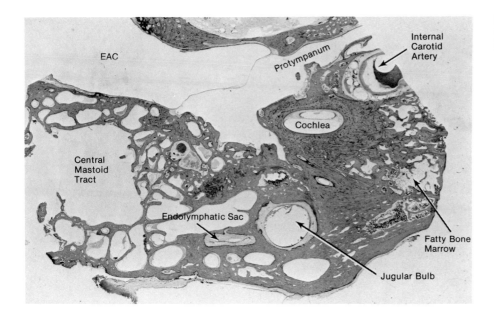

Labels on figure: EAC, Protympanum, Internal Carotid Artery, Cochlea, Central Mastoid Tract, Endolymphatic Sac, Fatty Bone Marrow, Jugular Bulb

FIG. 7.17: The jugular bulb may fail to reach the level of the hypotympanum (female, age 78 years).

The inferior petrosal sinus runs in the inferior petrosal sulcus at the petro-occipital suture line and connects the cavernous sinus with the jugular bulb. Its tributaries consist of the internal auditory veins and veins from the pons, medulla, and inferior aspect of the cerebellum.

The petrosquamous sinus is variably present; it occupies the petrosquamous junction and drains into the lateral sinus.

Emissary veins connect the extracranial veins with the cranial sinuses. The mastoid emissary vein traverses the mastoid foramen and carries blood from the occipital or posterior auricular vein to the lateral sinus. It may be large and can be transected, causing troublesome bleeding during mastoid surgical procedures as when soft tissues are elevated to expose the cortical bone of the mastoid.

Occasionally a large vein is seen within the fallopian canal, a condition which may cause bleeding during explorative procedures on the facial nerve (Fig. 7.19).

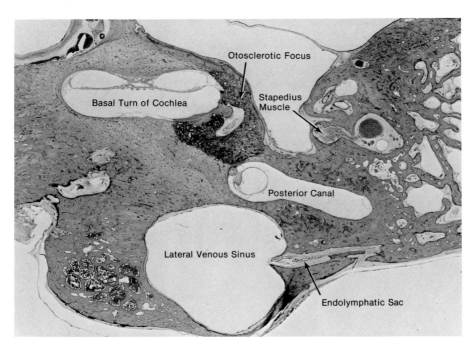

Labels on figure: Otosclerotic Focus, Basal Turn of Cochlea, Stapedius Muscle, Posterior Canal, Lateral Venous Sinus, Endolymphatic Sac

FIG. 7.18: In this ear the lateral venous sinus is located in an anterior position near the posterior canal and endolymphatic sac. An unrelated finding is obliteration of the round window niche by otosclerosis (female, age 82 years).

Vascular Anatomy   193

FIG. 7.19: The head of the malleus is in fibrous contact with the tegmen tympani but is not ankylosed to it. A large vein accompanies the facial nerve in the tympanic segment of the fallopian canal (male, age 70 years).

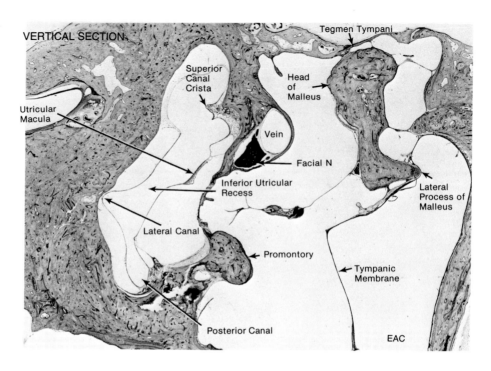

The internal jugular vein is a direct continuation of the lateral sinus. It begins at the base of the skull in the jugular foramen where it is dilated and is referred to as the jugular bulb; there is great variability in the dimensions of the jugular bulb, but it averages 15 mm in width and 20 mm in height (Graham, 1977). The right jugular bulb is usually somewhat larger than the left. In keeping with the inconstancy of venous structures, it may appear high in the middle ear, encroaching upon the tympanic annulus and round window niche, in which case it may cause conductive hearing loss (Moretti, 1976) (Figs. 7.20 to 7.22). The bony shell may be variably dehiscent (Figs. 7.23 to 7.25), with reported incidences of between 6 to 7% (Graham, 1977; Overton & Ritter, 1973).

FIG. 7.20: The jugular bulb lies in its normal position in the floor of the hypotympanum with its bony wall intact (female, age 77 years).

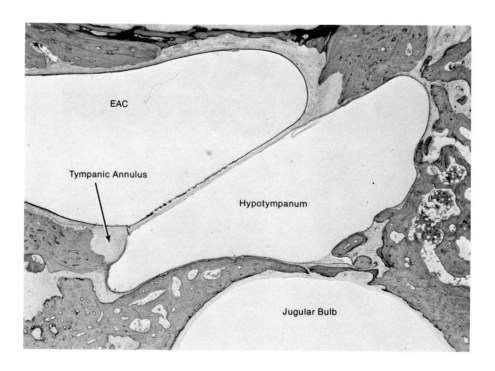

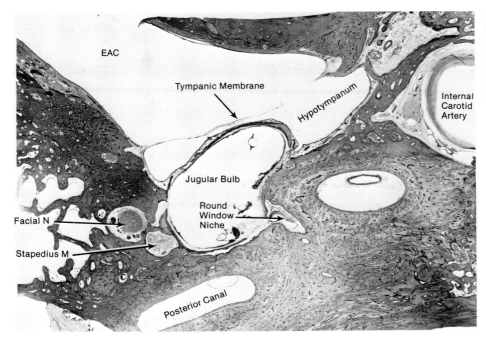

A high jugular bulb is susceptible to injury during surgical procedures in which the tympanic membrane is elevated from its sulcus. A high jugular bulb diminishes the depth of the hypotympanic space, which may increase the difficulty of establishing an aerated hypotympanum in tympanoplasty surgery. On otoscopic examination a high jugular bulb may be mistaken for a glomus body tumor.

The Vascular Supply to the Middle Ear

Nager and Nager (1953), in an exhaustive study of serially sectioned human temporal bones, elucidated the arterial supply of the middle ear and

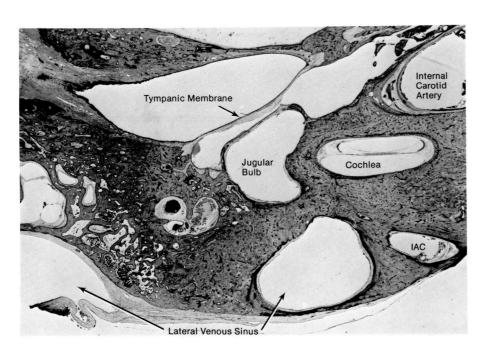

FIG. 7.22: In this ear the lateral venous sinus and the jugular bulb are located anteriorly. The mastoid is narrow (female, age 80 years).

FIG. 7.23: This case shows small dehiscences in the bony wall of the jugular bulb (male, age 45 years).

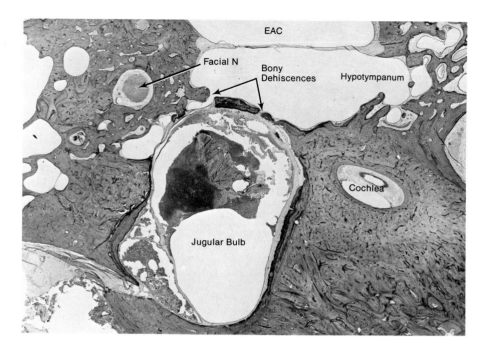

mastoid. On the whole their findings corroborated those of other investigators who had used dye perfusion techniques (Hyrtl, 1835; Nabeya, 1923a; Bast & Anson, 1949).

The blood supply of the middle ear stems from: 1) the external carotid artery by way of the ascending pharyngeal artery, the occipital artery (directly and via its posterior auricular branch), and the internal maxillary artery and its branches (the middle meningeal artery and accessory meningeal artery), 2) the internal carotid artery, and 3) the basilar artery via the subarcuate branch of the labyrinthine (internal auditory) artery.

From these three major sources stem the arteries which provide an extensively anastomotic vascular network for the middle ear and mastoid (Figs. 7.26 and 7.27). Those vessels which originate from the external carotid artery are: 1) the anterior tympanic artery, 2) the deep auricular artery, 3) the inferior tympanic artery, 4) the mastoid artery, 5) the stylomastoid artery, 6) the superficial petrosal artery, 7) the superior tympanic artery, and 8) the tubal artery.

FIG. 7.24: This section depicts a superiorly located jugular bulb impinging on the tympanic annulus. A jugular bulb in this location can be inadvertently opened during surgical elevation of a tympanomeatal flap (female, age 75 years). (See Fig. 7.25.)

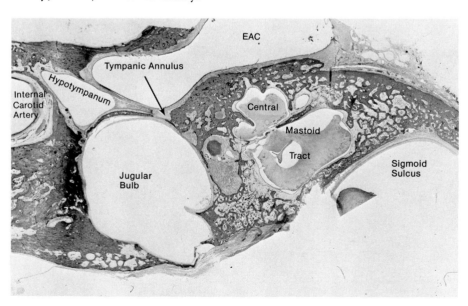

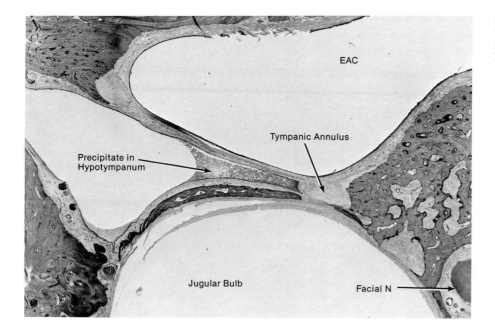

Fig. 7.25: Here is a higher magnification of Figure 7.24 showing the juxtaposition of the jugular bulb to the tympanic annulus (female, age 75 years).

The anterior tympanic artery (Fig. 7.26) arises from the mandibular segment of the internal maxillary artery and enters the petrotympanic (Glaserian) fissure, where it divides into three major branches: 1) The superior branch gains access to the middle ear through a short canal on the petrous side of the petrotympanic fissure; it supplies the mucosa and bone of the anterior and lateral epitympanic wall and the anterolateral aspect of the tegmen, as well as anastomosing with the superior tympanic artery through a branch which traverses the petrosquamosal fissure. 2) The posterior branch channels through the bone of the tympanic side of the petrotympanic fissure. It supplies the bone and mucosa of the posterolateral epitympanic wall, the lateral aspect of the tegmen tympani, and all but the medial wall of the aditus; it also provides the arterial network of the long process of the incus, lenticular process, incudostapedial articulation, and head of the stapes (Fig. 7.28). Through anastomotic linkages, the pos-

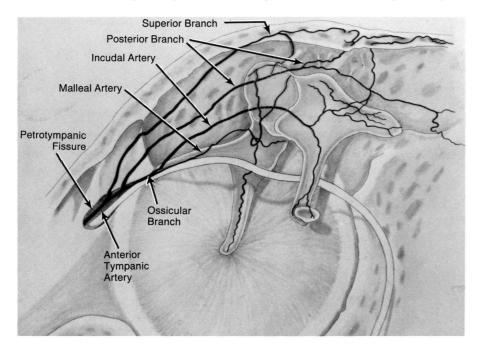

Fig. 7.26: The branches and distribution of the anterior tympanic artery are shown in this sketch. (After Nager & Nager, 1953.)

FIG. 7.27: This sketch shows the usual arterial supply of the middle ear and mastoid exclusive of the anterior tympanic and deep auricular arteries. (After Nager & Nager, 1953.)

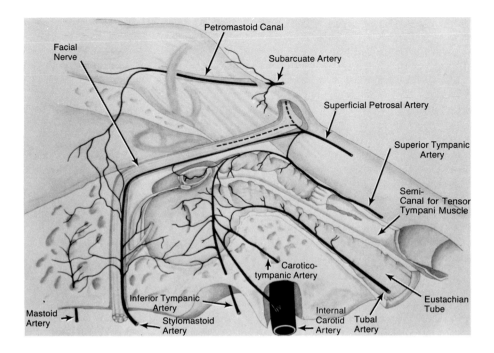

terior branch contributes to the peripheral vascular ring of the tympanic membrane. With a branch from the stylomastoid artery, it forms the descending artery in the mucosa on the medial aspect of the manubrium and supplies the medial surface of the tympanic membrane. The posterior and superior branches of the anterior tympanic artery anastomose to form the vascular network of the mucosa of the malleus and incus. 3) The ossicular branch (Fig. 7.26) enters the middle ear, either with the chorda tympani nerve or through its own canal, and divides to provide the two vessels which are the major blood supply for both the malleus and the incus. The malleal branch travels in the mucosa of the lateral malleal ligament and enters the malleus at the nutrient foramen, located in the anterolateral

FIG. 7.28: The usual arterial distribution to the lenticular process, incudostapedial articulation, and stapes is depicted. (After Anson et al., 1962; Alberti, 1963.)

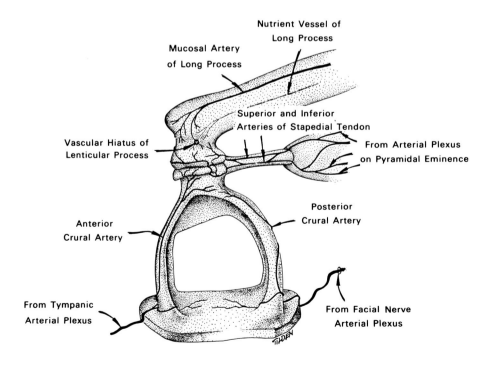

198   Anatomy of the Temporal Bone with Surgical Implications

region of its neck. It also supplies a twig to the lateral process of the malleus and, variably, may anastomose with the incudal branch. Either the ossicular artery or its malleal branch, depending upon the site of branching, sends a few twigs to nourish the anterior process of the malleus. The incudal branch pursues a less constant course, but usually runs across the lateral epitympanic wall in a mucosal fold to enter the incudal nutrient foramen, located laterally on the body of the incus. Having traversed their respective nutrient foramina, the malleal and incudal branches form complex vascular networks which ramify throughout their respective ossicles.

The deep auricular artery also arises from the mandibular branch of the internal maxillary artery, enters the temporal bone at the inferior aspect of the bony external auditory canal, and there divides into an anterior and a posterior branch. The anterior branch supplies the bone and skin of the anterior part of the external auditory canal, the peripheral vascular ring of the tympanic membrane, and the mucosa of the floor of the middle ear. The posterior branch supplies the bone and skin of the posterior part of the external auditory canal and the peripheral vascular ring of the tympanic membrane; it variably forms a vascular loop above the umbo which supplies the inferior part of the tympanic membrane.

The inferior tympanic artery (Fig. 7.27) stems from the ascending pharyngeal artery and traverses the inferior tympanic canaliculus in accompaniment with Jacobson's nerve to reach the anterior part of the floor of the middle ear. It scales the promontory in a bony groove or canal, remaining anterior to the round window. While on the promontory, it links with the caroticotympanic arteries and then with the superior tympanic artery anterior to the oval window. In conjunction with these vessels, it supplies the floor of the middle ear, the promontory, the tympanic orifice of the eustachian tube, the anteroinferior wall of the middle ear and the anterior part of the stapes.

The inferior tympanic artery plays a prominent role in providing blood supply for glomus body tumors of the middle ear. Other arteries which may supply this richly vascular neoplasm are branches of the stylomastoid artery, the caroticotympanic arteries, and branches of the occipital artery. Carotid arteriography not only shows the size and location of the neoplasm, but also reveals the major feeding arteries.

The mastoid artery is a branch of the occipital artery and supplies the vascular network of the posterior part of the mastoid bone.

The stylomastoid artery arises from the posterior auricular artery and joins the facial nerve at the stylomastoid foramen to travel superiorly in the fallopian canal; in its upward journey it gives off vessels which supply the bone and mucosa of the mastoid region, the floor and inferoposterior wall of the tympanic cavity, facial nerve fibers, the medial floor of the aditus, and part of the peripheral tympanic vascular ring. The posterior tympanic arteries are branches of the stylomastoid artery which supply the chorda tympani nerve as far as the iter chordae posterius, at which point they diverge to supply the posterior part of the vascular ring of the tympanic membrane. The largest branch of the stylomastoid artery supplies the stapedius muscle. The stylomastoid artery has anastomotic connections with branches of the posterior meningeal artery at the area of the intersection of Arnold's nerve and the facial nerve; it also sends branches which pass in the posterior malleal fold and join the posterior branch of the anterior tympanic artery to form a descending artery. The stylomastoid artery terminates by connecting with vessels from the superficial petrosal artery.

The superficial petrosal artery stems from the middle meningeal artery, just superior to the latter's entry into the cranial cavity via the foramen spinosum. It courses posterolaterally, sharing a groove in the middle cranial fossa with the greater superficial petrosal nerve, and supplies vessels to the dura as well as branches which anastomose with the subarcuate artery near the subarcuate fossa. Just before reaching the facial hiatus the superficial petrosal artery gives off an anastomotic branch to the adjacent superior tympanic artery and subsequently bifurcates. One of the resulting branches joins the facial nerve at the geniculate ganglion and then also bifurcates. One of these vessels supplies the facial nerve, the other heads medially to link with the facial branch of the labyrinthine (internal auditory) artery. The other major branch of the superficial petrosal artery skips the geniculate ganglion and descends between the facial nerve and the bony wall of its canal, supplying the bony labyrinth, the mucosa overlying the facial canal, and the posterior part of the stapes; its termination is marked by its anastomosis with the stylomastoid artery at the level of the oval window.

The superior tympanic artery also arises from the middle meningeal artery immediately superior to the foramen spinosum, and passes posterolaterally to enter the tympanic cavity with the lesser superficial petrosal nerve via the superior tympanic canaliculus. While in its canalicular course, the superior tympanic artery supplies the tensor tympani muscle, the medial part of the roof and wall of the epitympanum, and occasionally the posterior part of the stapes; it also anastomoses with the superior branch of the anterior tympanic artery, the superficial petrosal artery, and the stylomastoid artery. Emerging from its canaliculus, the superior tympanic artery descends with the lesser superficial petrosal nerve in a sulcus on the promontory and joins the inferior tympanic artery near the oval window; in this segment it sends a vessel to the anterior part of the stapes.

The tubal artery is a branch of the accessory meningeal artery. It courses in the wall of the eustachian tube and supplies the walls of the tube in its tympanic segment as well as the mucosa of the anterior part of the tympanic cavity and promontory. It terminates by anastomosing with branches of the caroticotympanic arteries.

The caroticotympanic arteries, usually two in number, arise from the internal carotid artery and are remnants of the embryonic hyoid artery (Fisch, 1982). They traverse the bone surrounding the carotid canal in separate canals and, in the middle ear, travel in the mucosa of the promontory. Before joining the inferior tympanic artery, the two caroticotympanic arteries supply the anteromedial wall of the middle ear from the floor to the tubal orifice.

The subarcuate artery usually is a branch of the labyrinthine (internal auditory) artery, but may originate from the anterior inferior cerebellar artery or as multiple branches from one or both of these vessels (Mazzoni, 1970). It enters the petromastoid canal and almost immediately sends off a branch which passes above the internal auditory canal to the petrous apex. As it courses posterolaterally, it sends vessels which supply the canalicular region of the bony labyrinth and the posterosuperior part of the wall of the vestibule. The subarcuate artery anastomoses with the superficial petrosal artery and the posterior meningeal artery; it terminates in the anteromedial wall of the mastoid antrum, dividing into two branches. One of these branches supplies the bone and mucosa of the anterior region of the mastoid as it descends to anastomose with vessels from the stylomastoid artery.

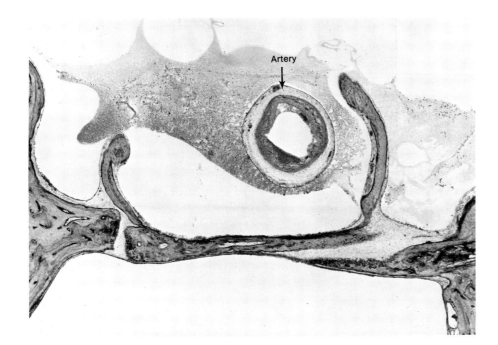

Artery

The second terminal branch supplies the superomedial part of the mastoid antrum and the wall of the superior petrosal sinus; it occasionally anastomoses with vessels from the mastoid branch of the occipital artery.

The persistent stapedial artery, first described by Hyrtl in 1835, represents the residua of the normal embryonic hyoid artery (see embryology of the stapedial artery, Chapter 9). Its incidence has been reported to be between 1 in 5,000 to 1 in 10,000 ears (Davies, 1967; Steffen, 1968). The persistent stapedial artery interferes with access to the oval window in reconstructive middle ear surgery (Baron, 1963). It arises from the internal carotid artery and passes through the floor of the middle ear to reach the posterior part of the promontory, where it ascends in a bony canal. It then passes through the obturator foramen of the stapes (Figs. 7.29 and 7.30) to

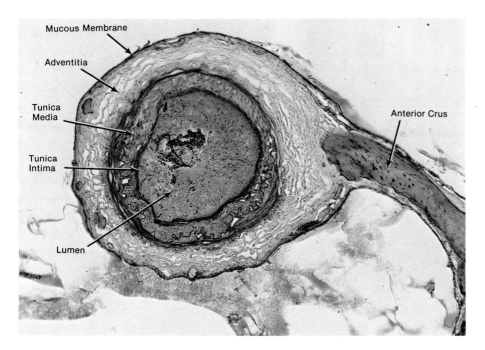

Mucous Membrane

Adventitia

Tunica Media

Tunica Intima

Lumen

Anterior Crus

FIG. 7.30: This view shows the histologic detail of a persistent stapedial artery (male, age 84 years). (See also Figure 7.31.)

enter the fallopian canal via a dehiscence near the cochleariform process. The artery soon leaves the fallopian canal by its own opening to pass anteriorly and superiorly in the middle cranial fossa (Altmann, 1947) (Fig. 7.31). The small artery that is frequently seen crossing the footplate in the vertical direction is not a persistent stapedial artery, but a branch from the adjacent tympanic or facial nerve arterial plexuses.

Aberrant branching of the stapedial artery may result in a stapedial anomaly. Steffen (1968) described a three-legged stapes which he suggests may be due to the stapedial artery giving rise to its supraorbital division (see embryology, Chapter 9, p. 253), or another branch at the site of the stapes. This supposition is based on the idea that the stapedial obturator foramen is a result of the passage of the stapedial artery through the embryonic, solid stapes.

The Vascular Supply to the Inner Ear

ARTERIES

The blood supply of the membranous labyrinth (Fig. 7.32) is predominantly derived from the labyrinthine (internal auditory) artery. This vessel usually arises as a branch of the anterior inferior cerebellar artery within the cranial cavity, but may stem as an independent branch of the basilar artery. Thus, the membranous labyrinth derives its arterial supply primarily from intracranial sources. It may not be entirely separated from the vasculature of the bony labyrinth and middle ear, however, for anastomotic branches which penetrate the endosteal layer of the bony labyrinth have been reported (Nager & Nager, 1953). The labyrinthine artery first supplies the nerves and dura of the internal auditory canal, the bone contiguous to the internal auditory canal, and the medial region of the inner ear. It then divides into two major branches, the common cochlear artery and the anterior vestibular artery (Mazzoni, 1972). The common cochlear artery divides to form the main cochlear and vestibulocochlear branches. Division of the vestibulocochlear artery results in the posterior vestibular artery and the cochlear ramus (Siebenmann, 1894; Shambaugh, 1903, 1905; Asai, 1908a, 1908b; Nabeya, 1923b).

FIG. 7.31: The persistent stapedial artery passes superiorly and anteriorly within the tympanic segment of the fallopian canal (male, age 84 years). Same case as shown in Figure 7.30.

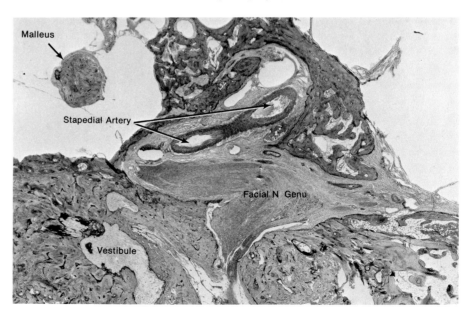

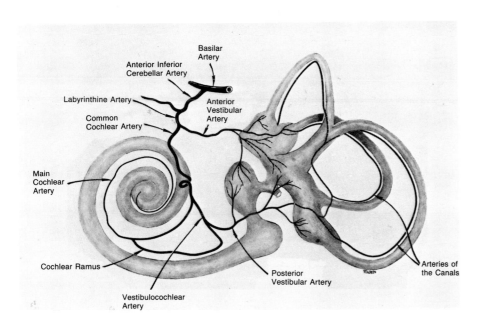

FIG. 7.32: The arterial system of the human membranous labyrinth is shown.

The main cochlear artery supplies the superior three-fourths of the cochlea and modiolus. As it enters the modiolus it sends out numerous primary and secondary arteries (Fig. 7.33). Further arborization of the cochlear artery gives rise to two sets of radiating arterioles; one set supplies the structures of the outer wall of the cochlea, the other supplies the inner wall (Smith, 1951).

The external radiating arterioles curl about the scala vestibuli in the intracochlear partition and distribute vessels to the walls of the scala vestibuli. Upon entering the apex of the spiral ligament, these vessels form four capillary networks: 1) the spiraling vessels located in that region of the spiral ligament which faces the scala vestibuli (vessels at Reissner's membrane, vessels of the scala vestibuli), 2) the capillary network of the stria vascularis, 3) the vessel of the spiral prominence, and 4) the vessels within the spiral ligament on the scala tympani side of the basilar crest. These latter vessels possess the morphologic characteristics of capillaries but function as collecting venules.

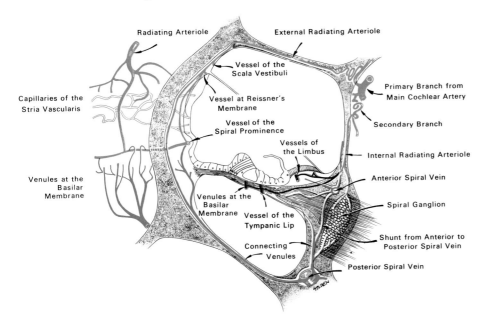

FIG. 7.33: The arterial supply and venous drainage of the cochlea are shown. (After Smith, 1951, 1954.)

FIG. 7.34: There is a large artery in the stria vascularis of the apical turn of the left cochlea. In both apical and basal directions this artery bifurcates and progressively dwindles to fuse with the capillary bed of the stria vascularis. The patient complained of pulsatile tinnitus in this ear (male, age 77 years). (Gulya & Schuknecht, 1984.)

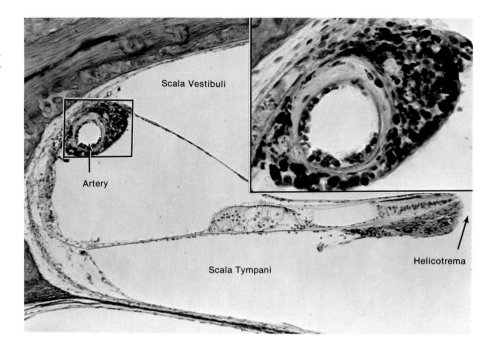

Although the capillary network of the stria vascularis is a tortuous, anastomotic network traveling in a spiral path, its boundaries are relatively straight and parallel (Smith, 1957). An abnormally large artery in the stria vascularis of a subject who complained of pulsatile tinnitus is shown in Fig. 7.34 (Gulya & Schuknecht, 1984).

The vessel of the spiral prominence generally receives a branch from each radiating arteriole and, although this vessel follows a spiral path paralleling that of the network of the stria vascularis, there are no interconnections between the two.

The internal radiating arterioles of the cochlear artery remain within the modiolus, supplying branches to the spiral ganglion as they course toward the base of the cochlea. They enter the vestibular lamina of the osseous spiral lamina, giving rise to the limbus vessels and the marginal vessels (Axelsson, 1968). The marginal vessels constitute two groups of independent arcades which serve as both arterial and venous channels; one group forms the vessel of the basilar membrane while the other comprises the vessel of the tympanic lip. Occasionally a vessel traverses a scala (Fig. 7.35).

The cochlear ramus of the vestibulocochlear artery supplies the basal one-fourth of the cochlea and adjacent modiolus, while the posterior vestibular branch supplies the macula of the saccule, the crista and membranous canal of the posterior canal, and the inferior walls of the utricle and saccule. The arteriolar ramifications are identical to those of the anterior vestibular artery.

The anterior vestibular artery supplies the entirety of the macula of the utricle, a small portion of the macula of the saccule, and the superior walls of both the utricle and saccule. The arterioles enter the stroma of the maculae along with the myelinated nerve fibers, and establish an extensive capillary network below the hair cell areas. The anterior vestibular artery also sends arterioles to the cristae and membranous ducts of the superior and lateral canals (Figs. 7.36 and 7.37). These arterioles enter the ampullae via osseous channels distinct from those of the nerve fibers. The capillary networks of the ampullary cristae and ampullary walls are supplied by several

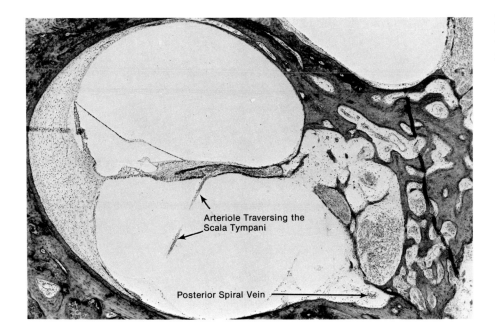

FIG. 7.35: In this cochlea an arteriole traverses the mid-portion of the scala tympani of the basal turn (male, age 8 months).

arterioles. Arteriolar ramification establishes capillary networks between the sensory epithelium and nerve fibers near the midline of each crista. Each canal is traversed throughout its length by one or two arterioles which sustain a system of loosely connected capillaries.

VEINS

The primary venous drainage of the cochlea is afforded by the anterior and posterior spiral veins (Figs. 7.38 and 7.39). The anterior spiral vein receives tributaries from the spiral lamina and scala vestibuli. The posterior spiral vein collects venous blood from the scala tympani, the outer wall of the scala media, and the spiral ganglion. There are several shunts from the anterior to the posterior spiral vein as they pass to the basal end of the cochlea where they join to form the common modiolar vein.

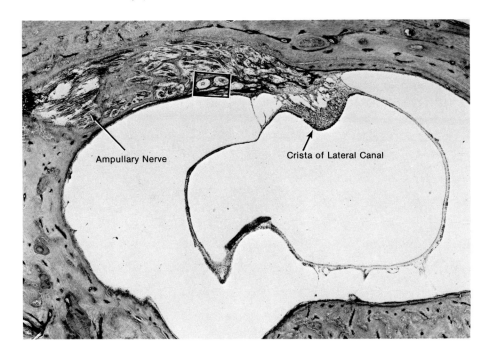

FIG. 7.36: The ampulla, crista, nerve, and vessel of the lateral canal are demonstrated. The artery is the ampullary branch of the anterior vestibular artery. The outlined area is enlarged in Figure 7.37 (female, age 92 years).

FIG. 7.37: The outlined area in Figure 7.36 is magnified to show the ampullary branch of the anterior vestibular artery (female, age 92 years).

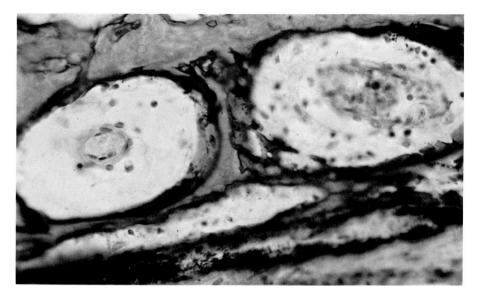

FIG. 7.38: This schematic drawing shows the venous drainage of the human membranous labyrinth.

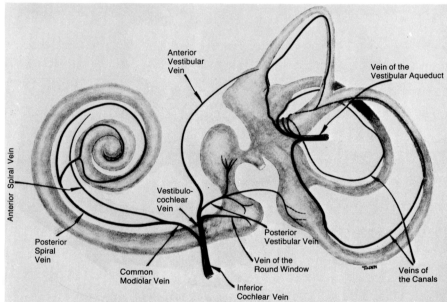

FIG. 7.39: The venous drainage of the cochlea is provided by the anterior and posterior spiral veins which join near the basal end to form the common modiolar vein (female, age 77 years).

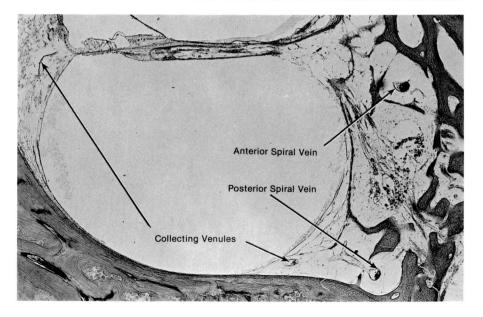

The utricle as well as the ampullae of the superior and lateral canals are drained by the anterior vestibular vein (Smith, 1953). The posterior vestibular vein receives blood from the saccule, the ampulla of the posterior canal, and the basal end of the cochlea. The vein of the round window joins with the confluence of the anterior and posterior vestibular veins to form the vestibulocochlear vein. The latter vessel unites with the common modiolar vein to become the inferior cochlear vein; it then traverses the bony canal of Cotugno (Cotunnio), located near the cochlear aqueduct, to empty into the inferior petrosal sinus. The membranous ducts are drained by channels which course towards their nonampullated ends to form the vein of the vestibular aqueduct; this vessel travels within the vestibular aqueduct or a paravestibular canaliculus to drain into the lateral venous sinus. A variably present vessel is the internal auditory vein (Bast & Anson, 1949). When present, it collects blood from the apical and middle turns of the cochlea and drains into the inferior petrosal sinus via the internal auditory canal.

8. Stereoscopic Views of the Temporal Bone

Surgical Dissection of the Temporal Bone (Reels III to VI)

Familiarity with the macroscopic anatomy of the temporal bone can be acquired by dissection of the fresh cadaver specimen with the aid of the operating microscope and appropriate surgical instruments. The following photographs (Figs. 8.1 to 8.28) complement stereo reels III through VI and present a logical approach to the step-by-step dissection of a right temporal bone. The sequence of dissection has relevancy for transmastoid surgical procedures only. It does not apply to transcanal procedures such as exploratory tympanotomy, stapedotomy, transcanal labyrinthectomy, ossiculoplasty, myringoplasty, etc. An organized sequence of dissection enables the maximum educational yield to be obtained from each specimen. The views are presented in surgical orientation with the anterior aspect of the ear located superiorly in the photographs.

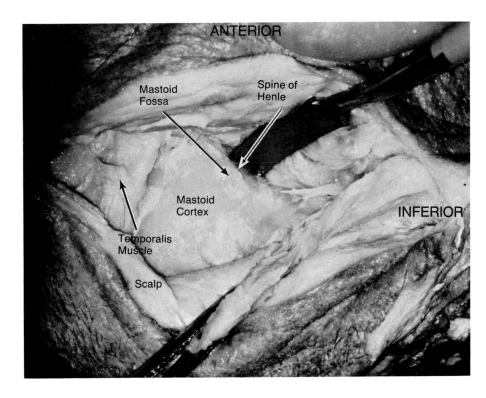

ANTERIOR

Mastoid Fossa

Spine of Henle

Mastoid Cortex

INFERIOR

Temporalis Muscle

Scalp

FIG. 8.1, Reel III—1: After the postauricular incision has been made, the muscle and periosteum are elevated to expose the mastoid cortex. The mastoid fossa and spine of Henle are identified.

FIG. 8.2, Reel III—2: Initial drilling is done in the mastoid fossa which overlies the mastoid antrum. Large burs are preferable at this stage.

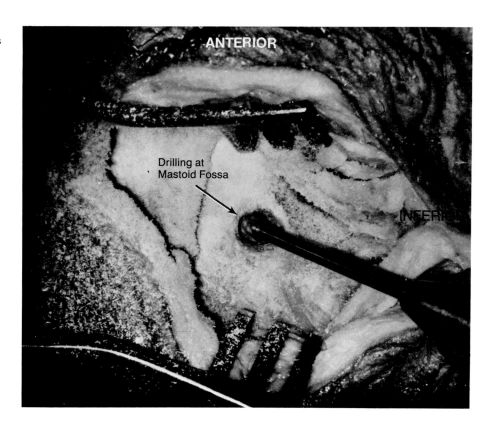

FIG. 8.3, Reel III—3: Koerner's septum, when present, is a plate of bone that extends downward from the mastoid tegmen for a variable distance. It represents the junction of the petrous and squamous portions of the mastoid. In this specimen it hides the lateral canal.

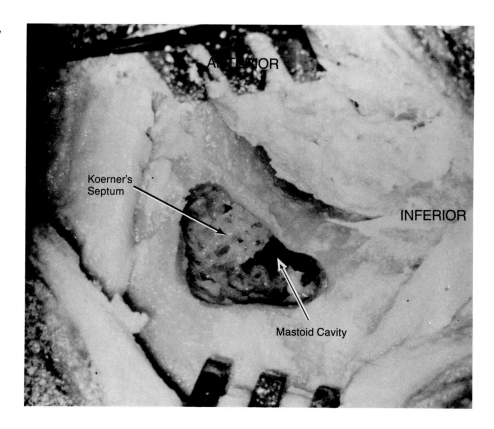

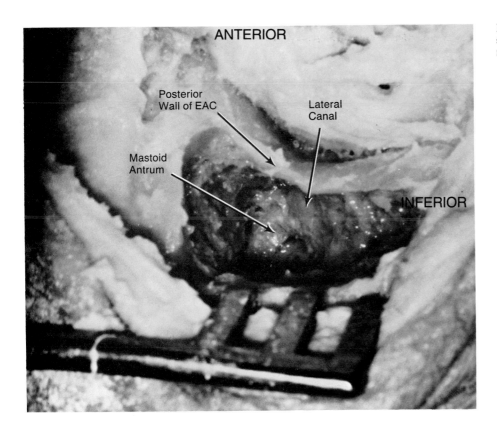

ANTERIOR

Posterior
Wall of EAC

Lateral
Canal

Mastoid
Antrum

INFERIOR

FIG. 8.4, Reel III—4: Once Koerner's septum has been removed, the prominence of the lateral canal is visualized.

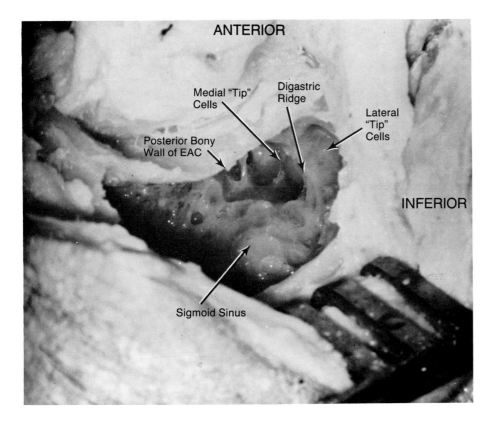

ANTERIOR

Medial "Tip"
Cells

Digastric
Ridge

Lateral
"Tip"
Cells

Posterior Bony
Wall of EAC

INFERIOR

Sigmoid Sinus

FIG. 8.5, Reel III—5: The mastoid tip is divided into medial and lateral compartments by the digastric ridge. The anterior portion of this ridge is located near the mastoid segment of the facial nerve.

FIG. 8.6, Reel III—6: The bony wall of
the lateral venous sinus (sigmoid sinus)
is seen as a protuberance of the posterior wall of the mastoid cavity, passing
anteroinferiorly towards the jugular
bulb. The sinodural angle represents the
junction of the tegmen (roof) of the
mastoid and the lateral venous sinus.

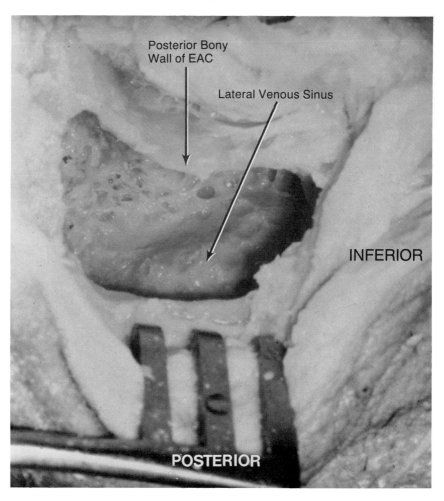

FIG. 8.7, Reel III—7: As bone is exenterated superiorly and anteriorly from
the antrum toward the epitympanum,
the incus comes into view.

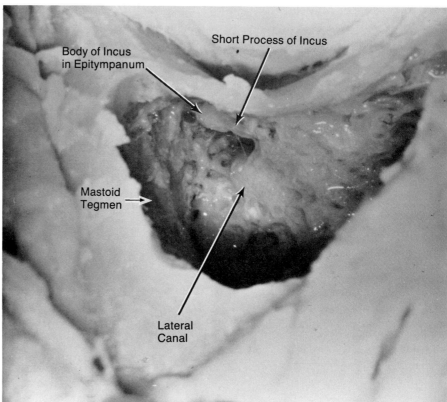

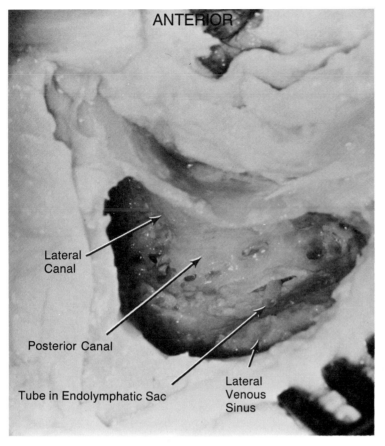

ANTERIOR

Lateral
Canal

Posterior Canal

Tube in Endolymphatic Sac

Lateral
Venous
Sinus

FIG. 8.8, Reel IV—1: The endolymphatic sac has been opened and a tube placed within its lumen. Note the anatomic relationship of the endolymphatic sac and the lateral venous sinus. Surgical procedures to drain the endolymphatic sac into either the subarachnoid space or mastoid cavity are known as *endolymphatic sacotomy* operations. Donaldson's line is a posterior extension of the plane of the lateral canal bisecting the posterior canal; the endolymphatic sac lies inferior to this line.

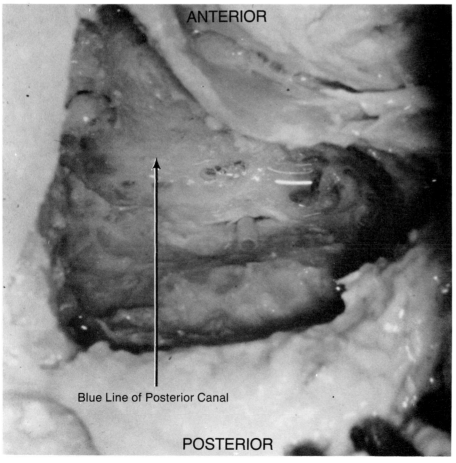

ANTERIOR

Blue Line of Posterior Canal

POSTERIOR

FIG. 8.9, Reel IV—2: The bone of the posterior canal has been thinned to create a blue line. The blueness is the result of light resorption (instead of reflection) at the site of the thinned bony wall.

FIG. 8.10, Reel IV—3: The extent of the mastoid exenteration shown here is known as a *simple mastoidectomy*. The bone of the lateral canal has been thinned to create a blue line.

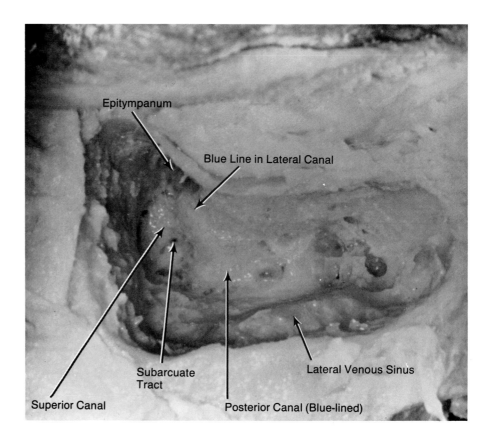

Epitympanum

Blue Line in Lateral Canal

Superior Canal

Subarcuate Tract

Posterior Canal (Blue-lined)

Lateral Venous Sinus

FIG. 8.11, Reel IV—4: The facial nerve has been partly uncovered by removing bone with a diamond bur. Exposing the trunk of the facial nerve throughout its course in the temporal bone is known as *facial nerve exploration*. The facial recess, which lies lateral to the facial nerve, is opened by drilling inferior to the short process of the incus and lateral to the plane of the facial nerve. The chorda tympani nerve is seen lateral and inferior to the facial recess. This surgical approach to the middle ear is known as *posterior tympanotomy* and is frequently used in association with intact canal wall procedures.

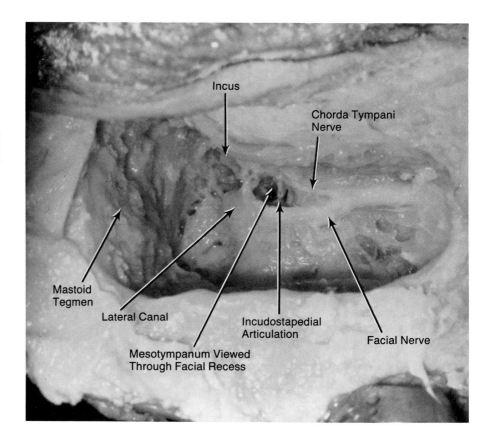

Incus

Chorda Tympani Nerve

Mastoid Tegmen

Lateral Canal

Mesotympanum Viewed Through Facial Recess

Incudostapedial Articulation

Facial Nerve

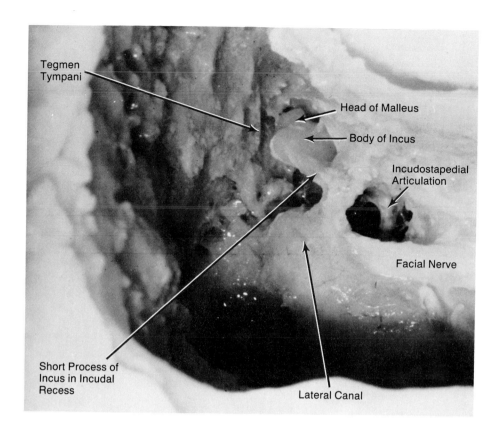

Tegmen
Tympani

Head of Malleus

Body of Incus

Incudostapedial
Articulation

Facial Nerve

Short Process of
Incus in Incudal
Recess

Lateral Canal

FIG. 8.12, Reel IV—5: Removal of
epitympanic bone exposes the body of
the incus and head of the malleus. This
surgical approach is known as *posterior
atticotomy*. The epitympanum is divided
into medial and lateral compartments
by these ossicles. The posterior incudal
ligament is seen.

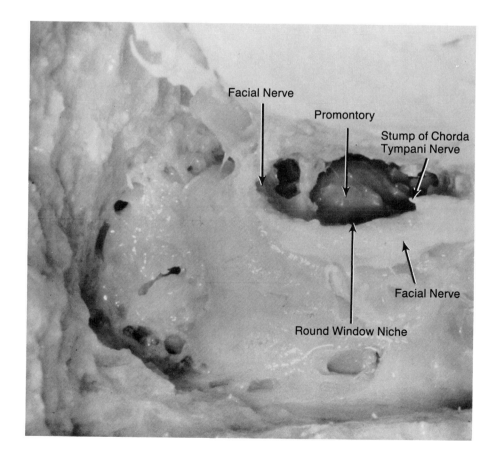

Facial Nerve

Promontory

Stump of Chorda
Tympani Nerve

Facial Nerve

Round Window Niche

FIG. 8.13, Reel IV—6: The posterior
tympanotomy has been extended to
expose the round window niche and
hypotympanum. This approach is also
used for the introduction of cochlear
implants through the round window.

FIG. 8.14, Reel IV—7: A blue line has been made on the superior canal. Making blue lines is not part of any surgical procedure, but as a dissection exercise it improves drilling skills and knowledge of the anatomic relationships of the canals to adjacent structures.

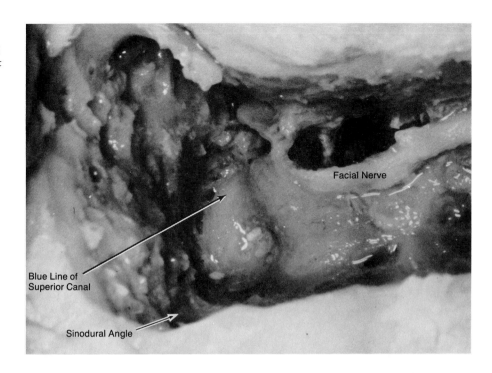

FIG. 8.15, Reel V—1: This overall view shows the anatomic relationships between the semicircular canals, facial nerve, ossicles, mastoid cavity, and middle ear. The exenteration, approximately as shown, is known as *intact-canal-wall tympanomastoidectomy*.

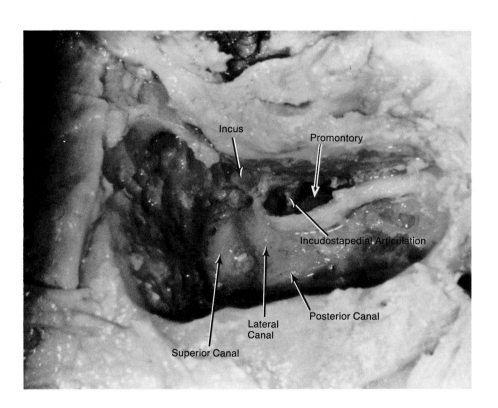

Anatomy of the Temporal Bone with Surgical Implications

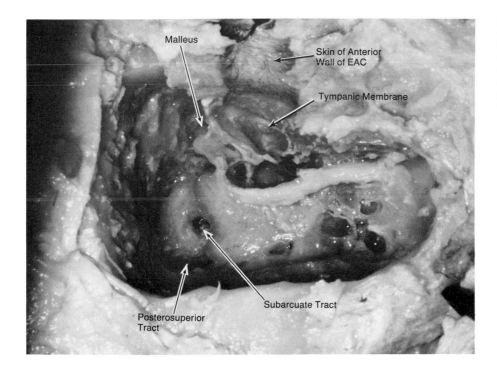

Malleus

Skin of Anterior
Wall of EAC

Tympanic Membrane

Subarcuate Tract

Posterosuperior
Tract

FIG. 8.16, Reel V—2: The posterior wall of the external auditory canal has been removed, exposing the tympanic membrane and the anterior wall of the external auditory canal (EAC). The subarcuate cell tract is evident, and the posterosuperior cell tract has been opened.

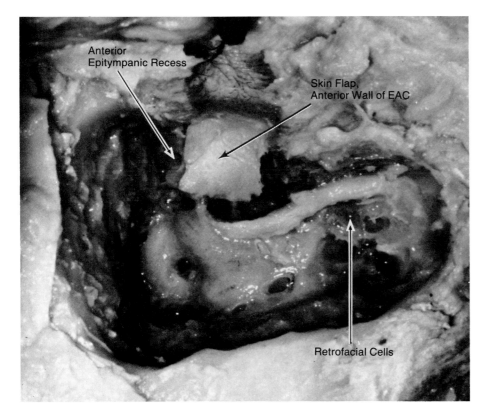

Anterior
Epitympanic Recess

Skin Flap,
Anterior Wall of EAC

Retrofacial Cells

FIG. 8.17, Reel V—3: The skin of the anterior wall of the external auditory canal (EAC) has been elevated as a laterally based, pedicled flap in preparation for thinning the bony wall to reduce its convexity.

Stereoscopic Views of the Temporal Bone   217

FIG. 8.18, Reel V—4: The convexity of the anterior wall of the external auditory canal has been removed to afford easy surgical access to the anterior aspect of the middle ear. The dissection shown here (exclusive of the facial nerve exposure) is the approximate extent of a *modified radical* (Bondy) *mastoidectomy* in which diseased tissue is removed from the mastoid and middle ear but the tympanic membrane and ossicles are left undisturbed.

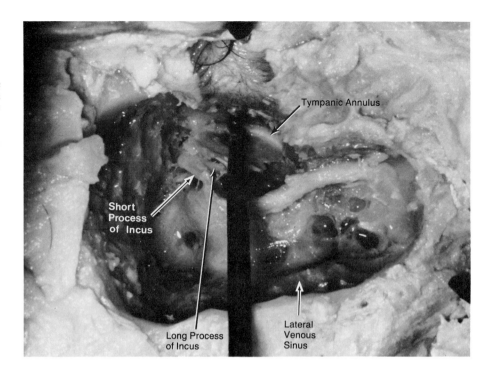

FIG. 8.19, Reel V—5: This is a high power view of the middle ear area seen in Figure 8.18.

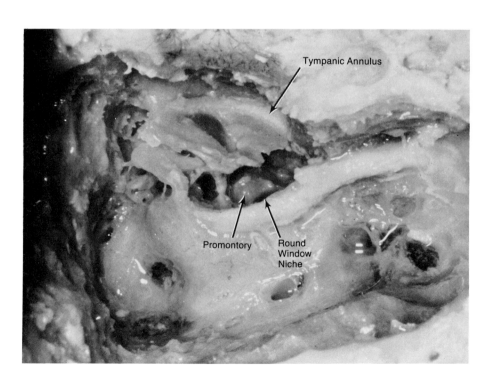

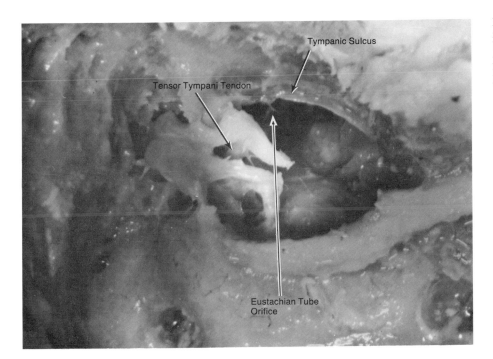

Tympanic Sulcus

Tensor Tympani Tendon

Eustachian Tube
Orifice

FIG. 8.20, Reel V—6: The tympanic membrane, including its annulus, has been removed to expose the anterior part of the mesotympanum, the protympanum, and the tympanic orifice of the eustachian tube.

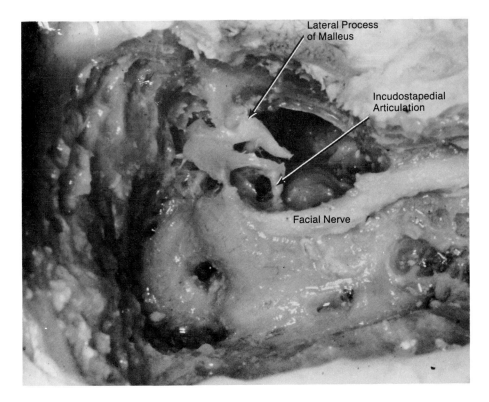

Lateral Process
of Malleus

Incudostapedial
Articulation

Facial Nerve

FIG. 8.21, Reel V—7: This view is the same as that shown in Figure 8.20, but at a lower magnification.

FIG. 8.22, Reel VI—1: The tensor tympani tendon is severed with scissors preparatory to removal of the malleus. The tympanic sulcus can be seen.

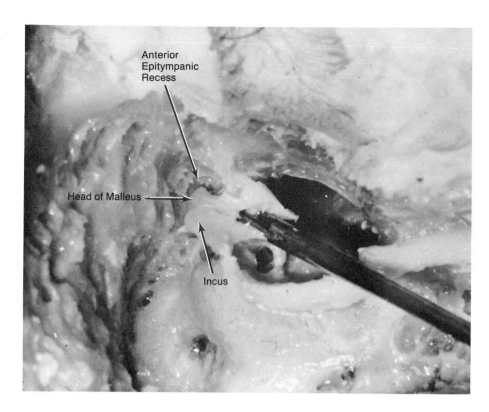

FIG. 8.23, Reel VI—2: The malleus and incus have been removed. The cochleariform process and tensor tympani tendon are seen. The exenteration to this stage (exclusive of the facial nerve exposure) is approximately that of a *radical mastoidectomy*.

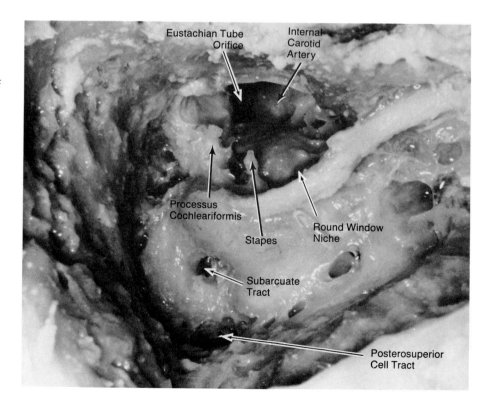

Anatomy of the Temporal Bone with Surgical Implications

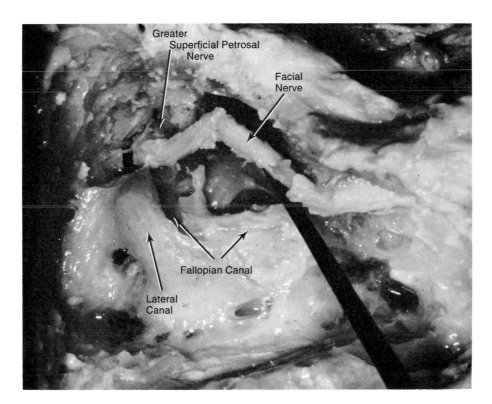

FIG. 8.24, Reel VI—3: The facial nerve has been lifted from its canal. During surgical removal of extensive cholesteatomas or neoplasms, it may be necessary to remove the nerve from its canal either temporarily or permanently, a procedure known as *transposition of the facial nerve.* The greater superficial petrosal nerve is visible as it exits anteriorly from the geniculate ganglion.

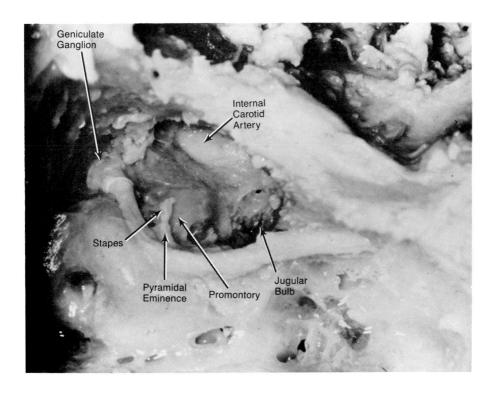

FIG. 8.25, Reel VI—4: The internal carotid artery has been exposed by removing overlying bone. The jugular bulb is seen in the hypotympanum.

FIG. 8.26, Reel VI—5: The semicircular canals have been opened.

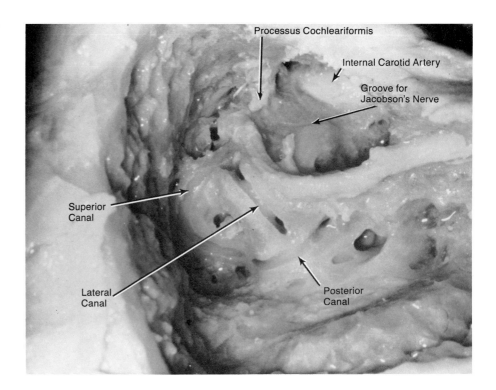

Processus Cochleariformis

Internal Carotid Artery

Groove for
Jacobson's Nerve

Superior
Canal

Lateral
Canal

Posterior
Canal

FIG. 8.27, Reel VI—6: Surgical removal of the semicircular canals leads to the vestibule and internal auditory canal (IAC). This procedure is known as the *translabyrinthine approach to the internal auditory canal* and is used for removal of neoplasms of the canal and cerebellopontine angle.

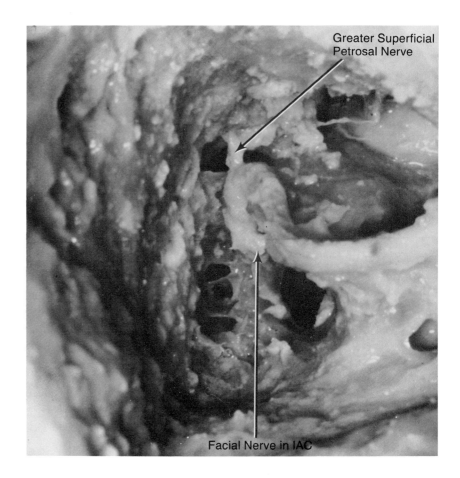

Greater Superficial
Petrosal Nerve

Facial Nerve in IAC

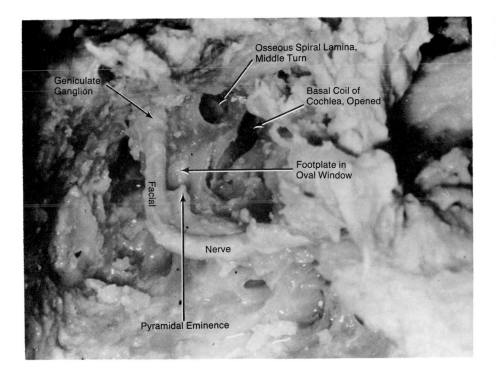

Geniculate Ganglion

Osseous Spiral Lamina, Middle Turn

Basal Coil of Cochlea, Opened

Footplate in Oval Window

Facial

Nerve

Pyramidal Eminence

FIG. 8.28, Reel VI—7: The basal and middle turns of the cochlea have been opened to expose the scalae and osseous spiral lamina.

Pathologic Conditions of the Temporal Bone (Reel VII)

With few exceptions, this text is limited to the presentation of normal anatomy and its variants. However, one of the reasons for learning normal anatomy is to develop the ability to recognize the abnormal. The photographs (Figs. 8.29 to 8.35) which accompany stereo reel VII illustrate several different pathologic entities. The photographs were taken from horizontal sections of celloidin-embedded temporal bones.

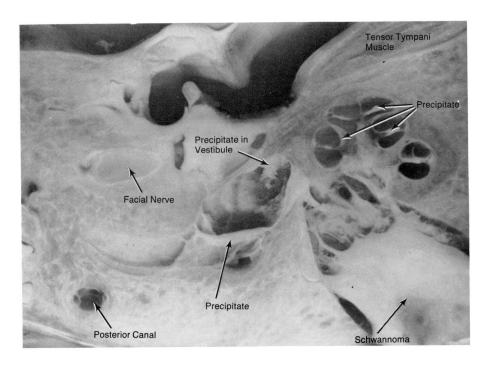

Tensor Tympani Muscle

Precipitate

Precipitate in Vestibule

Facial Nerve

Precipitate

Posterior Canal

Schwannoma

FIG. 8.29, Reel VII—1: Vestibular schwannoma (acoustic neurinoma). This person had an 18-year history of left-sided hearing loss and tinnitis; there was no history of vertigo or dysequilibrium. In the left ear there is a large vestibular schwannoma fully occupying the widened internal auditory canal. The cochlear and vestibular nerves are displaced inferiorly. There is a fibrinous precipitate in the endolymphatic and perilymphatic spaces (male, age 81 years).

FIG. 8.30, Reel VII—2: Sarcoma of the temporal bone. At the age of 24 the patient developed right serous otitis and was treated by introduction of a ventilation tube in the tympanic membrane. At the age of 26 she experienced multiple cranial nerve palsies and right hemiparesis. Physical examination showed a tumor mass in the inferior part of the middle ear which biopsy proved to be a chondromyxosarcoma. She died 12 days after attempted surgical removal. The petrous apex has been destroyed by the neoplasm; the tumor has also infiltrated the mesotympanum, hypotympanum, and infralabyrinthine regions. Compression of the eustachian tube causes the serous otitis media; pressure occlusion of the internal carotid artery accounts for the hemiparesis (female, age 27 years).

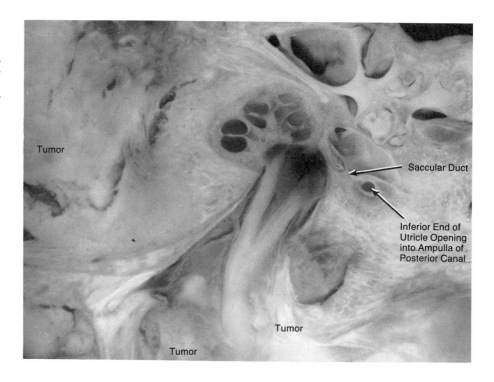

FIG. 8.31, Reel VII—3: Perforation of the tympanic membrane. There is a large posteroinferior perforation of the tympanic membrane with fibrous thickening of the anterior and inferior margins. The manubrium is medially displaced, presumably by the unopposed pull of the tensor tympani muscle. The inferior part of the external auditory canal (EAC) contains a plug of dried exudate and epithelial debris (male, age 69 years).

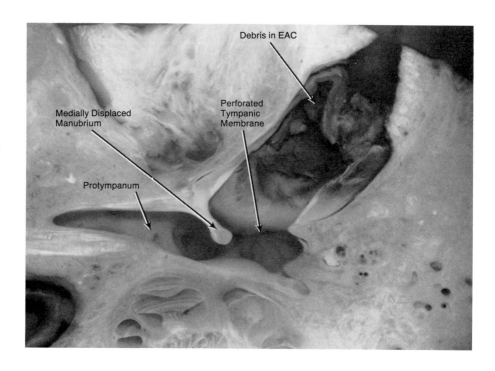

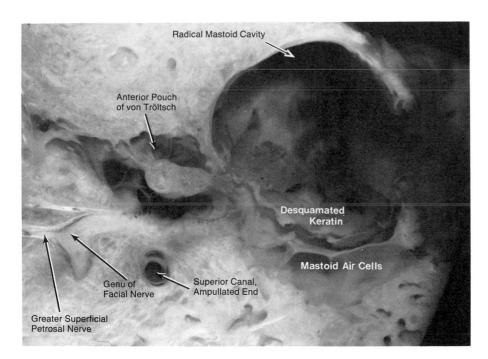

Radical Mastoid Cavity

Anterior Pouch
of von Tröltsch

Desquamated
Keratin

Mastoid Air Cells

Genu of
Facial Nerve

Superior Canal,
Ampullated End

Greater Superficial
Petrosal Nerve

FIG. 8.32, Reel VII—4: Radical mastoidectomy cavity. A surgical procedure including right modified radical mastoidectomy was performed for squamous cell carcinoma at age 71 years. The mastoid bowl contains desquamated keratin on a lining of squamous epithelium. The patient died of unrelated causes 9 years after surgery (male, age 80 years).

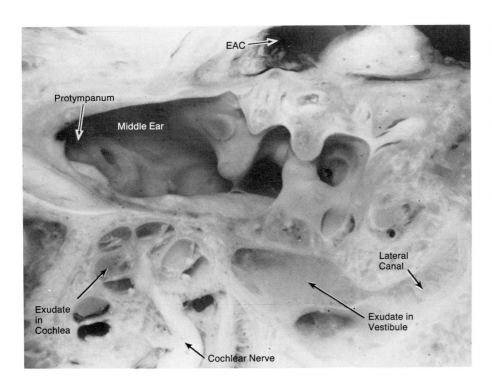

EAC

Protympanum

Middle Ear

Lateral
Canal

Exudate
in
Cochlea

Exudate in
Vestibule

Cochlear Nerve

FIG. 8.33, Reel VII—5: Purulent otitis media, meningitis, and labyrinthitis. This infant had repeated bouts of pneumonia and succumbed to acute pneumococcal meningitis at the age of 17 months. The precipitate in the middle ear is purulent fluid (otitis media). The cloudy fluid in all three turns of the perilymphatic scalae as well as in the vestibule and canals is characteristic of bacterial labyrinthitis; the precipitate around the nerve trunks in the internal auditory canal is the purulent cerebrospinal fluid of meningitis (male, age 17 months).

Stereoscopic Views of the Temporal Bone **225**

FIG. 8.34, Reel VII—6: Stapedectomy for otosclerosis. At the age of 45 this woman underwent right total stapedectomy followed by the implantation of a "fat-wire" prosthesis. She had an excellent hearing gain which persisted to the time of death 13 years later. There is a large vascular otosclerotic focus anterior to the oval window. The hook of the prosthesis is well attached to the long process of the incus. Its medial end extends to the posterior margin of the oval window instead of to the ideal central location (female, age 58 years).

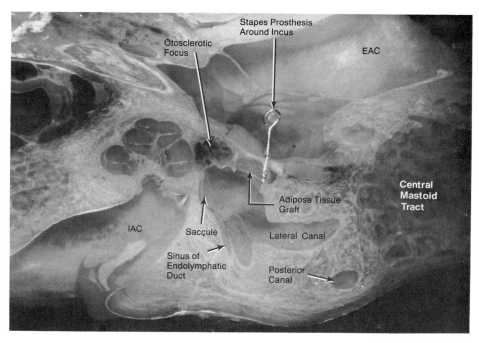

FIG. 8.35, Reel VII—7: Exostoses. These bony excrescences of the external auditory canal (EAC) are usually caused by refrigeration periostitis associated with swimming in cold water (male, age 80 years).

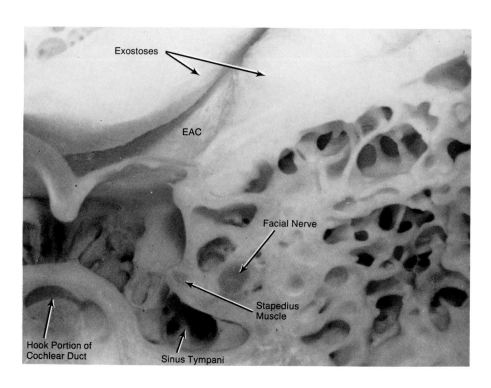

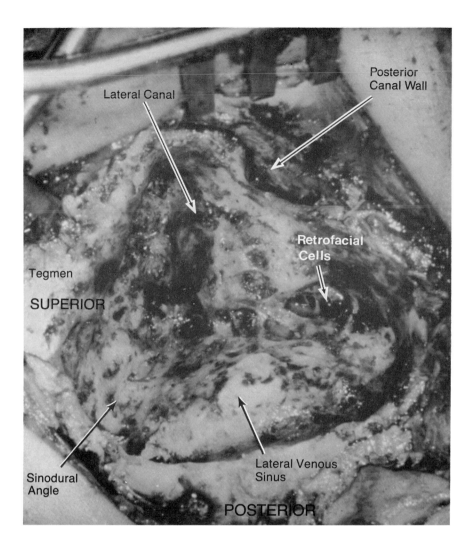

Lateral Canal

Posterior
Canal Wall

Retrofacial
Cells

Tegmen

SUPERIOR

Lateral Venous
Sinus

Sinodural
Angle

POSTERIOR

FIG. 8.36, Reel VIII—1: This photograph shows the operative field during a simple mastoidectomy on the right ear. In this procedure the mastoid is exenterated but the external auditory canal and middle ear are not entered (male, age 7 years).

Operative Views (Reels VIII and IX)

Surgery epitomizes applied anatomy. These operative views (Figs. 8.36 to 8.49) accompany stereo reels VIII and IX and depict disease entities encountered at various stages of surgery. All photographs are taken from the surgeon's view, thus the anterior aspect of the ear is located superiorly in the photographs.

FIG. 8.37, Reel VIII—2: This photograph was taken during the course of a tympanomastoidectomy on the right ear for chronic otitis media and cholesteatoma. The incus has been resorbed and the head of the malleus is surrounded by cholesteatoma. There is a perforation of the posterior half of the tympanic membrane (male, age 29 years).

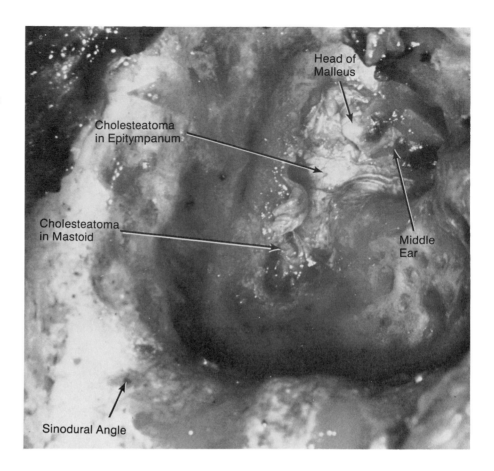

FIG. 8.38, Reel VIII—3: Same case as Figure 8.44. A cholesteatoma is seen in the middle ear and mastoid of this right ear. The incus and crural arch are absent and the malleus is enveloped by the cholesteatoma. As the operation proceeds, the posterior wall of the external auditory canal will be completely removed to gain access to the middle ear. The epitympanum has yet to be fully exteriorized (male, age 16 years).

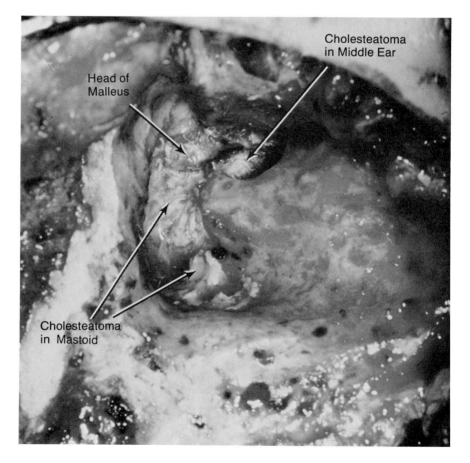

228   Anatomy of the Temporal Bone with Surgical Implications

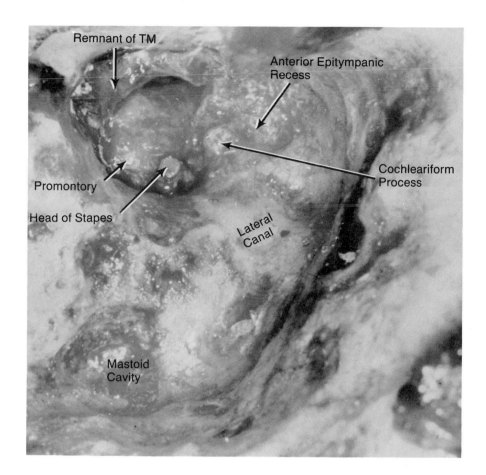

Remnant of TM

Anterior Epitympanic Recess

Promontory

Head of Stapes

Cochleariform Process

Lateral Canal

Mastoid Cavity

FIG. 8.39, Reel VIII—4: The photograph shows the tympanomastoid compartment of the left ear after surgical exenteration and removal of diseased tissues prior to reconstructive procedures (female, age 55 years). TM—tympanic membrane. (See Fig. 8.40.)

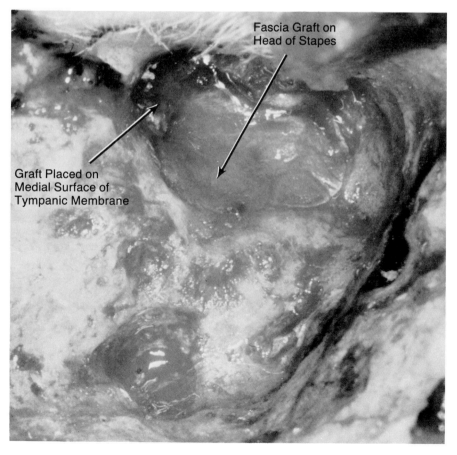

Fascia Graft on Head of Stapes

Graft Placed on Medial Surface of Tympanic Membrane

FIG. 8.40, Reel VIII—5: Same ear as Figure 8.39. A temporalis fascia graft has been introduced to bridge the tympanic space. The graft is placed in contact with the head of the stapes (female, age 55 years). This operation is a type III tympanoplasty.

FIG. 8.41, Reel VIII—6: This photograph was taken during tympanomastoidectomy on the right ear. The mastoid has been exenterated of diseased tissue and the posterior wall of the external auditory canal has been partially removed. Thick granular mucous membrane can be seen in the epitympanum surrounding the ossicles. An aural polyp protrudes from a hidden perforation in the tympanic membrane (male, age 39 years).

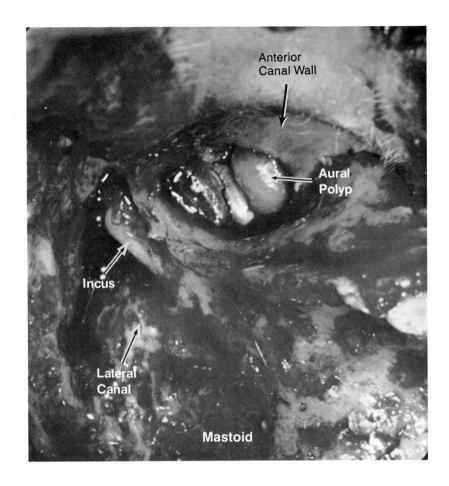

FIG. 8.42, Reel VIII—7: This photograph was taken during an intact-canal-wall tympanoplasty on the left ear. The skin of the posterior wall of the external auditory canal (EAC) has been elevated from the bony canal wall and displaced anteriorly along with the tympanic membrane to provide access to the middle ear (male, age 24 years).

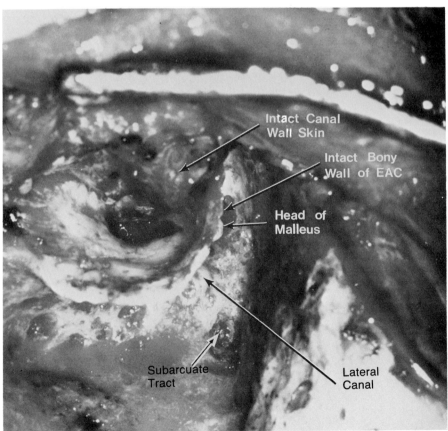

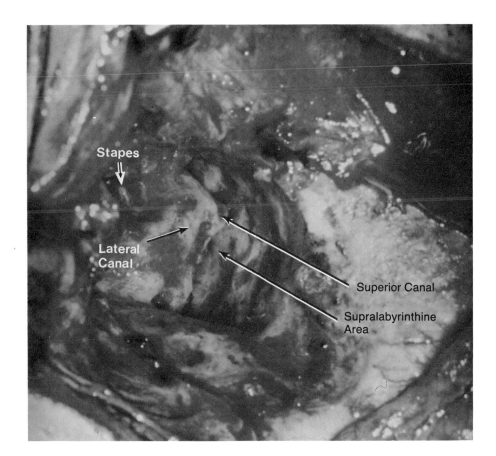

FIG. 8.43, Reel IX—1: This view shows an extensive surgical exenteration of the tympanomastoid compartment of the left ear for removal of an acquired cholesteatoma. The cholesteatoma had extended through the supralabyrinthine tract to the petrous apex (female, age 12 years).

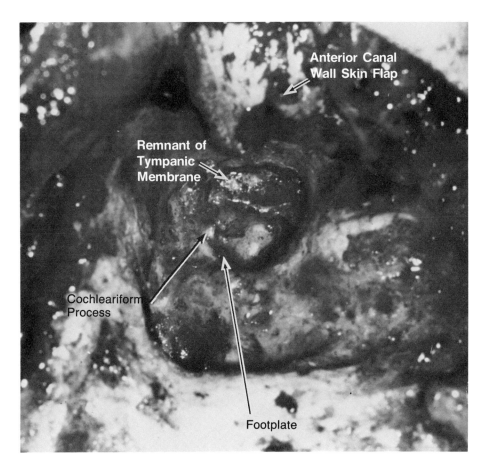

FIG. 8.44, Reel IX—2: Same case as Figure 8.38. Here we see the tympanomastoid compartment of the right ear after diseased tissues (cholesteatoma and granulations) have been removed preparatory to reconstructive procedures (male, age 16 years).

FIG. 8.45, Reel IX—3: This photograph taken during a surgical procedure shows a congenital cholesteatoma of the petrous apex of the left ear. The apex has been reached by drilling away the cochlear part of the bony labyrinth. The cholesteatoma cavity was permanently exteriorized to the external auditory canal (male, age 49 years).

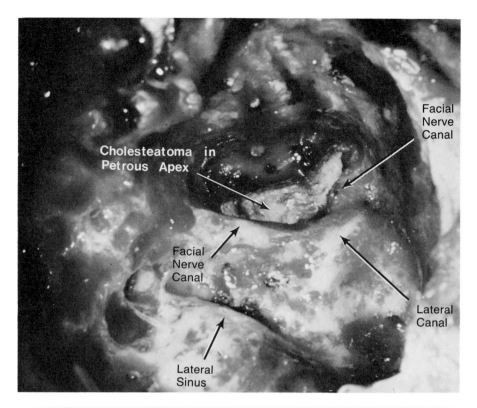

FIG. 8.46, Reel IX—4: The tympanomastoid compartment of the left ear has been thoroughly exenterated for the management of chronic otitis media and mastoiditis with cholesteatoma. In this case, since the ear was profoundly deaf, the entire compartment was obliterated with pedicled and free autogenous tissue grafts (female, age 52 years).

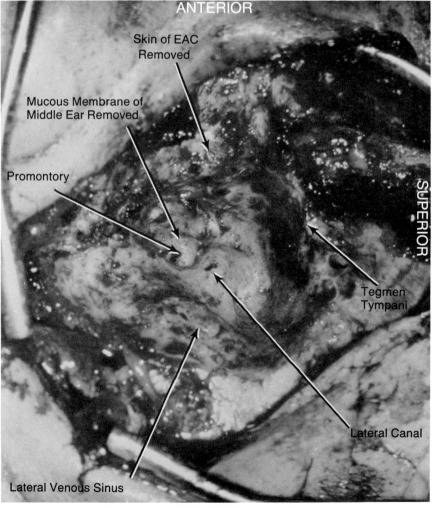

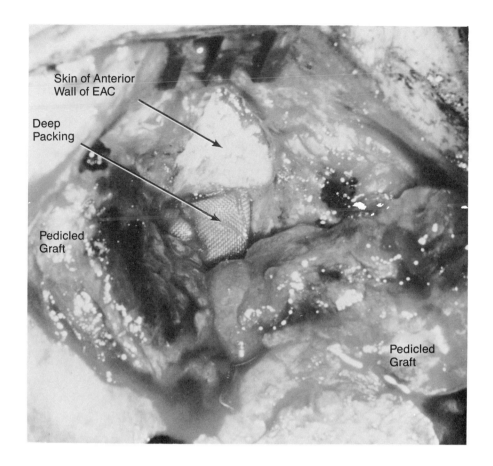

Skin of Anterior
Wall of EAC

Deep
Packing

Pedicled
Graft

Pedicled
Graft

FIG. 8.47, Reel IX—5: This view shows a late stage of a tympanomastoidectomy on the right ear. A packing, consisting of silk cloth strips and cotton, holds in place the tissue grafts used in reconstruction. Dual pedicled grafts composed of muscle, fascia, and periosteum are used to obliterate the mastoid cavity (female, age 58 years).

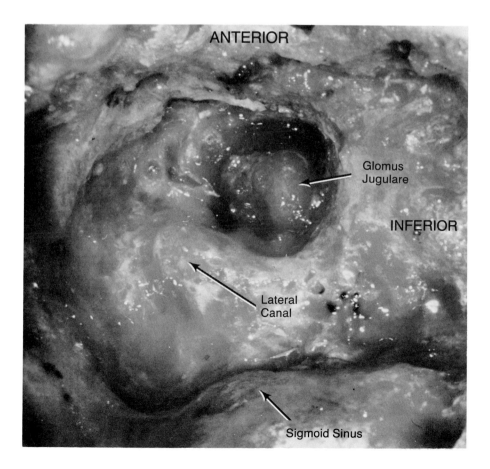

ANTERIOR

Glomus
Jugulare

INFERIOR

Lateral
Canal

Sigmoid Sinus

FIG. 8.48, Reel IX—6: This photograph taken during a surgical procedure on a right ear shows a glomus jugulare tumor occupying the mesotympanum and hypotympanum (female, age 63 years).

FIG. 8.49, Reel IX—7: This surgical
view of the right ear shows the opened
endolymphatic sac. A plastic tube was
placed in the opening to drain the sac
into the mastoid cavity for the allevia-
tion of vertigo caused by Ménière's disease (male, age 32 years).

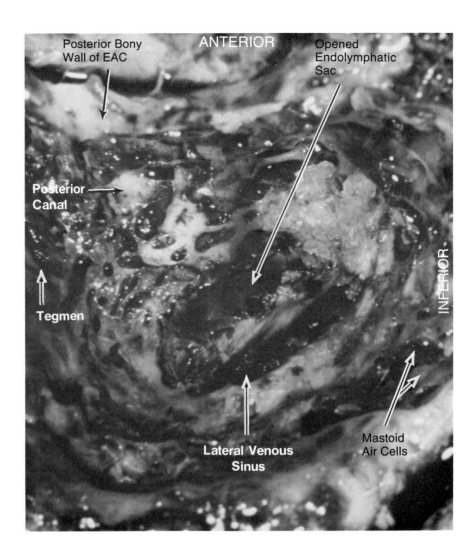

9. Phylogeny and Embryology

Throughout this book, we have presented photographic examples of variant anatomy that are clinically significant, particularly to the otologic surgeon. These variants (e.g. wide cochlear aqueduct, aberrant facial nerve, high jugular bulb, pneumatized incus) are not considered to be anomalies because of the frequency of their occurrence. However, they must be reckoned with and identified if the surgeon is to avoid complications.

Congenital malformations, on the other hand, are more severe but less frequent deviations in morphology and usually cause functional disorders. An anatomy book for clinicians would not be complete without a review of embryology which is essential to understanding the morphogenesis of most anomalies.

The understanding of anomalies of the ear is based on a knowledge of embryologic events such as the genesis of the pinna from the hillocks of His, the formation of the external auditory canal from the first branchial groove, the derivation of the ossicles from the first and second branchial arches, the formation of the ectodermal part of the membranous labyrinth from the primitive otic cyst, the genesis and maturing of the fissures and aqueducts of the otic capsule, etc. With the advent of microscopic reconstructive surgery some anomalies of the external and middle ears can now be corrected.

Kalter and Warkany (1983a, 1983b) have evolved a classification for the causes of malformation as follows: 1) simple genetic origin (caused by single major mutant genes), 2) interactions between hereditary tendencies and nongenetic, undefined factors, 3) chromosomal aberrations, 4) discrete environmental factors, and 5) all others (those with no identifiable cause).

The clinical manifestations of genetic and metabolic deafness, both isolated and in syndromes, may be found in a book by Konigsmark and Gorlin (1976). The morphogenesis of normal and malformed ears are described in a book edited by Gorlin (1980) and a chapter on histopathology of developmental defects of the ear can be found in a book by Schuknecht (1974).

Phylogeny

The auditory and vestibular systems of the mammalian ear represent phylogenetic salvage and modification of the branchial apparatus which serves primarily a respiratory function in aquatic and amphibious organisms. On the flanks of fish a water-motion sensing system, the lateral line, consists of a series of fluid-filled pits (ampullae) called neuromasts which are distributed from the head to the tail. These neuromasts are derived from epidermal placodes and are composed of hair cells bathed in fluid, encompassed by supporting cells, and innervated by cranial nerves VII, IX, and X. The head portion of the lateral line system gives rise to the first semicircular canal by a simple closing over of the lateral line groove; this development, first seen in the hagfish, represents the establishment of the first true vestibular mechanism (Guggenheim, 1948; Schuknecht & Belal, 1975).

The evolution of the membranous labyrinth to the form seen in man can be appreciated by comparing the following vertebrate series. In the Myxinoidea (hagfish, Fig. 9.1) of the vertebrate class cyclostomata, one finds the simplest ear comparable to that of man; it is analogous to the utricle and the superior and posterior semicircular ducts. There are two ampullae with cristae, as well as a macula communis which is recapitulated in the ontogeny of man. A primitive endolymphatic duct extends dorsally towards the skin.

In Petromyzontia (river lamprey, Fig. 9.2), also of the class cyclostomata, the situation is more intricate with a ventral saccule partially separated from the utricle. However, none of the cyclostomes develop a lateral canal.

The vestibular system of elasmobranchs (sharks, Fig. 9.3) has all three semicircular ducts. In addition, the saccule becomes distinct from the utricle and develops an outgrowth, the lagena. The endolymphatic spaces of the elasmobranchs communicate with the environment via an invagination

Fig. 9.1: Schema of the labyrinth of Myxinoidea (hagfish). This labyrinth is comparable to the mammalian utricle and the superior and posterior semicircular canals (After Guggenheim, 1948.)

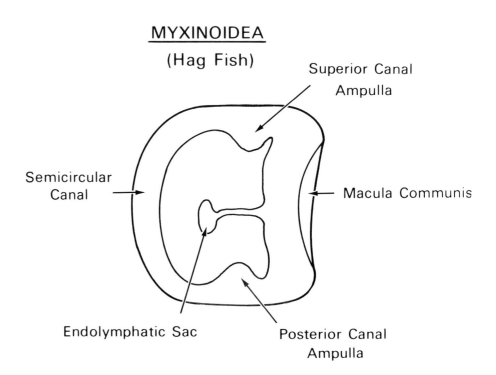

PETROMYZONTIA
(River Lamprey)

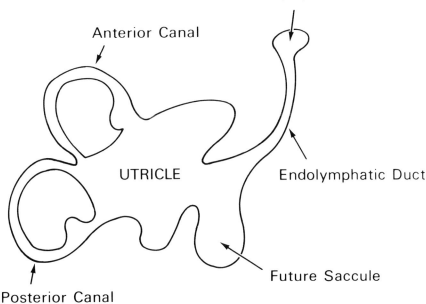

Endolymphatic Sac

Anterior Canal

UTRICLE

Endolymphatic Duct

Future Saccule

Posterior Canal

FIG. 9.2: Schema of the labyrinth of Petromyzontia (river lamprey). In this species the inner ear is still a purely vestibular organ with a utricle and two semicircular canals, but a saccule has appeared. (After Guggenheim, 1948.)

canal (not depicted in the diagram) so that sea water freely passes into and out of the endolymphatic chambers. For the first time the membranous labyrinth is enclosed in a cartilaginous capsule fused to the cranium.

In the lungfish (dipnoi) the invagination canal lies lateral to the endolymphatic duct which grows out from the saccule as an independent structure. Communication with the outside is maintained through the invagination canal; until this canal degenerates in the teleosts, the vestibular system is filled with sea water, not endolymph.

In the course of further evolution the lagena gives rise to the cochlear duct (Fig. 9.4). With these evolutionary modifications, the former neuro-

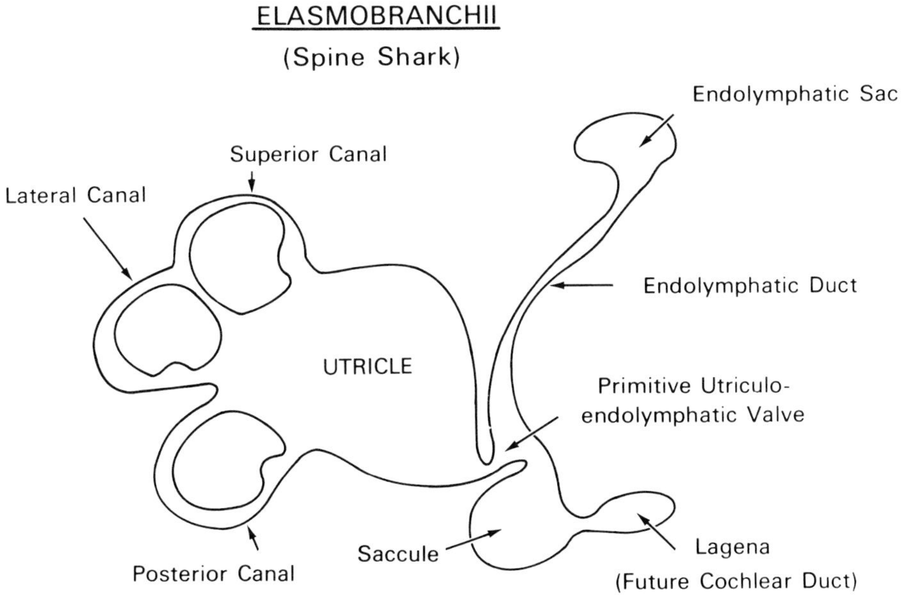

ELASMOBRANCHII
(Spine Shark)

Endolymphatic Sac

Superior Canal

Lateral Canal

UTRICLE

Endolymphatic Duct

Primitive Utriculo-
endolymphatic Valve

Posterior Canal

Saccule

Lagena
(Future Cochlear Duct)

FIG. 9.3: Schema of the labyrinth of Elasmobranchii (spine shark). A third (lateral) semicircular canal is now present as well as a distinct saccule and lagena. (After Guggenheim, 1948.)

FIG. 9.4: Schema of the mammalian labyrinth. Note the presence of the utriculo-endolymphatic valve and the development of the pars inferior (saccule and cochlear duct). (After Guggenheim, 1948.)

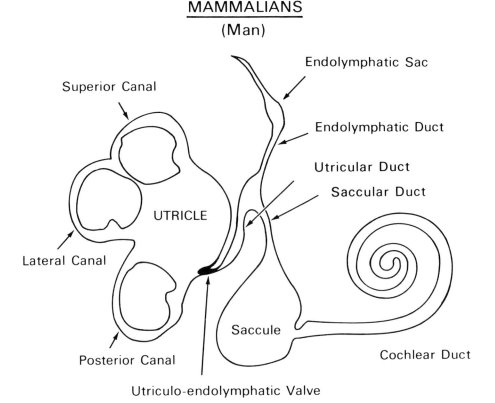

MAMMALIANS
(Man)

Superior Canal

Endolymphatic Sac

Endolymphatic Duct

Utricular Duct

Saccular Duct

UTRICLE

Lateral Canal

Saccule

Cochlear Duct

Posterior Canal

Utriculo-endolymphatic Valve

mast of the lateral line becomes the membranous labyrinth encased within the skull and, instead of abutting the fluid of the external environment, the sensory hair cells abut a fluid of the internal environment, endolymph. This enclosed system retains its function of detecting the motion of the organism for purposes of equilibrium.

A prerequisite to the development of auditory function is the ability to transduce sound pressure waves to fluid displacement through a sound transformer and impedance matching mechanism; these functions are provided by the external auditory canal, eustachian tube, and middle ear. The eusthenopteron, a crossopterygian fish, employed a specialized spiracular diverticulum to compensate for the acoustic impedance of air—the earliest middle ear (Van Bergeijk, 1966). The precursor of the mammalian tympanic membrane is hypothesized to be represented by a bilaminar membrane formed by the spiracular diverticulum. The inner layer of this membrane was derived from the endoderm of the diverticulum, while the outer layer originated from an ectodermal ligament which originally connected the diverticulum to the skull.

The phylogenetic origin of the mammalian ossicular system is complex and differs from that of all other vertebrates. According to the Reichert-Gaupp theory (Pye & Hinchcliffe, 1976), the mammalian stapes finds its ancestry in the columella auris of reptiles, the incus is derived from the quadrate of the upper jaw, and the malleus is derived from the articular of the lower jaw of ancestral vertebrates (Fig. 9.5). The mandible (dentary) evolved a new articulation with the squamosa, which in man is a part of the temporal bone. The gradual modification of the reptilian jaw is hypothesized to have occurred in the therapsids, mammal-like reptiles of the Triassic period. Through evolutionary transformation, the first mandibular arch gave rise to the jaws of all vertebrates and to the mammalian ossicles.

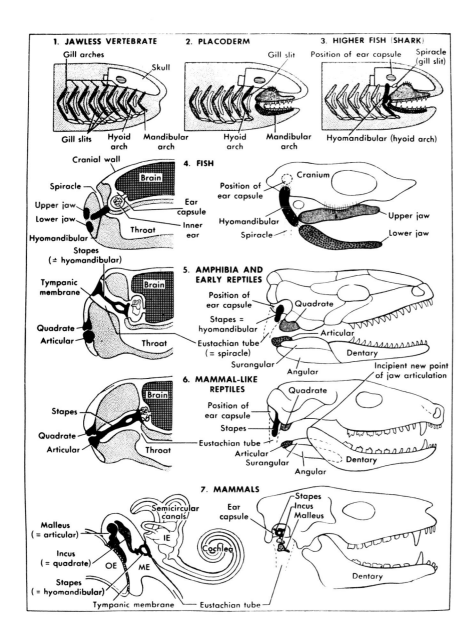

FIG. 9.5: The stapes finds its ancestry in the columella auris of reptiles, the incus in the quadrate of the upper jaw, and the malleus in the articular of the lower jaw of ancestral vertebrates. The mammalian ossicular system derives from the evolutionary transformation of the first mandibular arch. (Courtesy of Taylor, 1969.)

The jaws of the early vertebrates had ligamentous attachments to the cranium. As the hyoid (second branchial) arch moved forward it established the attachment of the otic capsular region to the jaw joint where it is known as the hyomandibular. Consequent to the anterior migration of the hyoid, the first gill slit (branchial cleft) migrated superior to the jaw joint and, as the spiracle, evolved into the eustachian tube. The outer surface of the spiracle was sealed by the tympanic membrane. With further migration the hyomandibular occupied the spiracle and developed into the stapes to provide its relationship with the oval window and inner ear. In the therapsids, however, the stapes lay in a deep recess sequestrated from the environment. Thus a mechanism for the conduction of sound to the stapes was needed.

Four bones comprised the lower jaw of amphibians and early reptiles (Van de Water et al., 1980): the dentary, the quadrate, the articular, and the angular (Fig. 9.5). The dentary (mandible) is the tooth-bearing component. The articular forms a joint with the quadrate and abuts the angular. With refinements in the masticatory apparatus which reduced the stresses on the jaw joint, the posterior elements of the jaw dwindled. As the lower jaw utilized an upper extension of the dentary to articulate with the skull (the future temporomandibular joint), the articular and quadrate bones became superfluous and were incorporated into the middle ear. The articular evolved into the malleus and the quadrate into the incus to provide the necessary connection of the stapes with the tympanic membrane (Tumarkin, 1968; Taylor, 1969).

Embryology

The development of the human ear has been the subject of numerous studies (Streeter, 1906; Anson, 1934, 1969, 1973; Bast, 1946; Davies, 1973; Pearson, 1984), yet many students of otology find it difficult to comprehend the developmental process and its time sequence. In an attempt to alleviate this difficulty, the material is presented in four time periods in fetal development as determined by availability of suitable specimens. These time periods are: 0 to 4 weeks, 4 to 8 weeks, 8 to 16 weeks, and 16 weeks and beyond. Within each period the developmental changes occurring within the various structures are presented. The reader has the option of following the sequential changes in one structure or of focusing on one particular time period.

The accompanying photomicrographs are arranged in developmental ages of approximately 8 weeks, 12 weeks, 16 weeks, and beyond (postnatal). Also presented is a summary of the unique ossification process of the otic capsule and a brief review of the steps in ossification. When integrating the reports of others, we noted some differences in opinion as to the fetal ages at which certain developments occur. For this reason we emphasize that the given fetal ages are approximations.

DEVELOPMENT TO FOUR WEEKS

The Membranous Labyrinth (0 to 4 weeks). The membranous labyrinth includes the cochlear duct with its organ of Corti, the utricle and saccule with their maculae, the semicircular ducts with their cristae ampullares, and the endolymphatic duct and sac. This interconnected system of epithelially lined ducts and chambers contains endolymph and is encased in

FIG. 9.6: The otic vesicle forms as an invagination of neural ectoderm (A, B). The first projection to appear is that of the endolymphatic appendage with the semicircular canals developing as flange-like outcroppings (C, D). Progression of development results in central obliteration of the canals and spiral lengthening of the cochlea (E, F). A = 22 days' gestation, B = 4 weeks, C = 4-1/2 weeks, D = 5-1/2 weeks, E = 6 weeks, and F = 8+ weeks. (After Streeter, 1906.)

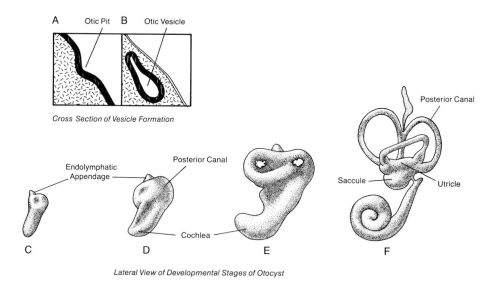

the otic capsule. The otic labyrinth begins its development from surface ectoderm (Fig. 9.6) at the end of the 3rd week of gestation (Huschke, 1824). A plaque-like thickening appears on the lateral aspect of the neural fold dorsal to the first branchial groove, in close relation to the hindbrain. The lining basement membrane of the primordial auditory placode is continuous with that of the rhombencephalic neural groove. In the course of the next few days, the cells in the placode elongate and begin to demonstrate a ciliary brush-border. The placode develops in close conjunction with the "acousticofacial ganglion." These ganglion cells, of neural crest origin, delaminate from the wall of the neural groove and migrate ventrally and laterally. Just before the 4th week (Fig. 9.6) the placode invaginates into the underlying mesenchyme to form the auditory pit. With dilation of the auditory pit a sac is formed; fusion of tissue at the mouth of this sac separates it from the surface, creating a structure called the otocyst (otic vesicle). Even as early as the 4th week of gestation, the endolymphatic appendage can be discerned on the dorsomedial aspect of the otocyst (Fig. 9.6). Concomitant with this development of the otocyst is the differentiation of mesenchymal tissue forming the cartilaginous capsule of the otocyst.

The Semicircular Ducts (0 to 4 weeks). By the 4th week of gestation the future semicircular ducts are two flange-like outcroppings of the utricular (dorsal) aspect of the auditory vesicle. They constitute the canalicular division of the otic capsule.

The Eighth Cranial Nerve and Ganglion (0 to 4 weeks). The so-called "acousticofacial primordium" is of neural crest origin and begins to develop during the 3rd week of gestation in close conjunction with the otic placode lateral to the hindbrain. The acousticofacial primordium was originally credited with giving rise to the geniculate ganglion of the VIIth nerve and the ganglion of the VIIIth nerve via a dorsoventral division. Current evidence (Batten, 1958; Van de Water & Ruben, 1976) supports the proposition, however, that only fibers of the VIIth nerve derive from this complex.

The statoacoustic nerve arises instead from cells of the anteromedial aspect of the otic placode; these cells migrate during the 4th week of gestation between the epithelium of the otic vesicle and its basement membrane. They then penetrate the basement membrane through minute defects to reach the region in which the VIIIth nerve ganglion forms (Batten, 1958; Pearson, 1984) (Fig. 9.7).

The cells of the acousticofacial primordium extend ventrally to the hyoid epibranchial placode (Fig. 9.7) where they give rise to the special visceral afferent (taste) fibers of the facial nerve. It is currently thought (Batten, 1958; Pearson, 1984) that cells of otic vesicle derivation are the anlage for the VIIIth cranial nerve ganglia. It now seems clear that these two ganglia, the VIIIth nerve and the geniculate ganglion, have independent and discrete identities (Batten, 1958).

The Otic Capsule (0 to 4 weeks). The otic capsule lies above the lateral extremity of the tubotympanic recess and consists of the cartilaginous mass which encompasses the inner ear. Eventually it forms the petrous portion of the temporal bone. The otic capsule develops in precartilage and by the end of the fourth week it can be discerned as an increase in cell density of the mesenchyme surrounding the otic vesicle.

Fig. 9.7: This drawing of a 6-week
embryo shows the relationship of the
otic vesicle to the acousticofacial primordium as well as the position of the
epibranchial placode. (After Gasser,
1967.)

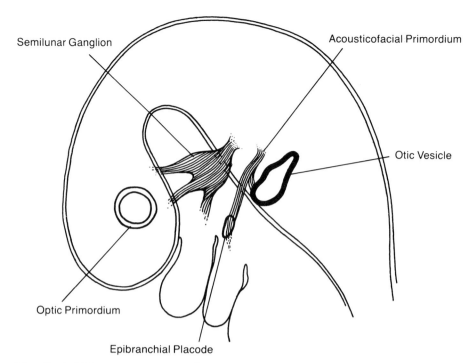

Semilunar Ganglion

Acousticofacial Primordium

Otic Vesicle

Optic Primordium

Epibranchial Placode

The Facial Nerve (0 to 4 weeks). Early investigations suggested that the facial nerve shared a common origin with VIIIth nerve (Fig. 9.7). In the 4-week embryo the so-called "acousticofacial primordium" (or acoustico-facial crest) can be seen attaching to the metencephalon rostral to the otic vesicle. More recent data (O'Rahilly, 1963) label the "acousticofacial pri-mordium" as purely facial and restrict it to giving rise only to general somatic sensory fibers and perhaps motor fibers of the facial nerve (Gasser, 1967; Pearson, 1984).

The Pinna (0 to 4 weeks). The first signs of auricular development occur as tissue condensations of the mandibular and hyoid arches at the distal portion of the first branchial groove in the 4th week of gestation. The specific contribution of the arches to the formation of the auricle is not definitely known, but some (Wood-Jones & Wen, 1934) believe that the entire auricle except the tragus develops from the hyoid (second branchial) arch and the anterior portion of the external acoustic meatus and the tra-gus are the sole contributions of the mandibular arch. Alternate theories (see Pinna 4 to 8 weeks, p. 249) favor a more or less equal contribution of both the mandibular and hyoid arches to the development of the auricle.

The Tympanomastoid Compartment (0 to 4 weeks). The middle ear com-municates with the mastoid air cells through the aditus ad antrum and with the pharynx by the auditory tube. The eustachian tube and middle ear cavity derive from the endodermal tissue of the dorsal end of the first pharyngeal pouch. This outpouching of the foregut is readily discernible in the 3-week embryo. The second pharyngeal pouch may also play a role in the development of the eustachian tube by merging with this evagination of the foregut. Most of the remainder of the middle ear structures (ossicles, muscles, tendons, etc.) arise from the mesoderm of the first and second branchial arches.

By the 4th week the dorsoventrally flattened terminal end of the first pharyngeal pouch has come into apposition with the infolding of the first branchial groove. This contact is short-lived because the mesoderm, which is destined to form the manubrium as well as a portion of the tympanic membrane (the tunica propria), grows in between these endodermal (first pharyngeal pouch) and ectodermal (first branchial groove) layers. The eustachian tube at this point is merely a slit-like tunnel.

The Malleus and Incus (0 to 4 weeks). The anlage of the ossicles has been the subject of much discussion. The consensus now holds that the ossicles have multiple origins. It is believed that the manubrium of the malleus and the long process of the incus derive from the hyoid visceral bar, while the head of the malleus and body of the incus differentiate from the mandibular visceral bar. The anterior process of the malleus, however, emerges from intramembranous ossification distinct from the visceral bars. In this context it is useful to draw a distinction between the mandibular and hyoid visceral bars as opposed to Meckel's and Reichert's cartilages (Pearson, 1984). Lying within the branchial arches is a condensation of mesenchymal tissue. With maturation it differentiates into cartilage and eventually becomes bone in some, although not all, regions. Visceral bar is the term used to describe the entire masses of condensed mesenchymal tissue, whereas the terms Meckel's and Reichert's cartilages refer only to the cartilage formed from the ventromedial portions of these mandibular and hyoid visceral bars, respectively.

At approximately 4 weeks of gestation (Fig. 9.8) areas of condensation of the mesenchyme appear at the dorsolateral ends of the mandibular and hyoid bars. An interbranchial bridge is formed which connects the upper end of the mandibular visceral bar to the central region of the hyoid visceral bar; it is this bridge that gives rise to the blastemae of the malleus and incus.

The Stapes (0 to 4 weeks). The stapes, like the malleus and incus, has a dual origin first described by Gradenigo in 1887. A stapedial "ring," which arises from mesenchyme of the hyoid visceral bar, gives rise to the capitulum, crura, and tympanic (lateral) surface of the footplate. The lamina stapedialis, which gives rise to the annular ligament and the labyrinthine (medial) surface of the footplate, develops from the otic capsule and retains some of its cartilaginous structure throughout life. A blastemal mass is all that is recognizable of the future stapes at the 4th week of gestation (Fig. 9.8). This blastema is composed of the condensed mesenchymal cells of the dorsolateral end of the hyoid visceral bar, adjacent to the facial nerve and the nascent stapedial artery.

The Arteries (0 to 4 weeks). In the 3rd week of gestation small vascular islands in the mesenchyme of the pharyngeal arches coalesce to form the six aortic arch arteries. These arch arteries originate ventrally from the unpaired aortic sac, course through the visceral arches, and terminate in the ipsilateral dorsal aorta. These arteries are never all co-existent. The first and second arteries dwindle and vanish even before the third and more caudally positioned arch arteries are completely developed. The paired dorsal aortae course cranially to supply the embryonic forebrain and midbrain as well as the inner ear. The auditory vesicle initially receives its blood supply from one or more dorsal branches of these aortae and later from the otic arteries which are branches of the primitive carotid artery.

Between 3 to 4 weeks the primitive carotid artery, derived as a cranial extension of the dorsal aorta, courses toward the optic vesicle to reach the first aortic arch where it fuses with its twin from the opposite side to form the basilar artery. The blood supply of the labyrinth becomes dependent upon the longitudinal neural arteries which are formed by fusion of the

FIG. 9.8: At 4-1/2 weeks to 6 weeks the chorda tympani nerve appears to progressively detach the malleus and incus from the hyoid visceral bar. The facial nerve deepens a groove on the blastemal mass of the stapes which eventually separates the blastema into a stapes primordium and laterohyale. The rotation of the structures of the stapes blastema with the laterohyale is the result of a combination of anterior (superior) growth of the stapes primordium with posterior (inferior) growth of the laterohyale. A = 4-1/2 weeks, B = 5-1/2 weeks, and C = 6 weeks. (After Pearson, 1984.)

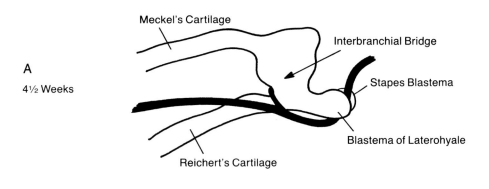

A
4½ Weeks

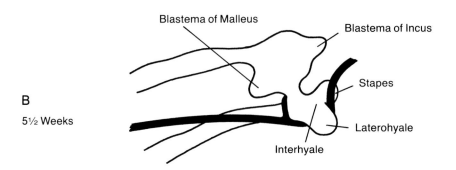

B
5½ Weeks

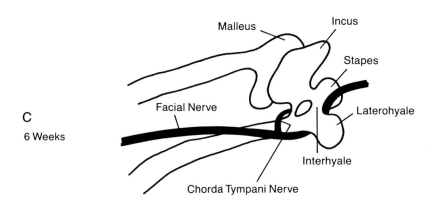

C
6 Weeks

neural arteries and the basilar arteries as the primitive otic artery fades away during the fourth week.

The first and second arch arteries disappear in fetal life, although the dorsal segment of the second arch artery may remain even into adulthood (see persistent stapedial artery, Chapter 7, p. 201), passing between the stapedial crura.

The third arch artery gives rise to the carotid arterial system; an offshoot from its ventral aspect gives rise to the external carotid artery. The common carotid artery develops from that portion of the third arch artery proximal to the origin of the external carotid artery. The internal carotid artery has dual origins; its proximal portion develops from the distal third arch artery while the remainder, encompassing its intracranial portion, develops from the dorsal aorta cranial to the third arch artery.

The Veins (0 to 4 weeks). Bordering the developing brain of the human embryo are simple channels which develop into the primary head sinus by the 3rd week of gestation. By the 4th week it has surrounded the Xth cranial nerve. The dorsolateral segments of the brain drain into this primary head sinus through the anterior, middle, and posterior dural plexuses. The latter two channels drain the auditory vesicle. The vascular ring around the Xth cranial nerve is only transient and by the end of the 4th week its medial aspect shrinks. The cranial aspect persists, however, and in part develops into the primitive myelencephalic vein, which in turn gives rise to the inferior petrosal sinus and the inferior cochlear vein. Meanwhile, the posterior and middle dural plexuses form anastomotic connections near the auditory vesicle.

DEVELOPMENT TO EIGHT WEEKS

The Membranous Labyrinth (4 to 8 weeks). As late as the 5th week of gestation, a small stalk may persist as the sole communication of the otocyst with the surface ectoderm. At 4 to 5 weeks of gestation the otic vesicle initiates dorsoventral elongation. Three folds begin to form which divide the vesicle into three major subdivisions: the endolymphatic duct and sac, the saccule and its cochlear duct, and the utricle with its semicircular ducts.

The first fold develops at the 5-week stage, as an inferiorly directed infolding which demarcates the future endolymphatic duct and sac as a dorsomedial projection from the utricular part of the vesicle (utriculosaccular chambers) (Fig. 9.9). A ventromedial projection is the precursor of the cochlear duct. At the same time, nerve fibers begin to extend from the statoacoustic ganglion to the subdivisions of the otic vesicle. A thickening of the medial wall of the otic vesicle forms the primordium of a common

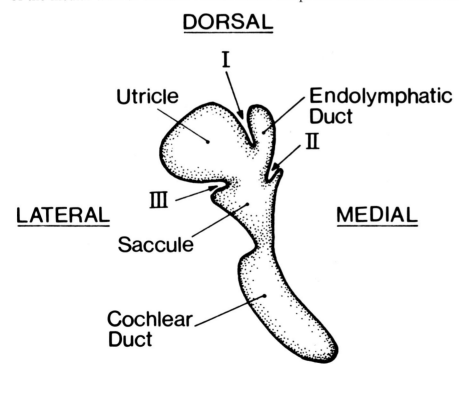

DORSAL

LATERAL

MEDIAL

VENTRAL

FIG. 9.9: Drawing after Bast and Anson (1949) of the developing otic labyrinth at 6 to 8 weeks. The nascent folds I, II, and III indent the otic vesicle to initiate the formation of the utricle, saccule, and endolymphatic duct.

macula (macula communis). This common macula soon divides into a superior segment which gives rise to the macula of the utricle and the ampullary crests of the superior and lateral semicircular ducts, and an inferior segment which forms the macula of the saccule and the ampullary crest of the posterior semicircular duct. By 6 weeks the primordial semicircular ducts (the canalicular division of the otic capsule) materialize as two flattened sacs; the lateral duct arises from a horizontal protuberance, while the superior and posterior semicircular ducts arise from a common outpouching.

The second of the three divisional infoldings appears on the medial aspect of the otic vesicle and is horizontally oriented at the junction of the saccule and ostium of the primordial endolymphatic duct.

The third fold is also horizontally oriented and is located on the lateral aspect of the utriculosaccular chamber. This infolding was called the utriculosaccular partition (cloison interutriculo-sacculaire) by Chatellier (1926) and Anson (1934), and is the fold primarily responsible for the separation of the utricle from the saccule. Initially, the medial and lateral horizontal infoldings are diametrically opposed, but by 8 weeks the medial shelf assumes a more caudal position with respect to the lateral ledge. The resultant structure has a Y-shaped configuration which connects the utriculosaccular division with the endolymphatic duct.

The Cochlear Duct (o to 8 weeks). In the 6-week embryo, the cochlear duct forms as a tubular diverticulum from the saccular portion of the otic vesicle (Fig. 9.6). This ventral projection coils with medial growth, completing one turn by the 6th week and its entire two and one-half turns by the 8th week. At this stage the communication of the cochlear duct with the saccule narrows to form the ductus reuniens. Even as the cochlear duct first appears, the organ of Corti can be seen as a placode of stratified epithelial cells in the wall of the cochlear duct (Figs. 9.30, 9.33, 9.40, and 9.43). Like the maculae and cristae, the organ of Corti appears early in gestation and attains maximum size by mid-term. At the region of the nascent organ of Corti, from base to apex, the epithelial cells of the cochlear duct differentiate into two ridges of tall, columnar cells. The cells of these ridges secrete the gelatinous cushion which forms the tectorial membrane. The smaller outer ridge differentiates into the organ of Corti, while the inner larger ridge gives rise to the spiral limbus. This metamorphosis spreads as a wave from the basal to the apical aspect of the cochlea. By the 8th week differentiation of the epithelium and subjacent mesenchyme at the outer wall of the cochlear duct initiates the development of the stria vascularis (Fig. 9.43). The modiolus, the tympanic and vestibular scalae, and the enveloping otic capsule begin to differentiate at about the 8th week.

The Utricle and Saccule (o to 8 weeks). The utricle in association with the semicircular ducts makes up the pars superior of the membranous labyrinth. This phylogenetically older segment of the membranous labyrinth develops earlier in the ontogeny of the fetus (Figs. 9.29 and 9.34). The saccule in association with the cochlear duct makes up the phylogenetically younger pars inferior (Figs. 9.30 and 9.35).

During the 7th week of gestation, the constriction between the saccule and the cochlear duct forms the ductus reuniens and in the ensuing week the three infoldings of the otic vesicle deepen to create the adult forms of the utricle, saccule, and endolymphatic duct (Fig. 9.9). The macula of the utricle, like the other sense organs, differentiates from the simple epithelium of the wall of the membranous labyrinth at those areas where the sensory nerves enter. Between the 7th and 8th weeks of development the simple epithelium is transformed into a complex pseudostratified type.

The Semicircular Ducts (4 to 8 weeks). At the 6-week stage the two arching flanges undergo partial obliteration of their cavities through fusion and disintegration of opposing epithelial walls (Fig. 9.6). The void is filled by mesenchymal tissue. The peripheral aspect of each flange retains its lumen, thereby creating the semicircular duct. This process occurs first in the superior semicircular canal and soon after in the posterior and the lateral canals. The ampullae are the dilated ends of the three semicircular ducts which open into the utricle; those of the superior and lateral canals are located on their anterior limbs (crura) while that of the posterior canal is found on its inferior limb (crus). By the 7th week of gestation a ridge-like structure formed by neuroepithelial cells appears within the ampullae at a point where the vestibular nerve fibers enter (Figs. 9.29, 9.32, and 9.36). These future cristae ampullares are oriented perpendicularly to the direction of endolymph flow. The nonampullated ends of the semicircular ducts also empty into the utricle. Because the posterior and superior ducts fuse to form a common duct (crus commune) a total of five crura (rather than six) enter the utricle.

The Endolymphatic Duct (0 to 8 weeks). The endolymphatic duct is first seen as a dorsomedial projection from the otic vesicle, known as the endolymphatic appendage, at approximately the 6th week of gestation (Fig. 9.9). Although it is a narrow tube at its vestibular end, it widens out distally into a sac-like configuration. With lateral development of the otic vesicle, the distal end of the endolymphatic appendage assumes a relatively more medial position and by the 8th week it is a large fusiform sac with a thin epithelial lining, rippled by low rugae.

The Eighth Cranial Nerve and Ganglion (4 to 8 weeks). Between the 4th and 5th weeks the statoacoustic ganglion divides into superior and inferior segments sending nerve fibers to the various areas of the otic vesicle. The superior division supplies the utricular macula and the cristae of the superior and lateral semicircular ducts. At 5 to 6 weeks the inferior segment further subdivides into upper and lower portions; the upper segment innervates the saccular macula and the crista of the posterior semicircular duct and the lower segment supplies the organ of Corti.

At approximately 6 weeks the nerve fibers to the posterior ampulla are splayed out, but later appear as one compact nerve. Streeter (1906) hypothesized that the streamlining may be related to the incorporation or atrophy of temporary fibers to sensory structures found in this area in lower forms (e.g. crista neglecta).

By the end of 7 weeks the pars superior has enlarged greatly and its nerve supply has become defined as discrete branches. By the end of 8 weeks the nerves approximate the adult condition. The vestibular nerve, a derivative of the upper part of the statoacoustic ganglion, now consists of a superior and inferior division with its ganglion on its trunk. The cochlear nerve likewise resembles that of the adult with its compactly arranged spiraling fibers.

Differentiation into sensory neuroepithelium and supporting cells occurs where neural contact is established. In a review of organogenesis of the ear, Van de Water and Ruben (1976) suggest, however, that neuronal contact may not be required for the initial differentiation of the sensory structures of the internal ear but may be of importance in maintenance of sensory structures, once differentiated. Hilding (1969) found that hair cells were differentiated before the appearance of synapses; he was unsure as to whether nerve fibers influenced differentiation.

The Otic Capsule (4 to 8 weeks). In the 5th week the condensation of mesenchyme occurs everywhere except in the region of the developing endolymphatic duct. It envelops the membranous labyrinth in the 6th week and begins to assume a cartilaginous character. A small area on the medial wall fails to be included in the mesenchymal condensation; it marks the future location of the internal acoustic meatus. The condensed mesenchyme, except for its lack of blood vessels, is identical to embryonic connective tissue elsewhere in the developing embryo. As the 6th week closes, precartilage (compacted mesenchyme which is assuming the character of embryonic cartilage) differentiates into the first true cartilage of the otic capsule. This process is not completed until approximately the 8th week. At this time the membranous labyrinth has attained its adult shape, although adult size is not reached until approximately midterm. Even as the outer zone of precartilage is becoming true cartilage, dedifferentiation of already formed cartilage is taking place, forming a loose, vascular reticulum of mesenchyme immediately adjacent to the epithelium of the otic vesicle.

The Perilymphatic Spaces (0 to 8 weeks). The perilymphatic (periotic) labyrinth occupies the space between the membranous labyrinth and the inner periosteal layer of the otic capsule. The development of this composite tissue and tissue-fluid space from the mesodermal tissue surrounding the membranous labyrinth occurs rapidly between the 8th and 24th weeks of development. The same general scheme is followed in the cochlear, canalicular, and vestibular portions of the labyrinth. As with development of the otic capsule, a process of retrogressive change in precartilage is involved; instead of differentiating to mature cartilage, it dedifferentiates into a loose, vascular reticulum. This process begins at approximately the 8th week with rarefaction of the precartilage surrounding the membranous ampullae of the semicircular ducts (Fig. 9.32). Also during the 8th week a loose vascular reticulum is seen lining the utricle, saccule, and proximal part of the cochlear duct (Fig. 9.34); it is the first evidence of the development of the perilymphatic (periotic) cistern of the vestibule (Fig. 9.31). An area of rarefaction in precartilage just under the round window initiates the beginning of the scala tympani.

The Capsular Channels (0 to 8 weeks). In the 7-week embryo a rarefaction of the otic capsular precartilage in the region of the medial wall of the basal turn of the cochlea, just medial to the developing round window and extending to the posterior cranial fossa, is the primordial cochlear aqueduct. With further development its contained periotic duct will provide a route of communication between the scala tympani and the subarachnoid space.

The reticular tissue contained by the cochlear aqueduct is continuous with that encompassing the IXth cranial nerve, the dura, and the inferior petrosal sinus. Hence, the round window niche, occupied by loose mesenchymal connective tissue and vessels, is also continuous with posterior fossa dura via the cochlear aqueduct.

The Facial Nerve (4 to 8 weeks). At 4 to 5 weeks the cells of the "acousticofacial primordium" at the level of the epibranchial placode begin to transform into the neuroblasts of the geniculate ganglion (Gasser, 1967). This ganglion which develops independently of the motor fibers (Fisch as quoted by Jahrsdoerfer, 1981) is well defined by 6 weeks.

The facial division of the "acousticofacial primordium" undergoes a division at 4 to 5 weeks into a caudal portion which gives rise to the main trunk of the facial nerve and a rostral portion which passes ventral to the first pharyngeal pouch to enter the mandibular arch. This rostral portion is the chorda tympani nerve which at this time is comparable in size to the main trunk of the facial nerve (Gasser, 1967). The distal termination of the chorda tympani nerve is in the same region as the termination of a branch of the mandibular nerve (the lingual nerve) and coincides with the area in which the submandibular ganglion develops at about 6-1/2 weeks. By the seventh week a definite union has been established between the lingual and chorda tympani nerves just proximal to the ganglion (Gasser, 1967).

The nervus intermedius (nerve of Wrisberg) develops from the geniculate ganglion and is present as a discrete entity by approximately 7 weeks. It courses as one or two bundles of fibers between the VIIth and VIIIth nerves to the brain stem and even at this stage is much smaller than the main trunk of the VIIth nerve (Gasser, 1967).

The greater superficial petrosal nerve, which is the second branch of the facial nerve to develop (Rabl, 1887), stems from the most ventral aspect of the geniculate ganglion; it is present at 5 weeks and is well developed by 6-1/2 weeks.

The Facial Canal (0 to 8 weeks). In the 8-week fetus the facial canal is a sulcus located on the tympanic wall of the posterior part of the otic capsule. The future canal, like the rest of the otic capsule, is still cartilaginous and houses the developing stapedius muscle, facial nerve, and vascular channels.

The Pinna (4 to 8 weeks). During the 5th and 6th weeks, the condensations seen at the 4-week stage now form six ridges, known as the hillocks of His (1885) (Figs. 9.10 to 9.12). Controversy surrounds the significance

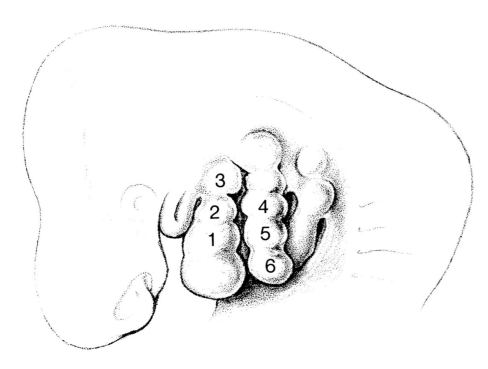

FIG. 9.10: The auricle develops from hillocks 1 to 3 of the first branchial arch and hillocks 4 to 6 of the second branchial arch at approximately 6 weeks (see Figs. 9.11 and 9.12). (After Levine, 1983.)

FIG. 9.11: The original six hillocks of His are further developed at approximately 7 weeks (see Figs. 9.10 and 9.12). (After Levine, 1983.)

FIG. 9.12: The adult auricle is shown with derived parts from the six hillocks of His indicated by numbers 1 to 6 (see Figs. 9.10 and 9.11). (After Levine, 1983.)

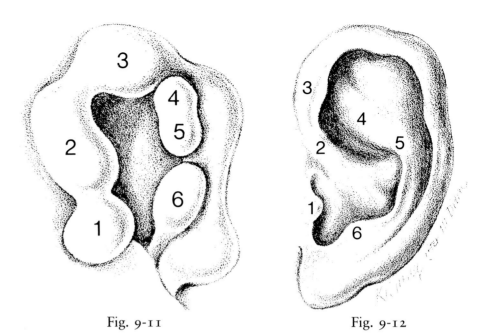

Fig. 9-11   Fig. 9-12

of these hillocks in the development of the pinna. Some authors believe that they are coincidental rather than integral to the process. Most authorities believe, however, that these six hillocks do bear upon the final configuration of the pinna.

Hillocks 1, 2, and 3, of mandibular arch origin, are innervated by the auriculotemporal branch of the Vth cranial nerve. Hillocks 4, 5, and 6 are of hyoid arch origin and are innervated by the small cutaneous branch of the VIIth nerve as well as the branches of the cervical plexus, in particular the greater auricular and lesser occipital nerves.

The adult homologues of these hillocks as described by Anson and Donaldson (1980), His (1885), and Arey (1974) are depicted in Figure 9.12. Streeter (1922) and Pearson (1984) suggest a different scheme. They propose that the first hillock forms the tragal region, the second establishes the crus of the helix, and the third is responsible for the major part of the helix. They suggest that hillock 4 gives rise to the anthelix, hillock 5 to the antitragus, and hillock 6 to both the future lobule and most of the inferior aspect of the helix. In a total departure from these theories, Wood-Jones and Wen (1934) propose that only the tragus is derived from the mandibular arch and that the remainder of the auricle is of hyoid arch origin.

Initially these ridges are closely situated along the first branchial groove but are separated as the groove develops to eventuate in the formation of the cymba conchae, the cavum conchae, and the incisura intertragica.

As the end of the 6th week approaches, the hillocks give rise to the two folds of the pinna, those of mandibular arch origin forming the anterior fold and those of the hyoid arch forming the posterior fold. These folds then fuse at the upper end of the first branchial groove. During the 2nd month of development, because of mandibular and facial growth, the pinna is displaced dorsolaterally from its original ventromedial position. After the 7th week, cartilage develops from the mesenchyme of the folds.

The External Auditory Canal, Tympanic Membrane, and Tympanic Ring (0 to 8 weeks). The external auditory canal is derived from the dorsal part of the first branchial groove which deepens during the 2nd month of gestation and forms a funnel-shaped depression located between the mandibular and hyoid arches. Between the 4th and 5th weeks the ectoderm of the first branchial groove transiently impinges upon the endodermal lining of the tubotympanic recess. By the 6th week ingrowth of mesoderm breaks this contact (Fig. 9.32). At 8 weeks, with extension of the inferior portion of the first branchial groove toward the middle ear, a narrow tunnel is established, the primary (primitive) canal. This primary canal corresponds to the future fibrocartilaginous portion of the adult canal.

The Tympanomastoid Compartment (4 to 8 weeks). Between the 4th and 6th weeks the tympanic cavity undergoes progressive expansion to keep pace with the developing cartilaginous otic capsule. Beginning at 7 weeks the tubotympanic recess becomes constricted at its midpoint due to the rapid growth of the second branchial arch. Hammar (cited by Proctor, 1967) defined the region of the tubotympanic recess lateral to this constriction as the primary tympanic cavity and the region lying medially as the primordial eustachian tube.

By the end of 8 weeks the approximation of the lateral aspect of the tympanic cavity to the first branchial groove (the future external auditory canal) is broken by the ingrowth of mesodermal tissue destined to form the pars propria of the tympanic membrane as well as the manubrium of the malleus (Fig. 9.13). Concomitantly the mesenchyme surrounding the middle ear thins out, allowing for progressive expansion of the middle ear space. The process of cavitation is present initially only in the inferior half of the middle ear cavity and attains completion only late in fetal life.

The superior periotic process develops as a projection of the otic capsule, and as it stretches forward over the ossicles it forms the lateral portion of the tegmen tympani; at this time, a plate of mesenchymal tissue is the sole component of the medial aspect of the tegmen.

Also at this time, growth of the fetal head has contributed to the narrowing and elongation of the medial aspect of the tubotympanic recess so that it now forms the eustachian tube.

The Malleus and Incus (4 to 8 weeks). Between 4 and 8 weeks cartilaginous models of the incus and malleus derive from the aggregated mesenchyme of the interbranchial bridge. The development of the chorda tym-

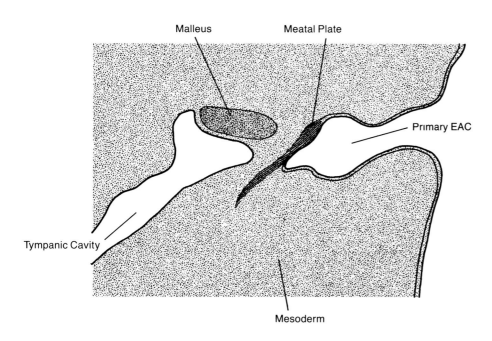

FIG. 9.13: By 9 weeks the ectoderm of the first branchial groove extends toward the middle ear, forming the primitive external auditory canal. The meatal plate is the result of surface ectodermal ingrowth, and extends from the external auditory canal (EAC) to the inferior wall of the tympanic cavity. (After Anson & Donaldson, 1981.)

pani nerve is closely involved in the steps of differentiation of these ossicles; this nerve forms a fixed point for growth of the ossicles as it sweeps around the ventral aspect of the combined incudal and malleal primordia (the interbranchial bridge) (Fig. 9.8).

Between the 5th and 6th weeks the primordial malleus and incus grow rapidly in size; however, the chorda tympani nerve lags behind and at 6 weeks seems to separate the incudal and malleal blastemae from the hyoid visceral bar. During the 6th week, precartilage forms in the future ossicles as well as in Meckel's and Reichert's cartilages. Rapid transformation into true cartilage occurs during the 7th week and the short process of the incus establishes contact with the otic capsule (Fig. 9.31). By the end of the 8th week the form of the cartilaginous malleus closely approximates that of the adult; however, there is still continuity between the malleus and Meckel's cartilage at a time when the incus is already separated from Reichert's cartilage. Different from the malleus, which has no continuity with hyoid arch derivatives in the adult, the incudal articulation with the stapes represents a persistent link to the hyoid arch structure. The re-establishment of this continuity is theorized to occur by proliferation of blastemal cells of the long process of the incus towards the stapes as the chorda tympani nerve is severing the link between the incus and the hyoid visceral bar (Fig. 9.8). The primordium of the long process has nearly reached the head of the stapes by the time this primary link has been broken. Fusion occurs at the site of future joint development. At the junction of Meckel's cartilage with the malleus there is an area of membranous bone formation which marks the future anterior process of the malleus (processus Folianus). Meanwhile, dense mesenchyme separates the malleus and incus at the area of their future articulation (Fig. 9.30).

The Stapes (4 to 8 weeks). During the 5th and 6th weeks the solid blastemal mass of the stapes develops a ring-like configuration about the stapedial artery. The first step in this transformation is the creation of a groove in the stapes blastema at its area of contact with the stapedial artery during the 5th week. In the following week the grooved stapedial mass fuses around the artery, forming the stapedial ring; the central defect housing the stapedial artery is the obturator foramen. During the same period the facial nerve tunnels another groove which divides the primordium of the stapes into the stapes proper and the laterohyale, bridged by the interhyale (Fig. 9.8). With posteroinferior expansion of the primordium of the laterohyale and the anterosuperior expansion of the stapes, these structures seem to rotate about the facial nerve so that the laterohyale eventually comes to rest posterior to the stapes (Fig. 9.8).

During the 7th week, several events occur in stapedial evolution. The laterohyale extends to meet the otic capsule as cells of the interhyale condense at the proximal end of the hyoid bar. The stapedial ring enlarges to approach the otic capsule at the region of the future oval window, and the long process of the incus impinges upon the head of the stapes. As is true for the incus and the malleus, blastemal tissue now differentiates into cartilage. For the stapes this process is coordinated with that of the adjacent otic capsule. There is a depression at the point where the stapes abuts the otic capsule. During the 8th week, while the remainder of the otic capsule is undergoing cartilaginous differentiation, the tissue at this junction (future bases of crura and footplate) changes to dense fibrous tissue (the lamina stapedialis of the otic capsule) (Fig. 9.31). This tissue gives rise to the vestibular (medial) surface of the stapes footplate. The tissue at the rim of the footplate condenses to form the annular ligament, but this does not occur until the footplate has reached its final size.

The Arteries (4 to 8 weeks). At 4 to 5 weeks the cranial nerve roots and the aortic arch arteries correspond to each pharyngeal bar and pouch; this relationship is known as the "branchial" phase of development. The first and second aortic arch arteries have diminished, save for a dorsal fragment of the first arch artery (the mandibular artery). In their places are the hyoid artery, representative of the dorsal end of the second arch artery, and the ventral pharyngeal artery which ends at the mandibular nerve root.

Beginning in the 5th week, the stapedial artery develops from the proximal portion of the hyoid artery and courses through the primordial stapes into the mandibular bar (Fig. 9.14). The distal remnant of the ventral pharyngeal artery has become separated from its proximal portion. By the end of the 6th week, the stapedial artery, as the major branch of the hyoid artery, has reached the peak of its development; however, the distal end of the hyoid artery shrinks to a small twig coursing in a caudal direction along with the tympanic branch of the glossopharyngeal nerve. This hyoid twig along with the stem of the stapedial artery gives rise to the caroticotympanic branches of the adult internal carotid artery.

Immediately beyond the stapes, the stapedial artery (Fig. 9.14) sends off a cranial branch which forms its supraorbital division accompanying the ophthalmic branch of the Vth cranial nerve. The remainder of the stapedial artery runs ventrally with the mandibular division of the Vth cranial nerve to join the plexiform distal remnants of the ventral pharyngeal artery at the region of the mandibular root of the chorda tympani nerve; this anastomosis becomes the maxillomandibular division of the stapedial artery.

In this embryologic discussion we will use the term "internal auditory artery" as is customary. We have elsewhere preferred to use the term "labyrinthine artery" for the reason that it supplies the vestibular as well as the auditory part of the labyrinth.

In the 4- to 6-week period of development the internal auditory artery and anterior inferior cerebellar artery extend laterally from the basilar artery; as they are connected by a vessel running parallel to the basilar artery,

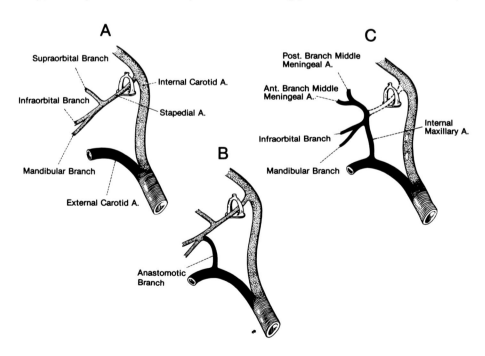

FIG. 9.14: These drawings show in sequence the developmental changes in the stapedial artery in human embryos of 6 weeks (A), 7 weeks (B), and 7+ weeks (C). (After Altmann, 1947; Davies, 1967.)

a vascular ring is formed around the abducens nerve. Atrophy of part of this ring determines the origin of the internal auditory artery with respect to the anterior inferior cerebellar artery (Fig. 9.15). If the lateral aspect of the ring degenerates, the internal auditory artery and anterior inferior cerebellar artery arise separately from the basilar artery; however, if the cranial aspect of the ring is interrupted, the internal auditory artery develops as a branch of the anterior inferior cerebellar artery.

In the 7-week embryo the stapedial artery through its supraorbital division is the primary blood supply to the orbit (except the globe); this division branches into supraorbital, frontal, anterior ethmoid, and lacrimal arteries. An anastomosis now begins to develop between the supraorbital division of the stapedial artery and the primitive ophthalmic artery; this anastomosis forms proximal to the division of the ophthalmic artery into its three optic branches and dorsal to the optic nerve. Meanwhile, an anastomotic linkage forms between the external carotid artery and the maxillomandibular branch of the stapedial artery which will give rise to the internal maxillary artery and middle meningeal arteries, as well as the inferior alveolar and infraorbital arteries. The stem of the stapedial artery, located between the internal carotid artery and the origin of the supraorbital division, undergoes atrophy and the external carotid artery system takes over the area previously supplied by the supraorbital and maxillomandibular divisions of the stapedial artery. Tandler (1898) suggested that the anterior tympanic artery, a branch of the internal maxillary artery, represents the remains of the withered stem of the stapedial artery. Altmann (1947) proposed that the superior petrosal artery is another remnant of the stem of the stapedial artery.

By the end of the 8th week, the subarcuate artery develops as a branch of either the internal auditory artery or the anterior inferior cerebellar artery and supplies part of the developing mastoid and labyrinthine capsule. It traverses the subarcuate fossa.

The Veins (4 to 8 weeks). In the 5th week the bilaterally symmetrical cardinal system of veins drains into the sinus venosus (the caudal chamber of the heart). The anterior cardinal veins on either side drain caudally from

FIG. 9.15: Two different developmental sequences determine the origin of the labyrinthine artery. If vascular atrophy occurs at point A, it will arise from the anterior inferior cerebellar artery (AICA) or if atrophy occurs at point B, it will arise from the basilar artery. (After Altmann.)

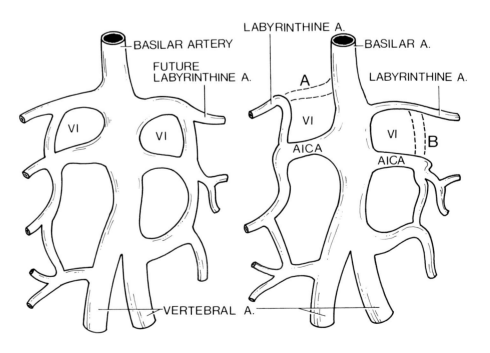

the head and join the posterior cardinal veins carrying blood from the caudal portion of the embryo. This union results in bilaterally symmetrical venous channels known as the ducts of Cuvier or the common cardinal veins which empty into the lateral horns of the sinus venosus. At this stage the anterior cardinal veins penetrate the skull at an opening which will become the jugular foramen. The segment of the anterior cardinal vein superior to this opening contributes to the sigmoid portion of the lateral venous sinus and the segment inferior to the opening becomes the internal jugular vein (Graham, 1977). Meanwhile the primary head sinus assumes a position lateral to the Xth cranial nerve.

Although the stem of the anterior dural plexus disappears, the portion which has an anastomosis with the middle dural sinus forms the transverse sinus. One of its tributaries is the primitive metencephalic vein which later becomes the superior petrosal sinus. The stem of the middle dural plexus persists as the pro-otic sinus. During the 8th week of development a medial extension of the pro-otic sinus joins the myelencephalic vein, forming a plexiform cranial extension known as the inferior petrosal sinus.

Temporal Bone (0 to 8 weeks). The adult temporal bone is made up of five major components, namely the squamous part (squama), the petrous part (petrosa), the tympanic bone, the mastoid process, and the styloid process. However, of these five components, the mastoid and styloid processes do not fully develop until after birth. Both the squama and the tympanic bone are products of membranous bone development. The petrous portion is represented by the cartilaginous otic capsule until 20 weeks of gestation at which time ossification proceeds; the styloid process also is preformed in cartilage.

It is not until the 8-week stage that one can first discern development of the squama of the temporal bone as commencing from an ossification center which extends into the zygomatic process.

DEVELOPMENT TO 16 WEEKS

The Membranous Labyrinth (8 to 16 weeks). Between 8 and 9 weeks migration of the vertical shelf downward initially brings it into contact with the medial fold (Fig. 9.16), and later it veers laterally to overlap the ridge from the lateral wall. As a result the utricle now connects only indirectly to the saccule through the utricular and saccular ducts. Further migration of the medial horizontal shelf in a ventral direction delineates the saccule from the utriculosaccular duct. The free edge of the dorsal vertically oriented infolding persists as the utriculo-endolymphatic valve of Bast.

Also in this time period, rugosities develop in the proximal portion of the endolymphatic duct. Between 10 and 12 weeks the adult configuration of the membranous labyrinth is completely achieved.

The Cochlear Duct (8 to 16 weeks). Having completed its requisite two and one-half turns by the 8- to 10-week stage, further growth of the cochlear duct occurs in caliber only and is essentially completed by midterm. The caliber of the cochlear duct is less than that of the neighboring scala tympani and scala vestibuli. The osseous spiral lamina stretches from the modiolus between the scalae to the inner margin of the cochlear duct (Figs. 9.44 and 9.51). The original round shape of the cochlear duct (Fig. 9.30) changes to oval by 11 weeks (Fig. 9.44) and to triangular by

FIG. 9.16: Drawing of the developing otic labyrinth in a human embryo at 9 weeks. The progressive deepening of folds I, II, and III transforms the original primitive utricular sac into the adult utricle, saccule, and endolymphatic duct (see Fig. 9.9). This embryologic process mimics that of the phylogenetic development of the otic labyrinth (see p. 236). Fold I gives rise to the utriculo-endolymphatic valve. (After Bast, 1949.)

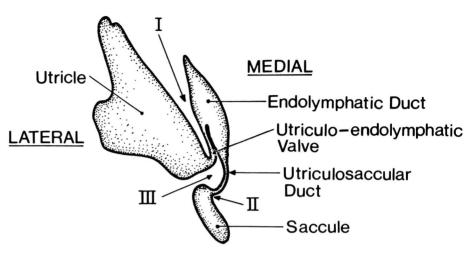

DORSAL

I

Utricle

MEDIAL

LATERAL

Endolymphatic Duct

Utriculo-endolymphatic Valve

Utriculosaccular Duct

III

II

Saccule

VENTRAL

16 weeks (Fig. 9.48). Three walls are thus defined: the anterior wall forms the vestibular (Reissner's) membrane by fusion with the wall of the scala vestibuli, the posterior wall forms the basilar membrane through union with the wall of the scala tympani, and the spiral ligament constitutes the outer wall. In the 11-week fetus, at the region of the future basilar membrane, the stratified epithelium of the cochlear duct flattens into a simple columnar epithelium. Further development results in a pseudostratified mound of cells and a vaguely discernible tectorial membrane along its free edge. By 14 weeks the epithelium of the anterior wall has progressed to a cuboidal architecture. At the basal end of the cochlear duct the epithelium of the future organ of Corti shows swelling and disjunction of the cells at the area of the outer hair cells. In the 16-week fetus the cochlear duct has attained its final triangular configuration (Fig. 9.51). The epithelium of the posterior wall (basilar membrane) continues its differentiation into the organ of Corti and the tectorial membrane. The epithelium of the outer wall undergoes differentiation into the stria vascularis with the spiral ligament acting as a foundation. Meanwhile the cellular differentiation of the organ of Corti spreads apically. The cochlear nerve traverses tissue which will become the osseous spiral lamina, the outer free margin of which acts as an anchor for the inner angle of the cochlear duct (Fig. 9.44).

The Utricle and Saccule (8 to 16 weeks). With further progression of the infoldings of the membranous labyrinth, the vertically oriented fold (Fig. 9.16) forms the utriculo-endolymphatic valve. In the 10- to 12-week stage the maculae show sensory cells with tufted free margins and supporting cells (Fig. 9.44). The now forming otolithic membrane appears as a gelatinous cushion overlying the epithelium of the maculae and is superficially studded with rhombic crystals of calcium carbonate, the otoconia. By the 14- to 16-week stage, the individual components of the maculae are almost fully differentiated to resemble the adult structure, yet the surrounding otic capsule is still largely cartilaginous.

The Semicircular Ducts (8 to 16 weeks). Progressive growth in ductal diameter and arch of curvature occurs throughout this period. The simple squamous epithelium of the cristae, now pseudostratified, progressively differentiates into the sensory hair cell and supporting cell populations of the adult cristae by the 10th to 12th weeks of gestation; the hair cells have cilia at their free margin. By the 15th week, the cristae are sickle-shaped in structure and there is a well-developed cupula in which are embedded the bristle-like projections of the sensory hair cells (Figs. 9.36 and 9.54).

The Otic Capsule (8 to 16 weeks). At 9 weeks the precartilage bordering the developing membranous labyrinth dedifferentiates into loose reticular mesenchyme, permitting growth of the labyrinth (Fig. 9.17). As precartilage dedifferentiates to reticulum, adjacent cartilage dedifferentiates to precartilage in preparation for yet further expansion. On the outer (advancing) aspect of the enlarging semicircular canals, cartilage dedifferentiates to precartilage and precartilage dedifferentiates into a mesenchymal reticulum. On the inner (trailing) edge of the canal, mesenchymal reticulum once more differentiates to precartilage which in turn redifferentiates into cartilage. The formation of the periotic space surrounding the otic labyrinth also involves the dedifferentiation of the immediately adjacent precartilage.

In the first phase of growth of the otic labyrinth, the inner zone of precartilage gradually forms three layers: an inner zone of dense areolar tissue which envelops the epithelium of the otic labyrinth (the membrana propria), a center zone of loose, arachnoid-like tissue which is the fluid-filled (periotic) space, and an outer zone of dense tissue which forms the perichondrium of the otic capsule. The dedifferentiation of precartilage to a reticulum first appears in the tissue between the stapes and utricle. In the second phase, between 9 and 10 weeks, the latticework of the reticulum of the center zone coalesces to form the first periotic space proper. The third and final stage begins with formation of perichondrium in the 12th week and proceeds to the beginning of ossification of the cartilage surrounding the membranous labyrinth by the 16th week (Figs. 9.46 and 9.51). Despite the small size of the otic capsule, ossification involves 14 centers which

FIG. 9.17: The semicircular canals undergo growth in the arc of curvature and in cross-sectional diameter. (After Pearson, 1984.)

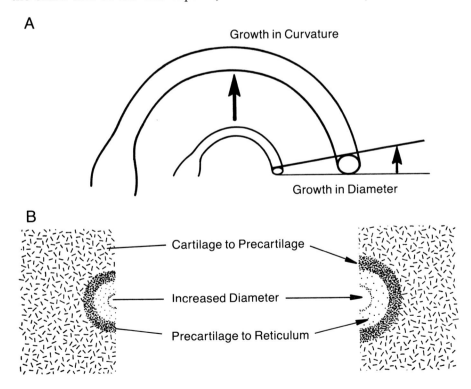

A

Growth in Curvature

Growth in Diameter

B

Cartilage to Precartilage

Increased Diameter

Precartilage to Reticulum

appear in succession and enlarge to fuse with other centers (see p. 271). The first such ossification center appears at approximately 16 weeks on the outer aspect of the capsule at the origin of the basal turn of the cochlea. Ossification is completed only shortly before birth.

The Perilymphatic Space (8 to 16 weeks). Vacuole formation in the reticulum (periotic mesenchyme) is the next step in the hollowing-out of space for the perilymphatic system. By the 10th week this process is relatively advanced, especially at the lateral region of the saccule and utricle, resulting in a mesothelially lined cavity separating the saccule and adjacent utricle from the stapedial footplate (Fig. 9.40). The periotic tissue immediately begins to develop fibers for the support of the saccular and utricular walls and their vascular and neural supply. The development of the periotic spaces in the canalicular region lags behind. By the 12th week the primitive reticulum surrounding the cochlear duct and nascent spiral lamina is extensively vacuolized with the interfibrillar spaces coalescing to form the scalae. However, the first periotic space to clearly develop is the perilymphatic cistern of the vestibule, adjacent to the oval window; this step occurs by late in the 12th week. The scala tympani differentiates soon thereafter in the region of the round window with the scala vestibuli forming slightly later as an outpouching of the perilymphatic cistern near the oval window (the area of the basal coil of the cochlea). The central boundaries of the developing scalae are smooth, but their peripheries are irregular, growing to keep up with the overall expansion of the cochlea. The osseous spiral lamina develops as membrane bone within the connective tissue between the periotic scala tympani and scala vestibuli, lengthening to meet the separately formed modiolus (also membrane bone). By 16 weeks the primordial reticulum surrounding the canalicular part of the periotic labyrinth also becomes highly vacuolated. At this same stage fibrils appear within the reticulum to support the passage of blood vessels and nerves entering from the internal auditory canal.

The Capsular Channels (8 to 16 weeks). By the 9th week the inferior cochlear vein (vein at the cochlear aqueduct) becomes apparent in the cochlear aqueductal syncytium. Also, a cartilaginous bar begins to stretch from the area of the round window niche and ampulla of the posterior canal toward the gap of the cochlear aqueduct which eventually forms the floor and medial rim of the round window.

The Fissula Ante Fenestram (0 to 16 weeks). In the 9th week the fissula ante fenestram is first noticed as a strip of precartilage in the lateral wall of the still cartilaginous otic capsule. Gradually it enlarges and by the 14-week stage its mesenchyme which consists of perilymphatic connective tissue is in continuity with the connective tissue of the middle ear, the stapediovestibular joint, and the vestibule. The fissula ante fenestram connects the inner and middle ear spaces as it traverses the bony partition of the otic capsule. Vascular channels enter the fissula from the middle ear.

The Fossula Post Fenestram (0 to 16 weeks). The fossula post fenestram is an evagination of vestibular periotic tissue into the lateral wall of the otic capsule at the posterior aspect of the oval window. The fossula develops in about two-thirds of embryos and usually is without a communication to the middle ear.

The Facial Nerve (8 to 16 weeks). In the 8th week a branch of the facial nerve to the stapedius muscle is evident as the stapedius muscle becomes distinctly separated from the facial nerve (Figs. 9.30 and 9.31).

Between 12 and 13 weeks the nervus intermedius develops communications with the motor root of the facial nerve and the cochlear nerve. Originating from the dorsomedial aspect of the facial nerve are two branches which fuse and then connect with the superior ganglia of the vagus and glossopharyngeal nerves; this connection results in a nerve which passes through the primitive tympanomastoid fissure to innervate the subcutaneous tissue of the external auditory canal (Gasser, 1967). By the 15th week the geniculate ganglion is developed to the form present at birth.

The External Auditory Canal, Tympanic Membrane, and Tympanic Ring (8 to 16 weeks). During the 9th week, a solid cord of epithelial cells called the meatal plate or plug, which represents an ingrowth from the fundus of the primitive external auditory canal, extends toward the lower wall of the tympanic cavity (Fig. 9.13); at its terminus this ectodermal plate forms a disc-like swelling (Altmann, 1950). The mesenchyme between the meatal plate and the epithelial cells of the tympanic cavity forms the fibrous layer of the lamina propria of the tympanic membrane. The inner mucosal layer of the tympanic membrane is derived from the endodermal tissue of the tympanic cavity (the tubotympanic recess). The first of four small ossification centers of the membrane bone of the tympanic ring appears at approximately 9 weeks. There is continued expansion of the solid external auditory canal with cranial growth until approximately the 12th week, at which point the bony tympanic ring has formed at the periphery of the tympanic membrane. Once the four ossification centers have fused, there is rapid growth so that the tympanic ring is almost fully developed by the 16th week. A fault known as the notch of Rivinus remains at the superior cranial aspect of the ring. While the tympanic membrane elsewhere inserts into a sulcus in the tympanic ring, superior to the notch of Rivinus it attaches directly to the petrous bone.

The Tympanomastoid Compartment (8 to 16 weeks). The tympanic cavity gradually expands so that by the 12th week it extends over the medial surface of the inferior two-thirds of the tympanic membrane as well as the lateral wall of the middle ear. Dissolution of the mesenchyme of the middle ear progresses to eventually reach the epitympanic recess. With the differentiation of the ossicles and their associated muscles, there is dissolution of much residual mesenchyme, facilitating the expansion of the tympanic cavity. In the process the middle ear structures become ensheathed in a lining mucosa similar to the development of the abdominal visceral peritoneum.

By 16 weeks, growth of the tympanic process of the squamous part of the temporal bone has defined the anterior wall of the epitympanic cavity and contributed to the lateral wall of the tympanic cavity proper. A major component of the floor of the middle ear is formed by a bony lamella developing either as an offshoot from the petrous pyramid or as a separate bone between the pyramid and tympanic ring. The tympanic membrane and the osseous tympanic ring determine the lateral boundary of the middle ear.

Frazer (cited by Proctor, 1969) suggests an alternative concept as to the origin of the middle ear cavity. Frazer's scheme involves forward growth of the third branchial arch to form the primitive tympanic cavity. The third arch then contacts the first arch at the anterior wall of the recess which results in the formation of the anterior and medial walls of the tympanic cavity. In this concept the second branchial arch and second branchial groove form the floor of the tympanic cavity.

The Malleus and Incus (8 to 16 weeks). Between the 8th and 10th weeks the ossicles and Meckel's cartilage keep pace with overall embryonic growth, dwarfing the anterior malleal process which grows more slowly. These progressive and prodigious ossicular growths occur as cartilaginous models until approximately the 15th week of gestation, at which point maximal chondral size is attained and the adult morphology is fully manifest (Fig. 9.49). The incus initiates the ossification process at this time, being the first to lay down a thin layer of perichondrial bone. This first ossification center is located on the anterior surface of its long process and extends up the body of the incus. Soon thereafter the malleus shows its first signs of ossification—vacuolization of cartilage in the area of continuity with Meckel's cartilage. Bone formation in the malleus begins during the 16th week with the development of a plaque of perichondrial bone on the medial aspect of the neck of the malleus. Meanwhile, a complete perichondrial bony shell forms around the long process of the incus and vascular buds enter the calcifying cartilage. In both the malleus and incus, ossification progresses through the formation of perichondrial, endochondral, and intrachondral bone. Meckel's cartilage, although it continues to grow in size, shows early signs of degeneration on its surface which results in the formation of the anterior ligament of the malleus.

The Stapes (8 to 16 weeks). In the 9-week fetus a condensation of tissue has formed in the mesenchyme at the interhyale—the future stapedius muscle (Fig. 9.18). The tendon of the stapedius muscle is derived from the remainder of the interhyale, which maintains its connection with the head of the stapes. The laterohyale fuses to the otic capsule and participates in the development of the anterior wall of the facial nerve canal as well as the bone of the stapedial pyramid (pyramidal eminence). That portion of the anterior wall of the facial nerve canal which lies distal to the laterohyale is formed by Reichert's cartilage. However, in later development, intramembranous ossification forms a wall separating Reichert's cartilage from the contents of the facial nerve canal, which terminates its brief role in the structure of the facial canal wall (Bast et al., 1956). By the 9th week the

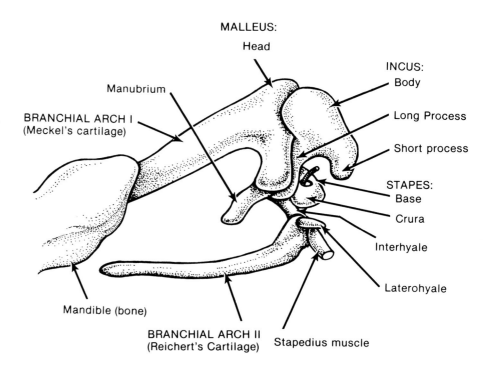

FIG. 9.18: This is a left lateral view of the derivation of the ossicles from their respective branchial arches at 8 to 9 weeks. The malleus is still in continuity with Meckel's cartilage. The interhyale, which develops from Reichert's cartilage, attaches to the stapes at the region of the incudostapedial articulation and establishes the site of the insertion of the stapedius tendon. An aggregation of cells adjacent to the medial and proximal aspect of Reichert's cartilage gives rise to the stapedius muscle. (After Hanson et al., 1962.)

MALLEUS:
Head

INCUS:
Body

Manubrium

Long Process

BRANCHIAL ARCH I
(Meckel's cartilage)

Short process

STAPES:
Base

Crura

Interhyale

Laterohyale

Mandible (bone)

BRANCHIAL ARCH II
(Reichert's Cartilage)   Stapedius muscle

stapes, like the malleus and incus (Fig. 9.41), is composed of cartilage and continued growth as a cartilaginous model occurs until approximately 15 weeks of gestation. Beginning in the 16th week, histologic differentiation and separation of the stapes from the otic capsule becomes apparent with an oval-shaped zone indicating the future annular ligament. Blood vessels appear in this region, coursing from the primordial facial nerve canal to both the footplate and the head of the stapes. In some specimens the first stapedial ossification center may be seen, although this does not usually occur until nearly the 18th week.

The Ossicular Muscles (0 to 16 weeks). The tensor tympani muscle is a derivative of the first branchial arch and therefore is innervated by the trigeminal (Vth cranial) nerve. The stapedius muscle is a derivative of the second branchial arch and is innervated by the facial (VIIth cranial) nerve. In the 8th week the primordial tensor tympani muscle is seen in the mesenchyme destined to become submucosal connective tissue lateral to the cochlea and the stapedius muscle has developed from tissue of the interhyale.

The Arteries (8 to 16 weeks). By the 10th week the site of origin of most of the vascular supply to the inner as well as external ear is readily discernible. The occipital artery branches into the posterior auricular branch and the stylomastoid artery, while it also supplies the endolymphatic sac. The inferior tympanic artery is recognizable as a branch of the ascending pharyngeal artery, as are the deep auricular and anterior tympanic arteries.

The Veins (8 to 16 weeks). In the 10-week fetus both the inferior petrosal sinus and the cavernous sinus are well developed. The superior petrosal sinus into which the internal auditory veins of the internal auditory canal drain is the last of the dural sinuses to appear. It is usually not until postnatal stages that its drainage into the cavernous sinus is established. By the 12th week the terminal segment of the superior petrosal sinus has evolved from the persisting proximal portion of the pro-otic sinus.

The Temporal Bone (8 to 16 weeks). The tympanic part of the temporal bone begins its development at about 9 to 10 weeks of gestation.

In the 9th week the squama and zygomatic process begin membrane bone formation. By the end of the 9th week, the superior wall of the middle ear emerges as a projection of the otic capsule; it is known as the superior periotic process. It grows forward over the ossicles forming the lateral aspect of the tegmen tympani. The medial part of the tegmen tympani consists of a fibrous tissue plate.

DEVELOPMENT AFTER 16 WEEKS

By the 20th week the membranous labyrinth is of maximum size and is housed within a bony capsule. By 25 weeks the inner ear displays an essentially adult configuration.

The Cochlear Duct (16+ weeks). During the 16th to 20th weeks the organ of Corti differentiates into its cellular components. At this time the inner ear has attained maximum size and the otic capsule forms a bony shell. Beginning at approximately the 19th week, the vascular supply of the cochlea is established by branches of the labyrinthine artery. The vessels pass through the cochlear modiolus, osseous spiral lamina, and walls of the scalae to form an end-vessel complex without anastomotic arborization.

FIG. 9.19: The inferior cochlear vein empties into the inferior petrosal sinus. The developing stapedius muscle is in close proximity to the stapes. The outlined area is enlarged in Figure 9.20 (fetus, age 17 weeks).

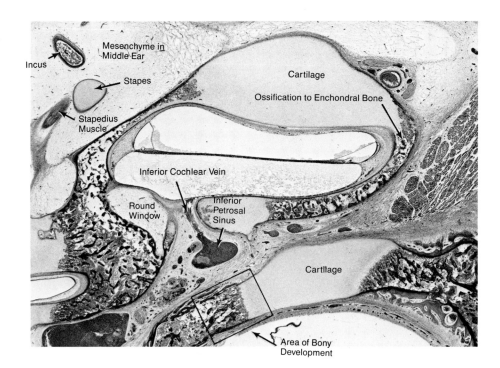

The blood supply of the membranous labyrinth remains discrete from that of the otic capsule, for although branches from the tympanic plexus penetrate the outer periosteal layer of the otic capsule, they do not pass through the inner periosteal layer. The stria vascularis is fully developed by the 20th week of gestation and the tunnel of Corti is present in all turns by the 21st week. By the 22nd week the inner and outer ridges of the primordial organ of Corti have differentiated from base to apex into recognizable inner and outer sensory cells, pillar cells, and cells of Hensen. Developing peripheral nerve fibers of the spiral ganglion have reached the sensory hair cells. In a scanning electron microscopic study of the development of the organ of Corti in fetuses between 18 and 20 weeks of gestation, Tanaka

FIG. 9.20: This higher power magnification of the outlined area in Figure 9.19 shows endochondral (enchondral) bone formation. Proceeding from right to left, notice that the cartilage cells sequentially multiply, hypertrophy, and undergo calcification; their lacunae are invaded by osteoblasts which lay down bone. Islands of cartilage that are not removed are known as globuli interossei or intrachondrial bone (fetus, age 17 weeks).

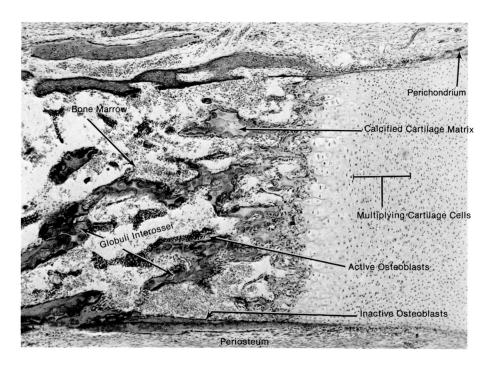

et al. (1979) found that afferent nerve endings were formed earlier than efferent ones. This observation suggests that the differentiation of the sensory cells of the organ of Corti is independent of efferent innervation. Deiters' cells with their tonofibril-rich cytoplasm also develop at this time. In the 24-week fetus a cellular reorganization occurs in the spiral limbus at the region of the insertion of the tectorial membrane; this reorganization accentuates an existing groove at the inner margin of the organ of Corti, the inner tunnel or inner spiral sulcus. The inner and outer pillar cells soon develop with their supportive tonofibrils. Cellular resorption is the mechanism of formation for both the outer tunnel and the space between the inner hair cells and outer hair cells. Gradual widening of the spaces between the outer phalangeal cells (so-called because of their resemblance to the bony phalanges of the hand) and the outer hair cells results in the formation of the spaces of Nuel.

The Semicircular Ducts (16+ weeks). The superior semicircular duct reaches its adult size by approximately 20 weeks of gestation. The posterior and then the lateral semicircular ducts follow closely in accordance with the order in which they were first created phylogenetically. Having already attained nearly adult structure, the cristae are fully developed at this time (Fig. 9.62).

The Endolymphatic Duct (16+ weeks). Originally a straight, tubal structure, by midterm the endolymphatic duct bends in a caudal direction. The endolymphatic duct originates from the junction of the saccular and utricular ducts and runs in the vestibular aqueduct parallel to the posteromedial aspect of the common crus. Its distal termination, the endolymphatic sac, shows its adult relationships as it lies adjacent to the lateral aspect of the sigmoid sinus into which its accompanying venous plexus empties. The endolymphatic sac is exceptional in that it continues to grow as the posterior cranial fossa expands; it may triple or even quadruple the size it was at midterm.

The Otic Capsule (16+ weeks). The ossification process of both the canalicular and cochlear regions of the otic capsule intensifies when the membranous labyrinth achieves full adult size. Between 16 and 20 weeks the cochlear part of the otic capsule completes growth. Even as early as the end of 16 weeks in some specimens, there may be fusion of the first three ossification centers superior to the round window (see p. 272). At this time successive ossification centers appear, 14 in all. Each ossification center, and the otic capsule as a whole, is trilaminar in structure. The external and internal periosteal layers are derived from the external and internal perichondrial membranes, respectively. They undergo transformation to periosteum with the deposition of calcareous material by osteoblasts and vascular bud invasion (Figs. 9.19 and 9.20). These layers develop Haversian systems exactly as in long bones elsewhere in the body. The intrachondrial (middle) layer is composed of both intrachondrial and endochondral bone. Intrachondrial bone represents persistent islands of calcified hyaline cartilage which house osteocytes in the originally cartilaginous lacunae and is the foundation upon which deposition of endochondral bone takes place. The initial step of the ossification process entails the invasion of chondral tissue by osteogenic buds which causes devitalization of the calcified cartilage. Vascular buds remove much of the calcified cartilage and the spaces created are soon occupied by bone. By 21 weeks the remaining islands of calcified cartilage become populated by osteoblasts to form intrachondral bone. On the outer surfaces of such islands osteoblasts deposit enchondral bone. Meanwhile, the modiolus begins to develop as membrane bone at the 20th to 21st week (Fig. 9.51). By the 21st week the final ossification center has appeared and fusion begins. There is no epiphyseal growth between the centers which fuse directly. Ossification lags in the canalicular region, allowing for continued growth of the semicircular ducts which is nearly completed by 24 weeks. The cartilage surrounding the semicircular canals then undergoes invasion and resorption by vascular buds from the vessels coursing beneath the arch of the superior semicircular canal in the subarcuate fossa. This process is soon followed by retreat of the vascular buds and trilaminar ossification similar to that seen in the cochlear region. The outer periosteal layer expands by internal and external lamellar bony deposition and in the central layer endochondral bone is laid down on the spicules of intrachondrial bone.

The modiolus is the central conical support for the coils of the cochlear canal and is unique in the otic capsule for its formation as membranous bone. Although its ossification is independent of the remainder of the otic capsule, it is attached to the outer cochlear wall by interscalar septa. It is traversed by the longitudinal and spiral modiolar canals which transmit both vessels and nerves. Beginning about the 23rd week the spiral lamina ossifies in the basal turn of the cochlea. By the 25th week the modiolus has become nearly completely ossified and the interscalar septa secure it to the cochlear wall. By 26 weeks the deposition of endochondral bone on the bars of intrachondrial bone diminishes the intervening marrow spaces to scattered, tiny vascular channels (somewhat like Volkmann's canals). This process accelerates to completion just before birth. Once formed, there is no further remodeling in either the intrachondrial or endochondral bone layers.

Several unique features in the development of the otic capsule deserve emphasis (Austin, 1977): 1) rapidity of growth, occurring primarily in the 15- to 21-week stages, 2) large number of ossification centers (14) despite the small size of the otic capsule, 3) fusion of ossification centers without intervening epiphyseal bone, 4) trilaminar histologic architecture of the otic capsule, 5) persistence of fetal architecture in the periosteal and endochondral bone areas without remodeling, and 6) independent appearance and ossification of each of the separate ossification centers and of each of the layers of their trilaminar structure.

The Perilymphatic Spaces (16+ weeks). Development of the perilymphatic space in the semicircular canal region lags behind that of the vestibule and cochlear scalae. The perilymphatic space of the semicircular canals achieves communication with the perilymphatic cistern of the vestibule by the 17th week (Fig. 9.48) and full development of the space is achieved by the 20th week. The final thinning of reticulum leaves an uninterrupted space, except for scattered trabeculae which stretch between the membranous labyrinth and the periosteum to provide support and conduits for vascular supply.

The Capsular Channels (16+ weeks). The term "cochlear aqueduct" refers to the channel in the otic capsule whereas the term "periotic duct" refers to its enclosed membranous duct which provides communication between the perilymphatic and subarachnoid spaces.

According to Spector et al. (1980), the primitive cochlear aqueduct in the 16- to 18-week embryo contains three structures: the tympanomeningeal fissure, the periotic duct, and the inferior cochlear vein. Their analysis of the 16- to 40-week period of development of these structures included four developmental stages: 1) at 20 weeks growth and ossification of the petrous apex relegates the inferior cochlear vein to a separate compartment (canal of Cotugno), 2) at 24 weeks the promontory and rim of the round window fuse with the capsule of the semicircular canals, obliterating the tympanomeningeal fissure (Figs. 5.9 and 5.10), 3) at 32 weeks progressive elongation of the cochlear aqueduct and its contained periotic duct occurs by a process of bone deposition on the medial aspect of the otic capsule at the petrous apex, and 4) by the 40th week arachnoid tissue has grown into the cochlear aqueduct to form a lining membrane and meshwork.

Between 32 and 40 weeks of gestation there is widening of the cranial opening of the cochlear aqueduct and periotic duct which completes the development of these structures.

The Facial Nerve (16+ weeks).   By the 17th week of gestation all of the neural connections of the facial nerve have been established.

The Facial Canal (8 to 16+ weeks).   The geniculate ganglion area of the canal is ossified partially in the membranous bone of the middle fossa plate and the squama of the temporal bone. In the 26-week fetus, as progressive ossification of the otic capsule takes place, a preliminary sulcus is gradually transformed into a true facial canal. Growth of periosteal bone is completed at the deep surface of the facial canal while the anterior superficial surface still is only partially closed. At 35 weeks the geniculate ganglion lies upon a bony plate which separates it from the epitympanum. Bone formation progresses along with continued morphogenesis of the contained structures so that the facial canal at full-term closely approximates that of the adult. The facial canal does not completely close at its cranial surface (facial hiatus) so that the perineural tissue of the geniculate ganglion maintains direct contact with the dura, a condition which may persist into adulthood.

The Pinna (16+ weeks).   The pinna (auricle) has attained adult configuration by the 20th week of gestation (growth continues, however, to age 9 years) (Fig. 9.21). First evident in about the 25th week of development is a tubercle occasionally appearing on the free margin of the helix known as

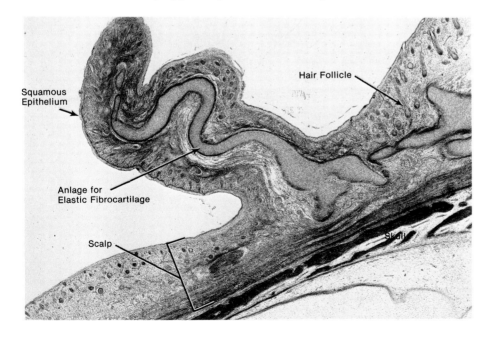

Squamous
Epithelium

Hair Follicle

Anlage for
Elastic Fibrocartilage

Scalp

Skull

FIG. 9.21: The developing pinna and scalp are shown. Skin appendages are present. The auricular cartilage is in an early stage of differentiation (fetus, age 17 weeks).

the Darwinian tubercle; this structure is the homologue of the tip of the auricle in lower mammals. The six extrinsic and three intrinsic muscles of the auricle develop from the mesoderm of the hyoid arch and, like other facial muscles, they are innervated by the VIIth cranial nerve.

The External Auditory Canal, Tympanic Membrane, and Tympanic Ring (16+ weeks). At approximately the 21st week the solid meatal plate begins to form a lumen beginning in its deepest portion. By the 28th week a canal is formed by disintegration of the central cells of the ectodermal plate. The remaining cells establish the epithelial lining of the bony external auditory canal. The ectodermal plate becomes the inner bony part of the external auditory canal; the most medial part of the plate also forms the superficial layer of the tympanic membrane. At approximately the 34th week the tympanic ring becomes fixed to the otic capsule commencing at its posterior aspect. The walls of the outer cartilaginous part of the meatus are formed by an extension of auricular cartilage; slit-like defects (fissures of Santorini) are present in that portion of the cartilage adjacent to the parotid gland and are of importance as channels of communication between the parotid gland and the external auditory canal. A gap between the bony and cartilaginous canals in their anterosuperior aspect is bridged by a fibrous membrane. Fusion of the tympanic ring to the otic capsule is not complete until birth. Up to 3 years after birth, progressive bone formation occurs in the remaining fibrous portion of the plate resulting in complete ossification of both the anterior and inferior walls of the external auditory canal. The superior wall of the external auditory canal is formed solely by the horizontal plate of the temporal squama while the floor grows in from the tympanic ring during early postnatal life. During early life, the tympanic membrane lies superficially in a nearly horizontal plane compared to the adult angulation of 50° to 60° from the horizontal plane. The tympanic ring also contributes to the formation of the mandibular fossa and the sheath of the styloid process. Atresia or stenosis of the external auditory canal is caused by failure of development of the first branchial groove, either from lack of epithelial ingrowth or failure of canalization of the meatal plate.

The Tympanomastoid Compartment (16+ weeks). During the period of 16 to 20 weeks of gestation the eustachian tube lengthens and areas of chondrification arise in the surrounding mesoderm to form the fibrocartilaginous part of the eustachian tube (Fig. 9.22).

At 21 weeks lateral growth of the loose connective tissue of the epitympanic recess marks the future antrum. As early as 24 weeks there is air cell formation in the petrous pyramid (apical cells) shortly after ossification of the otic capsule. Other air cell groups that form at about the same time are the pericarotid and peritubal cells, supracochlear cells (anterosuperior to the geniculate ganglion), and those of the wall of the tympanic cavity.

Ossification begins in the lateral and medial portions of the tegmen of the middle ear by 23 weeks; it is not complete until nearly the end of gestation.

At 29 weeks the periosteal layer of the otic capsule extends around the loose connective tissue of the antrum and fuses with the tympanic process of the squamous bone to form the mastoid process. By the next week, posteriorly directed evagination of the epitympanic space begins formation of the antrum which is well developed by the 35th week. As early as 33 weeks cavitation extends to the mastoid.

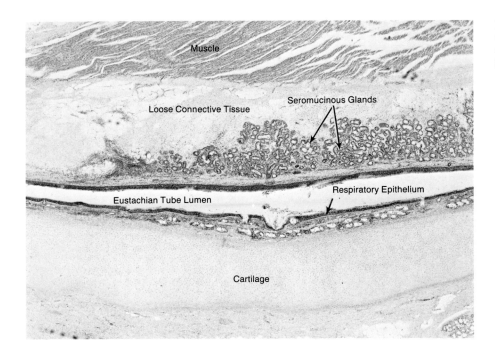

FIG. 9.22: The eustachian tube is patent, lined by respiratory epithelium, and richly supplied with seromucinous glands (male, age 5 months).

By 30 weeks the tympanic cavity has virtually completed its expansion; the epitympanum follows suit approximately 4 weeks later. The antrum of the infant is nearly as large as that of an adult, but the mastoid continues to grow for 5 to 10 years postnatally.

The Malleus and Incus (16+ weeks). By the end of the 17th week the original plaque of perichondrial bone has extended to the lateral aspect of the malleus so that the neck is completely encircled. Cartilaginous vacuolization by lacunar enlargement progresses rapidly beneath the perichondrial shell and endochondral ossification in the interior of the malleus results in areas of calcified cartilage. The center of the malleus is invaded by vascular buds during the next week and the calcifying cartilage is resorbed. The process permits the formation of bone marrow and trabeculae of intrachondrial bone (Fig. 9.49). This casing progressively envelops the head and proximal part of the manubrium during the 19th week and eventually sheaths the entire ossicle, leaving bare only ligamentous attachment sites on the articular surfaces and distal end of the manubrium.

Similarly the perichondrial shell of the incus envelops both the short and long processes. Endochondral bone forms a layer lining the inner surface of the perichondrial shell. Meanwhile, Meckel's cartilage regresses by dedifferentiation of cartilage cells to fibroblasts forming the anterior ligament of the malleus.

By the 20th week the ossicles have assumed their adult configuration. The membrane bone of the anterior process of the malleus fuses with the neck at about the 21st week (Fig. 9.55). Between the 21st and 24th weeks the ossification process extends to the tip of the manubrium by endochondral ossification. Also by endochondral ossification, the marrow cavities of the malleus and incus are gradually obliterated and by 26 weeks begin to undergo the lifelong remodeling process in which areas of bone are resorbed to be replaced by new bone. The degree to which primary bone is replaced by new bone is highly variable and does not seem age-dependent. At this stage, as regression of Meckel's cartilage continues, the only cartilage which remains is found in the area between the tympanic ring and the petrous portion of the temporal bone.

Nearly adult in structure by the 27th week and free from extraneous mesenchyme, the ossicles have become enveloped by mucous membrane which connects each to the walls of the tympanic cavity like the abdominal mesentery. The supporting ligaments and blood supply of the ossicles are located in these folds.

At 28 weeks endosteal bone with the periosteal shell render the ossicles bilaminar in structure. Deposition of endosteal bone occurs rapidly so that the histologic architecture of the malleus and incus in the early postnatal period closely mimics that of the adult (Figs. 9.55 and 9.57).

The Stapes (16+ weeks). Generally, ossification is initiated at the 18-week stage on the tympanic surface of the footplate and spreads to the adjacent surfaces of the crura and finally to the head. The perichondrial "shell" which occurs in the early stages of ossification of the other ossicles is incomplete in the stapes with numerous gaps on the obturator surface. At 20 weeks dissolution of the perichondrial bone and underlying calcified cartilage continues on the obturator surfaces of the crura in association with deposition of endosteal bone on the inner regions of the head and footplate. Endochondral bone forms a thin layer adherent to the permanently cartilaginous lamina stapedialis of the stapes footplate. As the footplate widens, the cartilaginous rim of the oval window dedifferentiates from cartilage to mesenchyme. This cartilage is continuous with that of the vestibular surface of the footplate and that of the fissula ante fenestram (Fig. 9.23). When adult size has been attained, the mesenchyme at the fenestral rim transforms to fibrous tissue to create the annular ligament which encircles the stapedial footplate and anchors it to the rim of the oval window.

During the 32nd week the mucous membrane of the expanding tympanic cavity penetrates the intercrural space as perichondrial bone is resorbed to create the obturator foramen. Unlike long bones which thicken and lengthen with body growth, the stapes loses substance in achieving its adult form and unlike the malleus and incus, the stapes does not enter into the remodeling process—the fetal bone persists throughout life.

Fig. 9.23: This photomicrograph shows the development of the annular ligament of the stapediovestibular articulation which involves the dedifferentiation of cartilage to precartilage and mesenchyme. Mesenchyme is the basis of the fibrous tissue of the adult annular ligament (fetus, near term).

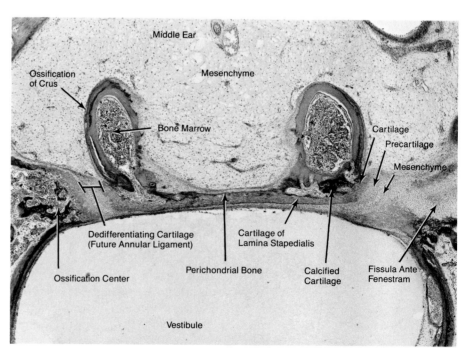

The Ossicular Muscles (16+ weeks). With ossification of the otic capsule, the semicanal of the tensor tympani muscle gradually encases the muscle in a bony shell which remains incompletely formed at term and throughout adult life (Fig. 9.56).

The Veins (16+ weeks). In late fetal life the distal segment of the pro-otic sinus joins the petrosquamous sinus. Even at birth, part or all of the pro-otic sinus may persist. Those segments which do remain are transformed postnatally into diploic channels and the cranial remnant is converted into the lateral wing of the cavernous sinus.

The Temporal Bone (16+ weeks). After 16 weeks, the postauditory process of the squama extends posterior to the tympanic ring forming the anterosuperior portion of the mastoid process. During the 20th to 24th week the petrous bone, composed of the cartilaginous otic capsule, begins rapid ossification from multiple centers (see p. 273). At this point the tympanic cavity and labyrinth have attained full size; however, the temporal bone, especially the mastoid process, continues to grow. At 25 weeks the floor of the middle ear develops, either as an independent bone located between the pyramid and the tympanic ring or as a bony lamellar projection of the petrous pyramid.

By the 29th week the tympanic process of the squama joins the antral segment of the periosteal otic capsule to form the lateral wall of the antrum. At term an ossification center forms at the dorsal aspect of Reichert's cartilage which fuses with the otic capsule to create the styloid eminence in the floor of the tympanic cavity and also part of the distal segment of the bony fallopian canal.

The external petrosquamous fissure demarcates the border between that part of the mastoid derived from the squama and the portion which arises from the petrosa. This fissure is visible in the newborn, but generally disappears by the 2nd year of life.

At birth the mastoid antrum is large with a thin shell of bone. The mastoid process develops as a prominence on the outer aspect of the petrous pyramid during the 1st year of life. As the mastoid grows, the antrum shrinks in relative size and assumes a more medial position, as does the facial nerve. The mastoid, although well developed by three years of age, does not achieve adult configuration for several more years.

Postnatally, the styloid process forms as an ossification center in the upper portion of Reichert's cartilage; concurrently, at its ventral aspect another ossification center appears which will become the lesser horn of the hyoid and the superior part of the body of the hyoid. The stylohyoid ligament represents the atrophied remnant of the intervening stylohyale. The fusion of the separate components of the temporal bone then becomes the major process in its further development.

Ossification

THE GENESIS AND GROWTH OF BONE

Bone is a connective tissue, the intercellular matrix of which becomes modified through the deposition of calcareous material. Two types of bone development are recognized, depending upon the type of connective tissue in which it occurs; intramembranous ossification occurs in mesenchyme and intracartilaginous ossification in a previously established cartilaginous model.

Intramembranous ossification is a method by which the flat bones of the skull, the clavicle, and the mandible ossify. The first step consists of mesenchymal condensation and increase in vascularity in the region where bone development is to occur. Certain cells of the connective tissue differentiate into osteoblasts and lay down osteoid, a blend of collagenous fibers and homogeneous matrix. Upon calcification, the osteoid becomes bone. Initially osteoblasts form a lining membrane on the surface of this bone, the osteogenic layer; it is at the inner surface of this layer that calcareous deposition occurs. Some of the cells of this osteogenic or cambium layer become trapped by the bony matrix, later to be recognized as osteocytes which occupy lacunae. The remainder of the osteogenic layer moves from the epicenter with the deposition of each successive layer of bone. The bone formed is insinuated between the vascular channels of the parent mesenchyme and consists of spicules of bone traversed by multiple blood vessels with their perivascular tissues. This bone is extant but a short time, for with growth of the individual, membrane bones also must shift and grow by selective resorption and deposition of bone.

There are three types of intracartilaginous bone: 1) perichondrial, 2) enchondral (synonomous with endochondral), and 3) intrachondral. The first two types are found in the majority of the long bones of the skeleton; however, intrachondrial bone is unique to the otic capsule and ossicles. Intracartilaginous bone formation differs from intramembranous bone formation in that it occurs in a pre-existing model of embryonic hyaline cartilage.

In the initial steps of enchondral bone development, the embryonic mesenchyme differentiates first into precartilage and then into a true hyaline cartilage model which mimics the final adult configuration. Growth in size, as exemplified in the ossicles and otic capsule, takes place primarily in such cartilage models; only after they attain adult size does ossification commence. The cartilage cells hypertrophy and calcareous salts are deposited on their intracellular matrix forming calcified cartilage.

At the same time the connective tissue (perichondrium) which surrounds the cartilaginous model gradually blends with the cartilage cells of the chondral layer. As ossification begins, the deep layer of the perichondrium differentiates into a layer of osteoblasts that deposit perichondrial bone on the subjacent ossifying cartilage. With the appearance of the perichondrial bone, the perichondrium is then more properly referred to as periosteum. The periosteal bone envelops the ossifying otic capsule.

At the time that perichondrial bone is being formed, highly cellular and vascular osteogenic buds enter the otic capsule to gain access to the cartilage lacunae which they enlarge and from which they remove the cartilage cells. Some of the cells of the osteogenic bud differentiate into osteoblasts which lay down bone in the enlarged cartilage lacunae. They remove some, but not all, of the calcified cartilage. The islands of calcified cartilage that remain are referred to as intrachondrial bone (cartilage islands, globuli interossei).

Osteoblasts form an enveloping membrane around the islands of calcified cartilage and deposit a bone known as enchondral or replacement bone.

The thin layer of periosteal bone that forms on the inner surface of the otic capsule is commonly known as the endosteal layer of bone. It develops after the cartilaginous otic capsule has been largely replaced by the osteogenic buds and intrachondrial bone has formed.

OSSIFICATION OF THE OTIC CAPSULE

There are 14 centers of ossification of the otic capsule which comprises the petrous portion of the temporal bone. According to Bast (1930), ossification centers arise in relation to nerve terminations, the internal auditory canal, and the semicircular canals; moreover, "ossification of a particular region of the otic capsule begins only after the part of the inner ear which it envelops has attained maximum size" (Bast, 1930). Initially, calcification of cartilage occurs, then osteogenic buds with their rich vascular supply invade the future ossification centers. The first three ossification centers appear at approximately 15 weeks' gestation (Fig. 9.24).

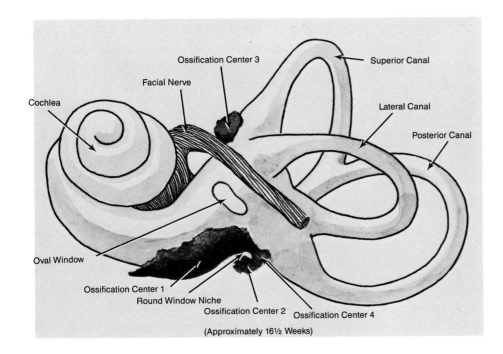

FIG. 9.24: Drawing showing ossification of the otic capsule at 16-1/2 weeks. (After Anson & Donaldson, 1981.)

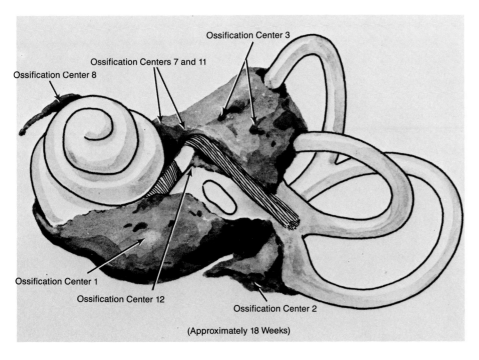

FIG. 9.25: Drawing showing ossification of the otic capsule at 18 weeks. (After Anson & Donaldson, 1981.)

FIG. 9.26: Drawing showing ossification of the otic capsule at 21 weeks. (After Anson & Donaldson, 1981.)

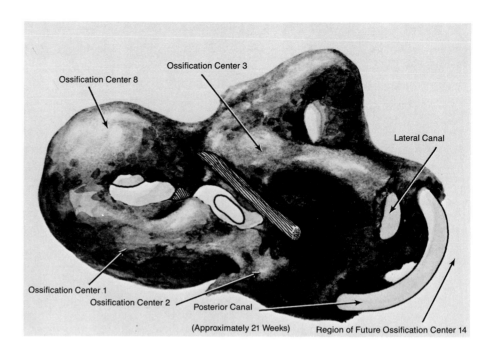

Ossification Center 3

Ossification Center 8

Lateral Canal

Ossification Center 1

Ossification Center 2

Posterior Canal

(Approximately 21 Weeks)

Region of Future Ossification Center 14

The first center appears at the outer aspect of the otic capsule as the basal turn of the cochlear duct sweeps over the round window. This center later joins with the eighth ossification center. The second center also appears on the outer aspect of the otic capsule inferior to the entrance of the posterior ampullary nerve to its crista. This center may appear concurrently with the first or may lag behind it. The third center also develops on the outer aspect of the otic capsule at the entrance of the superior division of the vestibular nerve. This center progressively enlarges, and by late in the 18th week practically encircles the VIIth cranial nerve, forming the initial facial canal.

The fourth center generally appears at about 16 weeks (Fig. 9.24). Located superior to the round window, it serves to connect the first and second centers. The fifth through the tenth ossification centers all begin to form at about 17 weeks. The fifth center appears on the outer aspect of the otic capsule as well as on the lateral wall of the internal auditory canal. It not only forms part of the roof of the internal auditory canal, but also fuses with the posterior aspect of the third center, completing a bony arch over the vestibular nerve. The sixth center is formed on the inner aspect of the otic capsule superior to the entry of the cochlear nerve branches to the cochlea; it also shields the cochlear nerve as it enters the superomedial aspect of the basal turn. This center also contributes in part to the medial wall of the internal auditory canal. The seventh center appears in the upper medial wall of the internal auditory canal in the outer part of the otic capsule. As this center fuses with the fifth center, the roof of the internal auditory canal is completed. Fusion with the sixth center completes the superomedial wall of the internal auditory canal. Thus, the fifth, sixth, and seventh centers all contribute to the formation of the bony walls of the internal auditory canal. The eighth center develops nearly concomitantly with the seventh center on the outer aspect of the otic capsule (Fig. 9.25).

Towards the end of the 17th week the ninth and tenth centers appear in close succession. The ninth center is situated at the outer aspect of the otic capsule at the inferomedial rim of the internal auditory canal. The tenth center develops at the posterior curve of the superior semicircular canal. The eleventh, twelfth, and thirteenth centers appear at 18 weeks in close proximity and therefore may not always arise as separate centers. The eleventh center develops in that portion of the otic capsule which lies superolateral to the cochlea, while the twelfth center arises between the cochlea and the superior division of the vestibular nerve. The thirteenth center appears just inferior to the twelfth center and, with an inferior extension, partly surrounds the vestibular nerve. Eventually fusion occurs with the second center.

The fourteenth and final ossification center appears at 20 to 21 weeks on the outer aspect of the otic capsule (Fig. 9.26), overlying a portion of the posterolateral part of the posterior semicircular canal. With the appearance of this center the ossification of the otic capsule is completed, save for the area of the fissula ante fenestram and an area covering the posterior and lateral semicircular canals. This latter area allows for the continuing growth of the canals and eventually ossifies to form the lateral aspect of the superior semicircular canal only when growth is completed at about 23 weeks. The area of the fissula ante fenestram usually starts its ossification in the 22nd or 23rd week.

Serial Embryologic Sections

The following photomicrographs (Figs. 9.27 to 9.62) show four developmental stages of the human ear. The first three series are from fetuses of approximately 8 weeks, 12 weeks, and 16 weeks of gestation, respectively. The ages of the fetal specimens were determined by crown-rump length correlated with gestational ages. These figures are compiled from averages and serve as approximations; therefore there may be individual variations. The fourth series is from an infant of approximately 5 months of age with retarded postnatal development caused by cerebrohepatorenal (Zellweger's) syndrome.

The first photomicrograph in each of the fetal series is a cranial overview, placing the ear into perspective with the rest of the head. Then five horizontal serial sections of the temporal bone are presented, progressing from superior to inferior levels. To the extent possible sections are presented at comparable levels. The higher power photomicrographs show in sequence the cochleae, utricles and saccules, and cristae ampullares.

FETUS A (8 WEEKS)

FIG. 9.27: Fetus A (8 weeks). This photomicrograph is an overview of a horizontal section of the head. The outlined area indicates the regions shown in Figures 9.28 to 9.32 passing sequentially from superior to inferior.

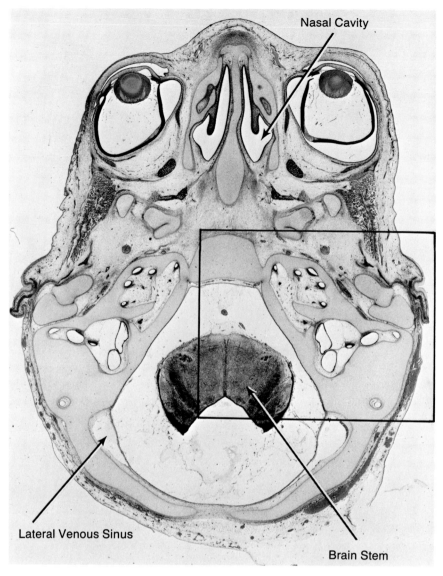

FIG. 9.28: Fetus A (8 weeks). The future middle ear cavity contains mesenchyme. The facial and vestibular nerves are seen passing from the brain stem to the internal auditory canal.

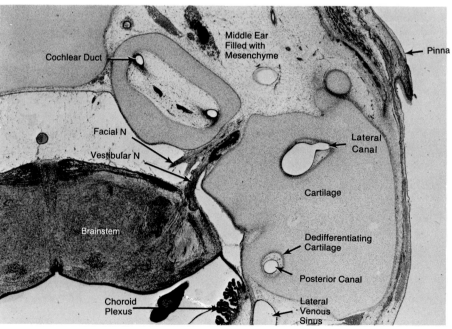

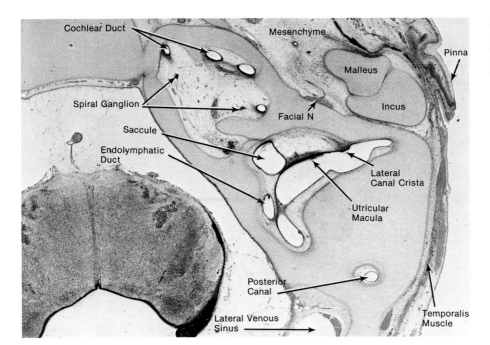

FIG. 9.29: Fetus A (8 weeks). This view shows the developing cartilaginous otic capsule and membranous labyrinth. The primitive cochlear duct and spiral ganglion are visible.

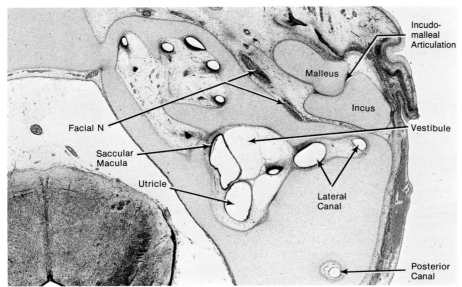

FIG. 9.30: Fetus A (8 weeks). The cochlear duct has its full two and one-half turns. The perilymphatic space of the vestibule is developing as reticulum is resorbed. (See Fig. 9.33.)

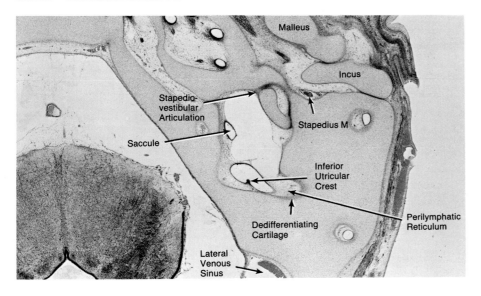

FIG. 9.31: Fetus A (8 weeks). The malleus and incus are seen. The normally massive cartilaginous footplate rests in the oval window.

Phylogeny and Embryology   **275**

FIG. 9.32: Fetus A (8 weeks). The tubotympanic recess is invading the mesenchyme of the middle ear. The ectoderm of the first branchial groove is approaching the mesodermal condensation of the future tympanic membrane.

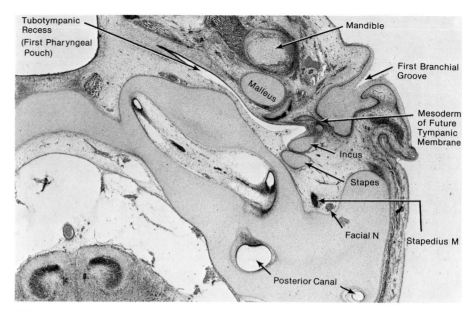

FIG. 9.33: Fetus A (8 weeks). This photomicrograph is a higher magnification of the cochlea appearing in Figure 9.31.

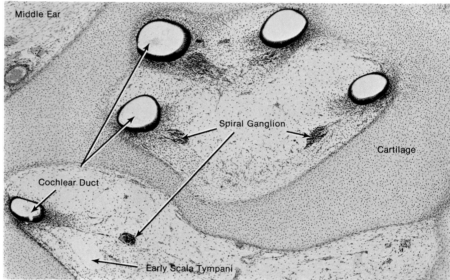

FIG. 9.34: Fetus A (8 weeks). The utricle is seen in high magnification. The sensory epithelium, otolithic membrane, and vestibular nerve bundles are visualized.

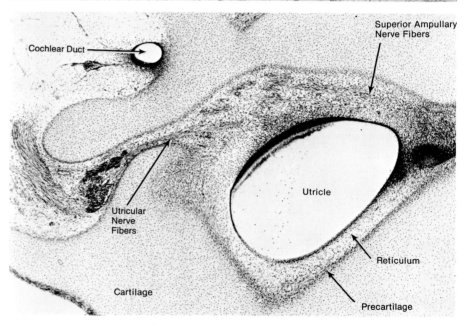

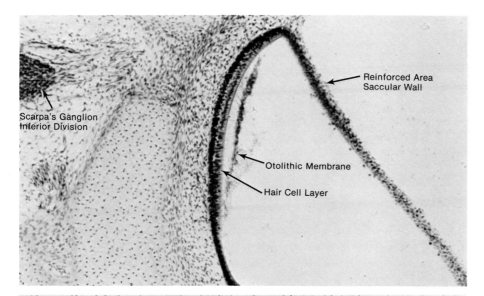

FIG. 9.35: Fetus A (8 weeks). This high magnification of the saccule shows an already well-formed sensory epithelium.

Reinforced Area
Saccular Wall

Scarpa's Ganglion
Inferior Division

Otolithic Membrane

Hair Cell Layer

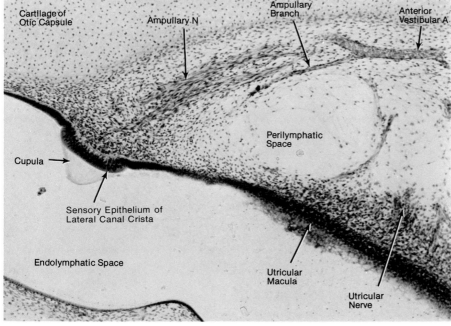

FIG. 9.36: Fetus A (8 weeks). The sensory epithelium and the cupula of the lateral canal are well developed. The endolymphatic space is fully developed and the perilymphatic space is forming by dissolution of reticulum.

Cartilage of
Otic Capsule

Ampullary N

Ampullary
Branch

Anterior
Vestibular A

Perilymphatic
Space

Cupula

Sensory Epithelium of
Lateral Canal Crista

Endolymphatic Space

Utricular
Macula

Utricular
Nerve

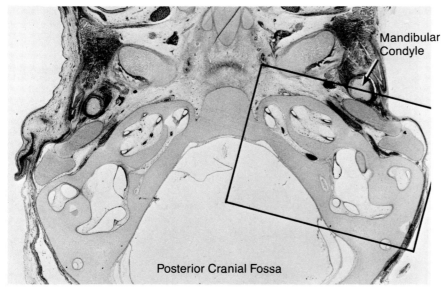

FETUS B (12 WEEKS)

FIG. 9.37: Fetus B (12 weeks). Shown here is an overview of a horizontal section of the head. The outlined area indicates the regions included in Figures 9.38 to 9.42.

Mandibular
Condyle

Posterior Cranial Fossa

FIG. 9.38: Fetus B (12 weeks). The internal auditory canal is well developed. Ossification has not yet begun. Facial nerve fibers are located in a sulcus in the middle ear.

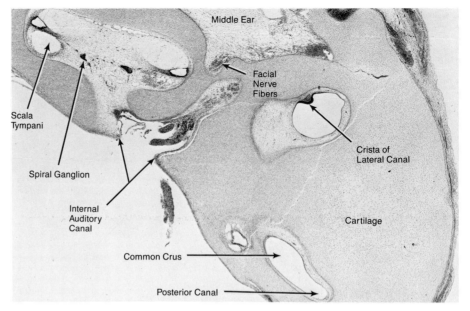

FIG. 9.39: Fetus B (12 weeks). The cochlear scalae are developing and the cochlear duct has assumed its characteristic triangular shape in the basal turn. The outlined area is magnified in Figure 9.43.

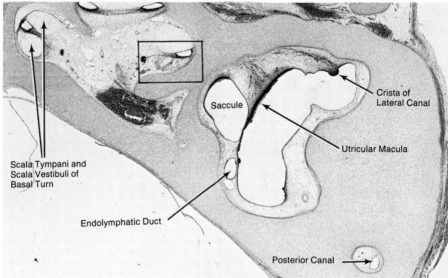

FIG. 9.40: Fetus B (12 weeks). The spiral ganglion is visible in the basal turn of the cochlea. The vestibule has expanded.

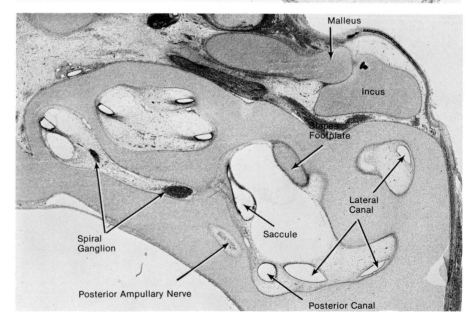

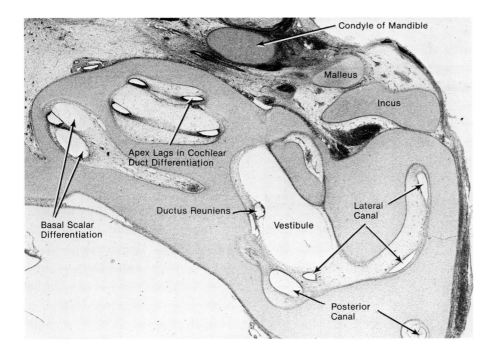

FIG. 9.41: Fetus B (12 weeks). Note that the cochlear duct in the basal turn already is nearly triangular in outline while the cochlear duct in the apex still possesses the more immature oval configuration.

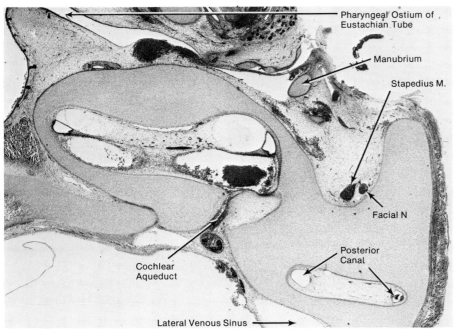

FIG. 9.42: Fetus B (12 weeks). The primitive cochlear aqueduct is seen extending from the scala tympani of the basal turn to the posterior cranial fossa near the inferior petrosal sinus.

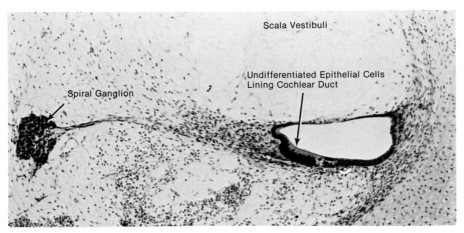

FIG. 9.43: Fetus B (12 weeks). This is a higher magnification of the cochlear duct and adjacent structures shown in the outlined area of Figure 9.39. The periotic reticulum shows greater resolution in the scala vestibuli than in the scala tympani. The spiral ganglion is well developed.

Phylogeny and Embryology   **279**

FIG. 9.44: Fetus B (12 weeks). At this stage the vestibular sense organs show greater differentiation than the cochlear duct.

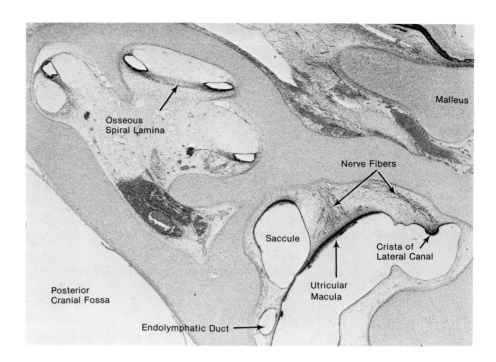

FETUS C (16 WEEKS)

FIG. 9.45: Fetus C (16 weeks). Shown is an overview of a horizontal section of the head. The outlined area indicates the regions included in Figures 9.46 to 9.50.

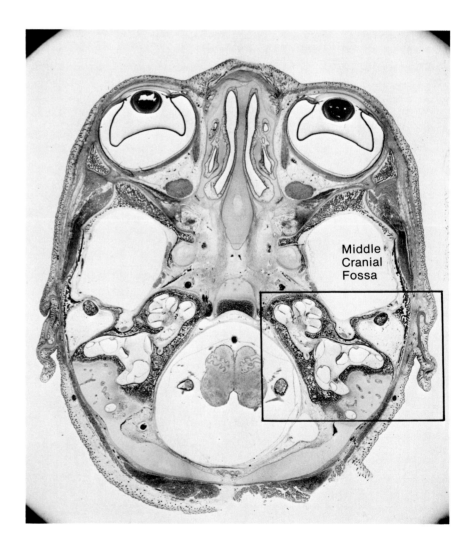

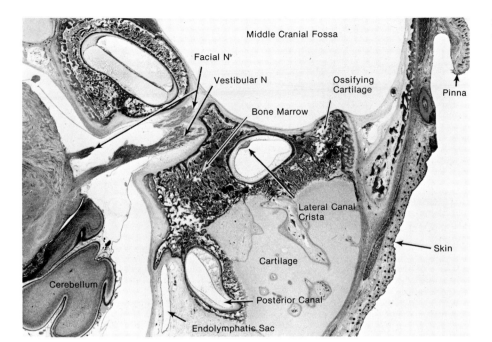

FIG. 9.46: Fetus C (16 weeks). The otic capsule is partly ossified.

Middle Cranial Fossa

Facial N⁰

Vestibular N

Ossifying Cartilage

Bone Marrow

Pinna

Lateral Canal Crista

Skin

Cartilage

Cerebellum

Posterior Canal

Endolymphatic Sac

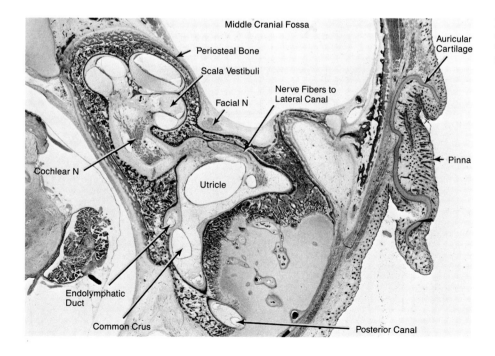

FIG. 9.47: Fetus C (16 weeks). Resolution of periotic reticulum proceeds toward development of the perilymphatic spaces.

Middle Cranial Fossa

Periosteal Bone

Auricular Cartilage

Scala Vestibuli

Nerve Fibers to Lateral Canal

Facial N

Cochlear N

Pinna

Utricle

Endolymphatic Duct

Common Crus

Posterior Canal

Phylogeny and Embryology **281**

FIG. 9.48: Fetus C (16 weeks). The stapes footplate is still cartilaginous. The periosteal, endochondral (enchondral), and endosteal layers of bone are seen in the cochlear capsule. The posterior part of the otic capsule is still largely cartilaginous, allowing for continued growth and expansion of the semicircular canals.

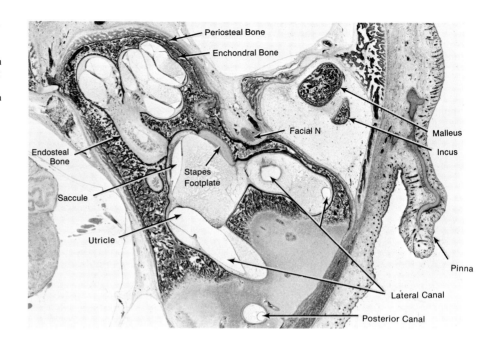

FIG. 9.49: Fetus C (16 weeks). The mesenchyme of the middle ear is undergoing resolution. The incus and malleus are partly ossified. At this stage the stapedial crura are larger than in the adult. Fibers of the tensor tympani muscle are seen. The fissula ante fenestram and fossula post fenestram are both visible.

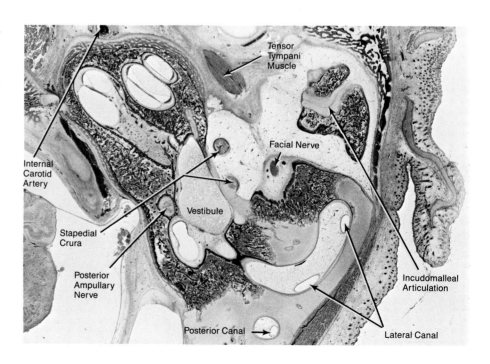

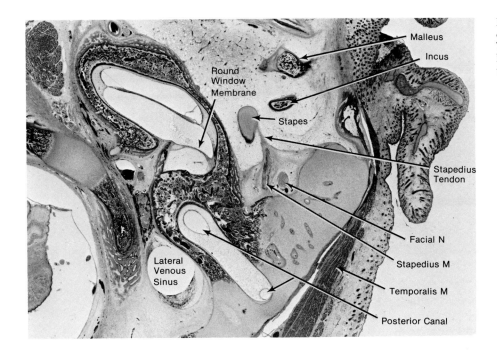

FIG. 9.50: Fetus C (16 weeks). The cochlear aqueduct is clearly defined. The stapedius muscle and its tendon have reached the cartilaginous head of the stapes.

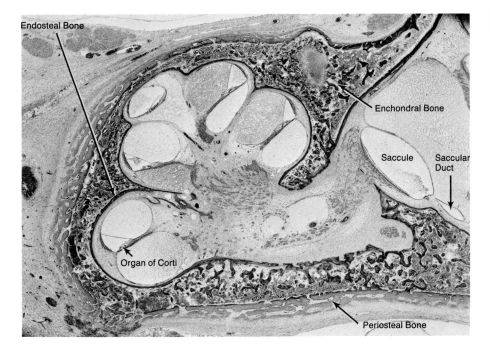

FIG. 9.51: Fetus C (16 weeks). The three layers of bone of the otic capsule are clearly visible. Structures of the cochlear duct (Reissner's membrane, stria vascularis, organ of Corti) are well developed. There is a fibrillar precipitate in the perilymphatic spaces which will disappear in later stages of development.

FIG. 9.52: Fetus C (16 weeks). The cytoarchitecture of the utricular macula is nearly mature. The perilymphatic reticulum has not yet completely resolved.

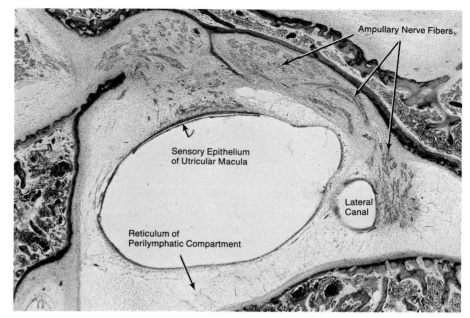

FIG. 9.53: Fetus C (16 weeks). The cribrose area for the saccular nerve bundles has not yet formed. There is a precipitate in the perilymphatic and endolymphatic compartments which indicates a high protein content.

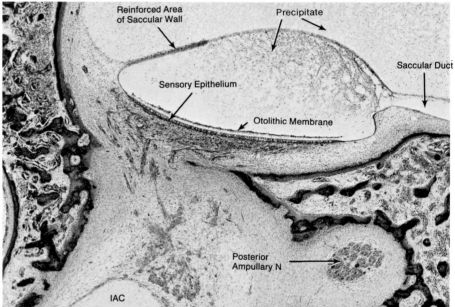

FIG. 9.54: Fetus C (16 weeks). The ampulla of the lateral canal and its crista show advance toward maturity. Perilymphatic reticulum remains.

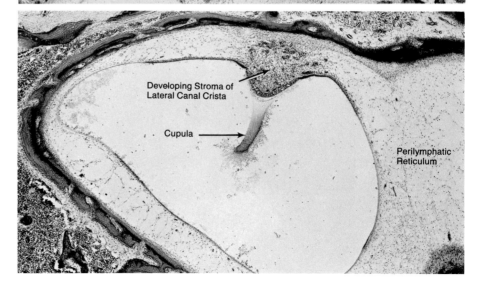

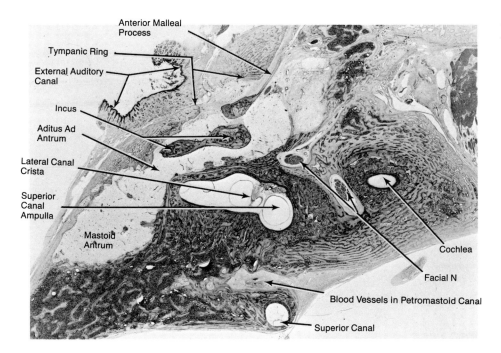

Anterior Malleal Process

Tympanic Ring

External Auditory Canal

Incus

Aditus Ad Antrum

Lateral Canal Crista

Superior Canal Ampulla

Mastoid Antrum

Cochlea

Facial N

Blood Vessels in Petromastoid Canal

Superior Canal

INFANT (5 MONTHS)

FIG. 9.55: Infant (5 months). The anterior process of the malleus extends into the petrotympanic fissure. Thin mesenchyme remains in the epitympanum and mastoid antrum.

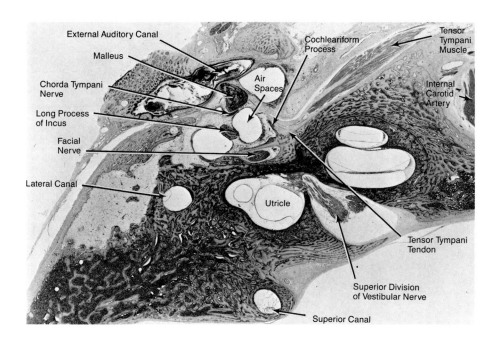

External Auditory Canal

Malleus

Chorda Tympani Nerve

Long Process of Incus

Facial Nerve

Lateral Canal

Cochleariform Process

Air Spaces

Utricle

Tensor Tympani Muscle

Internal Carotid Artery

Tensor Tympani Tendon

Superior Division of Vestibular Nerve

Superior Canal

FIG. 9.56: Infant (5 months). The superior part of the mesotympanum still contains mesenchyme but is partially pneumatized. The external auditory canal contains ceruminous and keratin debris.

FIG. 9.57: Infant (5 months). The middle part of the mesotympanum is fully pneumatized. The obturator foramen of the stapes still contains mesenchyme. The mastoid consists of bone trabeculae and marrow.

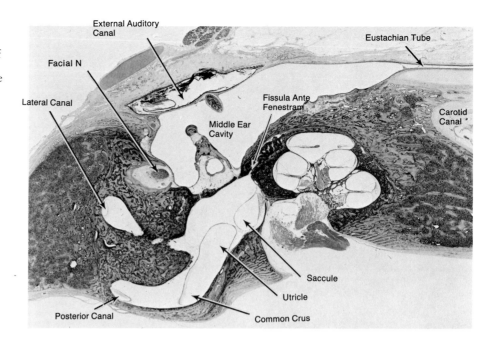

FIG. 9.58: Infant (5 months). The periosteal and endochondral (enchondral) layers of bone are well demarcated. The internal auditory canal is normal but flares at its ostium.

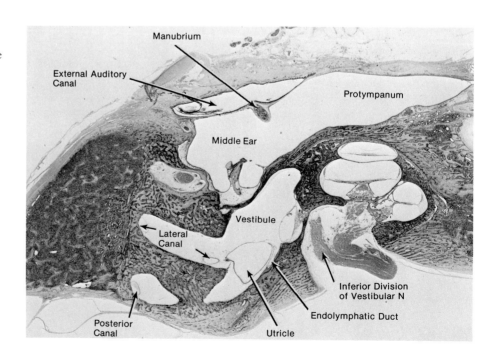

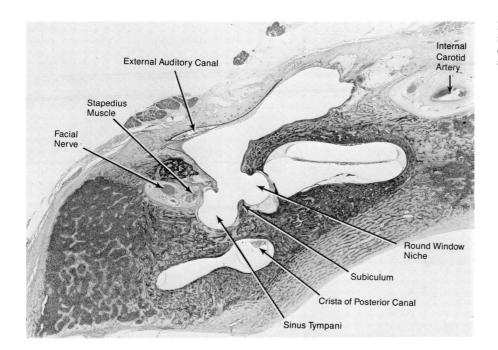

Labels for top figure:
External Auditory Canal
Stapedius Muscle
Facial Nerve
Internal Carotid Artery
Round Window Niche
Subiculum
Crista of Posterior Canal
Sinus Tympani

FIG. 9.59: Infant (5 months). The carotid artery is small at this age. The facial nerve and stapedius muscle occupy a common intraosseous space.

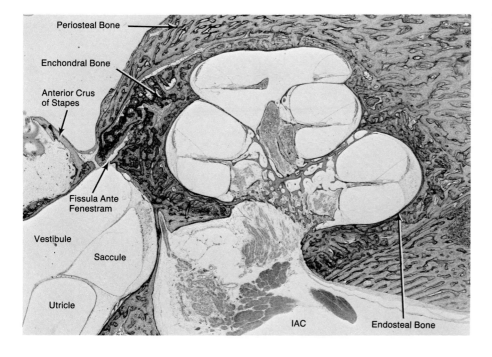

Labels for bottom figure:
Periosteal Bone
Enchondral Bone
Anterior Crus of Stapes
Fissula Ante Fenestram
Vestibule
Saccule
Utricle
IAC
Endosteal Bone

FIG. 9.60: Infant (5 months). The trilaminar structure of the bony labyrinth is well demonstrated. The membranous labyrinth appears normal. The attachment of the posterosuperior wall of the saccule to the anteroinferior wall of the utricle is a normal condition.

Phylogeny and Embryology 287

FIG. 9.61: Infant (5 months). The saccular branch of the inferior vestibular nerve, as it passes anteriorly through the cribrose area, normally tends to bypass the saccular macula; it then bends abruptly posteriorly to innervate it. The reinforced area of the saccular wall probably serves the function of protection against eddy currents in the perilymph which are generated by movements of the footplate.

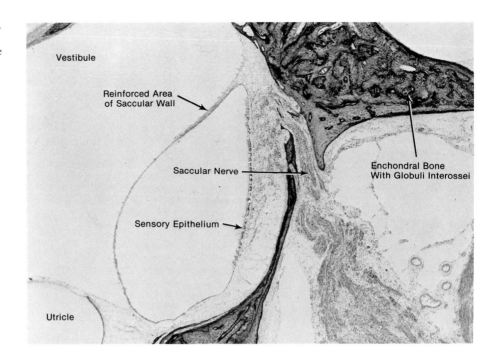

FIG. 9.62: Infant (5 months). This high power view shows the crista of the lateral canal. The sensory epithelium has undergone moderate postmortem autolysis. The rarefaction of the perilymphatic reticulum and the formation of the bony latticework of the cribrose area are evident.

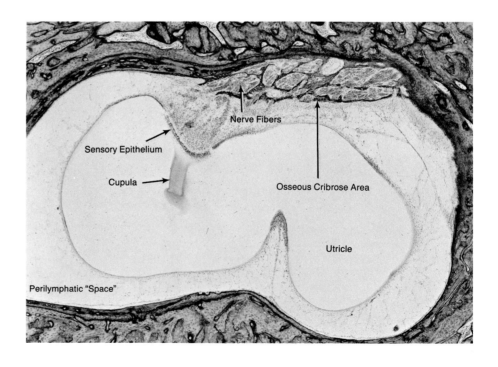

References

ADLINGTON P: The ultrastructure and the functions of the saccus endolymphaticus and its decompression in Ménière's disease. J Laryngol Otol 81:759, 1967.

ALBERTI PWRM: The blood supply of the incudostapedial joint and the lenticular process. Laryngoscope 73:605, 1963.

ALFORD BR, GUILFORD FR: A comprehensive study of the tumors of the glomus jugulare. Laryngoscope 72:765, 1962.

ALLAM AF: Pneumatization of the temporal bone. Ann Otol Rhinol Laryngol 78:49, 1969.

ALTMANN F: Anomalies of the internal carotid artery and its branches; their embryological and comparative anatomical significance. Report of a new case of persistent stapedial artery in man. Laryngoscope 57:313, 1947.

ALTMANN F: Malformations of the eustachian tube, the middle ear and its appendages. A critical review. Arch Otolaryngol 54:241, 1951.

ALTMANN F: Discussion. Otolaryngol Clin N Am 1:352, 1968.

ANGELBORG C, ENGSTRÖM H: The normal organ of Corti. In *Basic Mechanisms in Hearing*. Edited by AR Møller. New York, Academic Press, Inc, 1973.

ANSON BJ: The early development of the membranous labyrinth in mammalian embryos, with special reference to the endolymphatic duct and utriculo-endolymphatic duct. Anat Rec 59:15, 1934.

ANSON BJ: The labyrinths and their capsule in health and disease. Trans Am Acad Ophthalmol Otolaryngol 73:17, 1969.

ANSON BJ: Developmental anatomy of the ear. In *Otolaryngology*. Edited by MM Paparella, DA Shumrick. Philadelphia, WB Saunders Co, 1973.

ANSON BJ, DONALDSON JA: *The Surgical Anatomy of the Temporal Bone and Ear*. Philadelphia, WB Saunders Co, 1967.

ANSON BJ, DONALDSON JA: *Surgical Anatomy of the Temporal Bone*. 3rd. ed. Philadelphia, WB Saunders Co, 1981.

ANSON BJ, DONALDSON JA, WARPEHA RL, WINCH TR: A critical appraisal of the anatomy of the perilymphatic system in man. Laryngoscope 74:945, 1964.

ANSON BJ, DONALDSON JA, WARPEHA RL, WINCH TR: The vestibular and cochlear aqueducts: their variational anatomy in the adult human ear. Laryngoscope *75:*1203, 1965.

ANSON BJ, HARPER DG, HANSON JR: Vascular anatomy of the auditory ossicles and petrous part of the temporal bone in man. Ann Otol Rhinol Laryngol *71:*622, 1962.

ANSON BJ, WARPEHA RL, DONALDSON JA, RENSINK MJ: The developmental and adult anatomy of the membranous and osseous labyrinths of the otic capsule. Otolaryngol Clin N Am *1:*273, 1968.

ARENBERG IK, RASK-ANDERSEN H, WILBRAND H, STAHLE J: The surgical anatomy of the endolymphatic sac. Arch Otolaryngol *103:*1, 1977.

AREY LB: *Developmental Anatomy; A textbook and laboratory manual of embryology.* Philadelphia, WB Saunders Co, 1974.

ARNOLD F: *Der Kopftheil des vegetativen Nervensystems beim Menschen.* Heidelberg, Karl Groos, 1831.

ARNVIG J: Lymph vessels in the wall of the endolymphatic sac. Arch Otolaryngol *53:*290, 1951.

ASAI K: Die Blutgefässe des häutigen Labyrinthe der Ratte. Anat Hefte *36:*711, 1908a.

ASAI K: Die Blutgefässe im häutigen Labyrinthe des Hundes. Anat Hefte *36:*369, 1908b.

ASCHAN G: The anatomy of the eustachian tube with regard to its function. Acta Soc Med Upsal *60:*131, 1955.

AUSTIN DF: Anatomy and embryology. In *Diseases of the Nose, Throat, and Ear.* 12th ed. Edited by JJ Ballenger. Philadelphia, Lea & Febiger, 1977.

AXELSSON A: The vascular anatomy of the cochlea in the guinea pig and in man. Acta Otolaryngol (Stockh) Suppl *243:*1, 1968.

BALLANCE C: *Essays on the Surgery of the Temporal Bone.* London, Macmillan Company, 1919.

BARON SH: Persistent stapedial artery, necrosis of the incus, and other problems which have influenced the choice of technique in stapes replacement surgery in otosclerosis. Laryngoscope *73:*769, 1963.

BASEK M: Anomalies of the facial nerve in normal temporal bones. Ann Otol Rhinol Laryngol *71:*382, 1962.

BAST TH: The utriculo-endolymphatic valve. Anat Rec *40:*61, 1928.

BAST TH: Ossification of otic capsule in human fetuses. Contrib Embryol *121:*53, 1930.

BAST TH: Development of the aquaeductus cochleae and its contained periotic duct and cochlear vein in human embryos. Ann Otol Rhinol Laryngol *55:*278, 1946.

BAST TH, ANSON BJ: *The Temporal Bone and the Ear.* Springfield, Charles C Thomas, 1949.

BAST TH, ANSON BJ, RICHANY SF: The development of the second branchial arch (Reichert's cartilage), facial canal, and associated structures in man. Northwest U Med Sch Quart Bull *30:*235, 1956.

BATTEN EH: The origin of the acoustic ganglion in sheep. J Embryol Exp Morphol *6:*597, 1958.

BAXTER A: Dehiscence of the fallopian canal. An anatomical study. J Laryngol Otol *85:*587, 1971.

BEDDARD D, SAUNDERS WH: Congenital defects in the fallopian canal. Laryngoscope *72:*112, 1962.

BERGSTRÖM B: Morphology of the vestibular nerve. I. Anatomical studies of the vestibular nerve in man. Acta Otolaryngol (Stockh) *76:*162, 1973.

BIRKEN EA, BROOKLER KH: Surface tension lowering substance of the eustachian tube in non suppurative otitis media: an experiment with dogs. Laryngoscope 83:255, 1973.

BOETTCHER A: Über entwickelung und Bau des Gehörlabyrinthes nach Untersuchungen an Säugethieren. Nova Acta Acad Cesariae 35:1, 1869.

BOLZ EA, LIM DJ: Morphology of the stapediovestibular joint. Acta Otolaryngol (Stockh) 73:10, 1972.

BÖTNER V, ANCETTI A: La istomortologia dei ganglia timpanici nell'uomo. Min Otorhinolaryngol 6:106, 1956.

BREDBERG G, LINDEMAN H, ADES H, WEST R, Engström H: Scanning electron microscopy of the organ of Corti. Science 170:861, 1970.

BRÖDEL M: Three Unpublished Drawings of the Anatomy of the Human Ear. Philadelphia, WB Saunders Co, 1946.

BRUNNER H: Die Verbindungen der Gehörknöchelchen. Arch Augen Ohrenheilk 3:23, 1873.

BULL TR: Taste and the chorda tympani. J Laryngol Otol 79:479, 1965.

CABEZUDO LM: The ultrastructure of the basilar membrane in the cat. Acta Otolaryngol (Stockh) 86:160, 1978.

CARPENTER MB: Core Text of Neuroanatomy. 1st ed. Baltimore, Williams & Wilkins, 1972.

CHATELLIER HP: Evolution embryologique de l'appareil endolymphatique et du cloisonnement utriculo-sacculaire chez l'homme. Arch Anat Histol Embryol 5:49, 1926.

CHEATLE AH: Some Points in the Surgical Anatomy of the Temporal Bone from Birth to Adult Life. London, J and A Churchill Ltd, 1907.

CHILLA R, NICKLATSCH J, ARGLEBE C: Late sequelae of iatrogenic damage to chorda tympani nerve. Acta Otolaryngol (Stockh) 94:461, 1982.

CLEMIS JD, VALVASSORI GE: Recent radiographic and clinical observations on the vestibular aqueduct. (A preliminary report.) Otolaryngol Clin N Am 1:339, 1968.

CORTI A: Recherches sur l'organe de l'ouie des mammifères. Z Wiss Zool 3:109, 1851.

COTUNNIUS D: De Aqueductibus Auris Humanae Internae Anatomica Dissertatio. 4°. Neapoli, 1761.

CRUMLEY RL: Spatial anatomy of facial nerve fibers—a preliminary report. Laryngoscope 90:274, 1980.

DAVIES DG: Persistent stapedial artery: a temporal bone report. J Laryngol Otol 81:649, 1967.

DAVIES DG: Malleus fixation. J Laryngol Otol 82:331, 1968.

DAVIES J: Embryology and anatomy of the head and neck. In Otolaryngology. Edited by MM Paparella, DA Shumrick. Philadelphia, WB Saunders Co, 1973.

DAVIS H: Advances in the neurophysiology and neuroanatomy of the cochlea. J Acoust Soc Am 34:1377, 1962.

DEAVER JB: Surgical Anatomy: A Treatise on Human Anatomy in Its Application to the Practice of Medicine and Surgery. 3V roy 8°. Philadelphia, P Blakiston's Sons & Co, 1901–1903.

DE VRIES H: Struktur und Lage de Tektorialmembran in der Schnecke, untersucht mit neueren Hilfsmitteln. Acta Otolaryngol (Stockh) 37:334, 1949.

DIAMANT M: Otitis and pneumatisation of the mastoid bone. A clinical-statistical analysis. Acta Otolaryngol (Stockh) Suppl 41:1, 1940.

DICKINSON JT, SRISOMBOON P, KAMERER DB: Congenital anomaly of the facial nerve. Arch Otolaryngol 88:357, 1968.

Dobozi M: Surgical anatomy of the geniculate ganglion. Acta Otolaryngol (Stockh) *80*:116, 1975.

Dobson J: *Anatomical Eponyms*. 2nd ed. Edinburgh, E & S Livingstone Ltd, 1962.

Donaldson JA, Anson BJ, Warpeha RL, Rensink MJ: The perils of the sinus tympani. Trans Pac Coast Oto-Ophthalmol Soc *49*:93, 1968.

Duckert L: The morphology of the cochlear aqueduct and periotic duct of the guinea pig—a light and electron microscopic study. Trans Am Acad Ophthalmol Otolaryngol *78*:21, 1974.

Durcan DJ, Shea JJ, Sleeckx JP: Bifurcation of the facial nerve. Arch Otolaryngol *86*:619, 1967.

Duvall AJ, III: The ultrastructure of the external sulcus in the guinea pig cochlear duct. Laryngoscope *79*:1, 1969.

Dworacek H: Die anatomischen verhältnisse des Mittelohres unter operationsmikroskopischer Betrachtung. Acta Otolaryngol (Stockh) *51*:15, 1960.

Eggston AA, Wolff, D: *Histopathology of the Ear, Nose and Throat*. Baltimore, Williams & Wilkins, 1947.

Engström H: The cortilymph, the third lymph of the inner ear. Acta Morphol Neerl Scand *3*:195, 1960.

Engström H, Wersäll J: Structure and innervation of the inner ear sensory epithelia. Int Rev Cytol *7:535, 1958a*.

Engström H, Wersäll J: The ultrastructural organization of the organ of Corti and of the vestibular sensory epithelia. Exp Cell Res *5*:460, 1958b.

Epley JM: Reflexogenic vertigo treated by tensor tympani transection. Otolaryngol Head Neck Surg *89*:849, 1981.

Etholm B, Belal A Jr: Senile changes in the middle ear joints. Ann Otol Rhinol Laryngol *83*:49, 1974.

Fisch U: Transtemporal surgery of the internal auditory canal. Report of 92 cases, technique, indications and results. Adv Otorhinolaryngol *17*:203, 1970.

Fisch U: Carotid lesions at the skull base. In *Neurological Surgery of the Ear and Skull Base*. Edited by DE Brackmann. New York, Raven Press, 1982.

Flock Å: Electron Microscopic and electrophysiological studies on the lateral line canal organ. Acta Otolaryngol (Stockh) Suppl *199*:1, 1965.

Foley JO, DuBois FS: An experimental study of the facial nerve. J Comp Neurol *79*:79, 1943.

Fowler EP Jr: *Medicine of the Ear*. 1st ed. New York, Thomas Nelson & Sons, 1947.

Fowler EP Jr: Variations in the temporal bone course of the facial nerve. Laryngoscope *71*:937, 1961.

Friedmann I: Electron microscope observations on in vitro cultures of the isolated fowl embryo otocyst. J Biophys Biochem Cytol *5*:263, 1959.

Gacek RR: The macula neglecta in the feline species. J Comp Neurol *116*:317, 1961.

Gacek RR: Transection of the posterior ampullary nerve for the relief of benign paroxysmal positional vertigo. Ann Otol Rhinol Laryngol *83*:596, 1974.

Gacek RR, Radpour S: Fiber orientation of the facial nerve: an experimental study in the cat. Laryngoscope *92*:547, 1982.

Gaffney JG: Carotid-body-like tumors of the jugular bulb and middle ear. J Pathol Bacteriol *66*:157, 1953.

Garrison FH: *History of Medicine.* 4th ed. Philadelphia, WB Saunders Co, 1929.

Gasser RF: The development of the facial nerve in man. Ann Otol Rhinol Laryngol 76:37, 1967.

Ge X-X, Spector GJ: Labyrinthine segment and geniculate ganglion of facial nerve in fetal and adult human temporal bones. Ann Otol Rhinol Laryngol Suppl 85, 90:1: 1981.

Gerhardt HJ, Otto H-D: The intratemporal course of the facial nerve and its influence on the development of the ossicular chain. Acta Otolaryngol (Stockh) 91:567, 1981.

Glasgold AI, Horrigan WD: The internal carotid artery presenting as a middle ear tumor. Laryngoscope 82:2217, 1972.

Glasscock ME III, Dickins JRE, Jackson CG, Wiet RJ: Vascular anomalies of the middle ear. Laryngoscope 90:77, 1980.

Goldman NC, Singleton GT, Holly EH: Aberrant internal carotid artery. Arch Otolaryngol 94:269, 1971.

Goodhill V: External conductive hypacusis and the fixed malleus syndrome. Acta Otolaryngol (Stockh) Suppl 217:1, 1966a.

Goodhill V: The fixed malleus syndrome. Trans Am Acad Ophthalmol Otolaryngol 70:370, 1966b.

Goodhill V, Harris I, Brockman SJ, Hantz O: Sudden deafness and labyrinthine window ruptures. Audio-vestibular observations. Ann Otol Rhinol Laryngol 82:2, 1973.

Goodman RS, Cohen NL: Aberrant internal carotid artery in the middle ear. Ann Otol Rhinol Laryngol 90:67, 1981.

Gorlin RJ (ed): *Morphogenesis and Malformation of the Ear.* New York, Alan R. Liss, 1980.

Goycoolea MV, Carpenter A-M, Paparella MM, Juhn SK: Ganglia and ganglion cells in the middle ear of the cat. Arch Otolaryngol 106:269, 1980.

Gradenigo G: Die embryonale Anlage des Mittelohres: die morphologische Bedeutung der Gehörknöchelchen. Med Jahrb 83:61, 1887; 83:219, 1887.

Graham MD: The jugular bulb: its anatomic and clinical considerations in contemporary otology. Laryngoscope 87:105, 1977.

Graves GO, Edwards LF: The eustachian tube: a review of its descriptive, microscopic, topographic and clinical anatomy. Arch Otolaryngol 39:359, 1944.

Gray H: *Anatomy of the Human Body.* 27th ed. Edited by CM Goss. Philadelphia, Lea & Febiger, 1959.

Greisen O: Aberrant course of the facial nerve. Arch Otolaryngol 101:327, 1975.

Groves J: Facial nerve. Chapter 30 in *Scientific Foundations of Otolaryngology.* Edited by R Hinchcliffe, D Harrison. London, William Heinemann Medical Books Publication, 1976.

Guerrier Y: Surgical anatomy, particularly vascular supply of the facial nerve. In *Facial Nerve Surgery.* Edited by U Fisch. Birmingham, Aesculapius Publishing Company, 1977.

Guggenheim L: *Phylogenesis of the Ear.* Culver City, Murray & Gee, Inc, 1948.

Guild SR: A hitherto unrecognized structure, the glomus jugularis, in man. Anat Rec Suppl 2, 79:28, 1941.

Guild SR: Natural absence of part of the bony wall of the facial canal. Laryngoscope 59:668, 1949.

GUILD SR: The glomus jugulare, a nonchromaffin paraganglion, in man. Ann Otol Rhinol Laryngol 62:1045, 1953.

GUILFORD FR, ANSON BJ: Osseous fixation of the malleus. Trans Am Acad Ophthalmol Otolaryngol 71:398, 1967.

GULYA AJ, SCHUKNECHT HF: Letter to the editor. Am J Otol 5:262, 1984.

GUSSEN R: The stapediovestibular joint: normal structure and pathogenesis of otosclerosis. Acta Otolaryngol (Stockh) Suppl 248:1, 1969.

GUSSEN R: Pacinian corpuscles in the middle ear. J Laryngol Otol 84:71, 1970.

GUSSEN R: The human incudomalleal joint. Chondroid articular cartilage and degenerative arthritis. Arth Rheum 14:465, 1971.

HAGENS EW: Anatomy and pathology of the petrous bone: based on a study of fifty temporal bones. Arch Otolaryngol 19:556, 1934.

HALL GM, PULEC JL, RHOTON AL JR: Geniculate ganglion anatomy for the otologist. Arch Otolaryngol 90:568, 1969.

HAMILTON DW: The cilium on mammalian vestibular hair cells. Anat Rec 164:253, 1969.

HANSON JR, ANSON BJ, STRICKLAND EM: Branchial sources of the auditory ossicles in man. Part II: Observations of embryonic stages from 7 mm to 28 mm (CR length). Arch Otolaryngol 76:200, 1962.

HARADA T, SANDO I, MYERS EN: Microfissure in the oval window area. Ann Otol Rhinol Laryngol 90:174, 1981.

HARRIS WD: Topography of the facial nerve. Arch Otolaryngol 88:264, 1968.

HAYNES DR: The relations of the facial nerve in the temporal bone. Ann Roy Col Surg England 16:175, 1955.

HELD H: Die cochlea der Säuger und der Vögel, ihre Entwicklung und ihr Bau. *Handbuch der normalen und pathologischen physiologie.* Volume 11. Edited by A Bethe. Berlin, J Springer, 1926.

HENTZER E: Ultrastructure of the normal mucosa in the human middle ear, mastoid cavities, and eustachian tube. Ann Otol Rhinol Laryngol 79:1143, 1970.

HILDING DA: Electron microscopy of the developing hearing organ. Laryngoscope 79:1691, 1969.

HIRAIDE F, PAPARELLA MM: Histochemical characteristics of normal middle ear mucosa. Acta Otolaryngol (Stockh) 74:45, 1972.

HIS W: Die Formentwicklung des ausseren Ohres. Anat Menschl Embr pt. 3, 1885.

HOSHINO T, PAPARELLA MM: Middle ear muscle anomalies. Arch Otolaryngol 94:235, 1971.

HOUGH JVD: Malformations and anatomical variations seen in the middle ear during the operation for mobilization of the stapes. Laryngoscope 68:1337, 1958.

HOUGH JVD: Ossicular malformations and their correction. In *Proceedings of the Shambaugh Fifth International Workshop on Middle Ear Microsurgery and Fluctuant Hearing Loss.* Edited by GE Shambaugh, JJ Shea. Huntsville, Strode Publishers, Inc, 1977.

HOUSE JW, HITSELBERGER WE, McELVEEN J, BRACKMANN DE: Retrolabyrinthine section of the vestibular nerve. Otolaryngol Head Neck Surg 92:212, 1984.

HOUSE WF: Surgical exposure of the internal auditory canal and its contents through the middle, cranial fossa. Laryngoscope 71:1363, 1961.

HOUSE WF, BRACKMANN DE: Dizziness due to stenosis of the internal auditory canal. In *Neurological Surgery of the Ear.* Edited by H Silverstein,

H Norrell. Birmingham, Aesculapius Publishing Co, 1977.

HOUSE WF, CRABTREE JA: Surgical exposure of petrous portion of seventh nerve. Arch Otolaryngol *81*:506, 1965.

HUG JE, PFALTZ CR: Temporal bone pneumatization. A planimetric study. Arch Otorhinolaryngol *233*:145, 1981.

HUNT JR: The sensory field of the facial nerve: a further contribution to the symptomatology of the geniculate ganglion. Brain *38*:418, 1915.

HUSCHKE E: Über die Hörwerkzeuge. Beitr Physiol, p 35, 1824a.

HUSCHKE E: Ueber die Sinne. Beitr Physiol Naturgesch, Volume 1. Weimar, GHS pr Landes-Industrie-Compoirs, 1824b.

HYRTL J: Neue Beobachtungen aus dem Gebiete der menschlichen und vergleichenden Anatomie. Med Jahrb K K Österreich Staates *10*:446, 1836; also *19*:457, 1835.

IIDA H: Topographic anatomy of the middle ear. Pract Otolaryngol (Kyoto) *44*:420, 1951.

IURATO S: Submicroscopic structure of the membranous labyrinth. I. The tectorial membrane. Z Zellforsch *52*:105, 1960.

IURATO S: *Submicroscopic Structure of the Inner Ear.* Long Island City, Pergamon Press, 1967.

JAHRSDOERFER RA: The facial nerve in congenital middle ear malformations. Laryngoscope *91*:1217, 1981.

JAHRSDOERFER RA, RICHTSMEIER WJ, CANTRELL RW: Spontaneous CSF otorrhea. Arch Otolaryngol *107*:257, 1981.

JOHNSSON L-G, KINGSLEY TC: Herniation of the facial nerve in the middle ear. Arch Otolaryngol *91*:598, 1970.

JONES MF: Pathways of approach to the petrous pyramid. Ann Otol Rhinol Laryngol *44*:458, 1935.

KALTER H, WARKANY J: Medical progress. Congenital malformations: etiologic factors and their role in prevention (first of two parts). N Engl J Med *308*:424, 1983a.

KALTER H, WARKANY J: Congenital malformations (second of two parts). N Engl J Med *308*:491, 1983b.

KAPLAN J: Congenital dehiscence of the fallopian canal in middle ear surgery. Arch Otolaryngol *72*:197, 1960.

KAWABATA I, PAPARELLA MM: Fine structure of the round window membrane. Ann Otol Rhinol Laryngol *80*:13, 1971.

KELEMAN U: Über die Fissuren im knochernen innenohr. Arch Klin Exp Ohr Nas Kehlkopfheilk *137*:36, 1933.

KELEMEN G, LA FUENTE AD, OLIVARES FP: The cochlear aqueduct: structural considerations. Laryngoscope *89*:639, 1979.

KEMPE LF: Topical organization of the distal portion of the facial nerve. J Neurosurg *52*:671, 1980.

KESSEL J: Ueber Form- und Lageverhältnisse eigenthümlicher an der Schleimhaut des menschlichen Mittelohres vorkommender Organe. Arch Ohrenheilk *5*:254, 1870.

KIKUCHI J: Topographic anatomy of the temporal bone of Japanese. Jpn J Otolaryngol *13*:605, 1907.

KIMURA RS: Hairs of the cochlear sensory cells and their attachment to the tectorial membrane. Acta Otolaryngol (Stockh) *61*:55, 1966.

KIMURA RS: Distribution, structure, and function of dark cells in the vestibular labyrinth. Ann Otol Rhinol Laryngol *78*:542, 1969.

KITAMURA K, KIMURA RS, SCHUKNECHT HF: The ultrastructure of the geniculate ganglion. Acta Otolaryngol (Stockh) *93*:175, 1982.

KÖLLIKER A VON: Entwicklungsgeschichte des Menschen und der Höheren Thiere. Leipzig, W Engelmann, 1861.

KOLMER W: Gehörorgan. I. Das äussere Ohr. In *Handbuch Der Mikroskopischen Anatomie des Menschen.* Edited by W von Möllendorff. Berlin, J Springer, 1927.

KONIGSMARK BW, GORLIN RJ: *Genetic and Metabolic Deafness.* Philadelphia, WB Saunders Co, 1976.

KURÉ K, SANO T: Faserarten im N. facialis und die funktionelle Bedeutung der Ganglion geniculi. Z Zellforsch Mikroskop Anat 23:495, 1936.

LAPAYOWKER MS, LIEBMAN EP, RONIS ML, SAFER JN: Presentation of the internal carotid artery as a tumor of the middle ear. Radiology 98:293, 1971.

LATTES R, WALTNER JG: Nonchromaffin paraganglioma of the middle ear (carotid-body-like tumor; glomus-jugulare tumor). Cancer 2:447, 1949.

LAWRENCE M: Hair cell-tectorial membrane complex. Am J Otolaryngol 2:345, 1981.

LEMPERT J, WOLFF D: Histopathology of the incus and the head of the malleus in cases of stapedial ankylosis. Arch Otolaryngol 42:339, 1945.

LEMPERT J, WOLFF D, RAMBO JHT, WEVER EG, LAWRENCE M: New theory for the correlation of the pathology and the symptomatology of Meniere's disease. A research study of the vestibular endolymphatic labyrinth. Ann Otol Rhinol Laryngol 61:717, 1952.

LEVINE H: Cutaneous carcinoma of the head and neck: management of massive and previously uncontrolled lesions. Laryngoscope 93:87, 1983.

LIM DJ: Three dimensional observation of the inner ear with the scanning electron microscope. Acta Otolaryngol (Stockh) Suppl 255:1, 1969.

LIM DJ: Human tympanic membrane. An ultrastructural observation. Acta Otolaryngol (Stockh) 70:176, 1970.

LIM DJ: Fine morphology of the tectorial membrane: its relationship to the organ of Corti. Arch Otolaryngol 96:199, 1972.

LIM DJ: Functional morphology of the lining membrane of the middle ear and eustachian tube. An overview. Ann Otol Rhinol Laryngol Suppl 11, 83:5, 1974.

LIM DJ: Normal and pathological mucosa of the middle ear and eustachian tube. Clin Otolaryngol 4:213, 1979.

LIM DJ, HUSSL B: Macromolecular transport by the middle ear and its lymphatic system. Acta Otolaryngol (Stockh) 80:19, 1975.

LIM D, JACKSON D, BENNETT J: Human middle ear corpuscles—a light and electron microscopic study. Laryngoscope 85:1725, 1975.

LIM DJ, SHIMADA T, YODER M: Distribution of mucus-secreting cells in normal middle ear mucosa. Arch Otolaryngol 98:2, 1973.

LIM DJ, VIALL J, BIRCK H, ST PIERRE R: Symposium on prophylaxis and treatment of middle ear effusions. Laryngoscope 82:1625, 1972.

LINDSAY JR: Suppuration in the petrous pyramid. Ann Otol Rhinol Laryngol 47:3, 1938.

LINDSAY JR: Petrous pyramid of temporal bone. Pneumatization and roentgenologic appearance. Arch Otolaryngol 31:231, 1940.

LINDSAY JR: Pneumatization of the petrous pyramid. Ann Otol Rhinol Laryngol 50:1109, 1941.

LINDSAY JR: Osteomyelitis of petrous pyramid of temporal bone. Ann Surg 122:1060, 1945.

LITTON WB, KRAUSE CJ, ANSON BA, COHEN WN: The relationship of the facial canal to the annular sulcus. Laryngoscope 79:1584, 1969.

LIU YS, LIM DJ, LANG RW, BIRCK HG: Chronic middle ear effusions. Immunochemical and bacteriological investigations. Arch Otolaryngol 101:278, 1975.

LUNDQUIST P-G: The endolymphatic duct and sac in the guinea pig. An electron microscopic and experimental investigation. Acta Otolaryngol (Stockh) Suppl *201*:1, 1965.

LUNDQUIST P-G, KIMURA R, WERSÄLL J: Ultrastructural organization of the epithelial lining in the endolymphatic duct and sac in the guinea pig. Acta Otolaryngol (Stockh) *57*:65, 1964.

LUPIN AJ: The relationship of the tensor tympani and tensor palati muscles. Ann Otol Rhinol Laryngol *78*:792, 1969.

MAIN T, LIM D: The human external auditory canal secretory system—an ultrastructural study. Laryngoscope *86*:1164, 1976.

MATSUNAGA E: The dimorphism in human normal cerumen. Ann Hum Genet *25*:273, 1962.

MAY M: Anatomy of the facial nerve (spatial orientation of fibers in the temporal bone). Laryngoscope *83*:1311, 1973.

MAYER O: Über die Entstehung der Spontanfrakturen der Labyrinthkapsel und ihre Bedeutung für die Otosklerose. Z Hals Nas Ohrenheilk *26*:261, 1930.

MAYER O: Die Ursache der Knochenneubildung bei der Otosklerose. Acta Otolaryngol (Stockh) *15*:35, 1931.

MAYER O: Die Pyramidenzelleneiterungen. Z Hals Nas Ohrenheilk *42*:1, 1937.

MAZZONI A: Internal auditory canal arterial relations at the porus acusticus. Ann Otol Rhinol Laryngol *78*:797, 1969.

MAZZONI A: The subarcuate artery in man. Laryngoscope *80*:69, 1970.

MAZZONI A: Internal auditory artery supply to the petrous bone. Ann Otol Rhinol Laryngol *81*:13, 1972.

MAZZONI A: Vein of the vestibular aqueduct. Ann Otol Rhinol Laryngol *88*:759, 1979.

MELTZER PE: The mastoid cells: their arrangement in relation to the sigmoid portion of the transverse sinus. Arch Otolaryngol *19*:326, 1934.

MEURMAN Y: Zur Anatomie des Aquaeductus cochleae nebst einigen Bemerkurgen über dessen Physiologie. Acta Soc Med Fenn Duodecim (Ser B, Fasc No 1) *13*:1, 1930.

MIEHLKE A: Normal and anomalous anatomy of the facial nerve and an embryological study of the thalidomide catastrophe in Germany. Trans Am Acad Otolaryngol *68*:1030, 1964.

MIEHLKE A: Anatomy and clinical aspects of the facial nerve. Arch Otolaryngol *81*:444, 1965.

MIEHLKE A: *Surgery of the Facial Nerve.* 2nd ed. Philadelphia, WB Saunders Co, 1973.

MIRA E, DAL NEGRO F: Die histochemischen und histoenzymologischen Eigenschaften des Epithels der Übergangszone der Crista ampullaris. Arch Ohr Nas Kehlkopfheilk *193*:322, 1969.

MITCHELL GAG: Cranial extremities of sympathetic trunks. Acta Anat *18*:195, 1953.

MÖLLER J: Le septum de Körner. Acta Otolaryngol (Stockh) *14*:213, 1930.

MONIZ E: L'encephalographie artérielle son importance dans la localization des tumeurs cérébrales. Rev Neurol *342*:72, 1927.

MONTANDON P, GACEK RR, KIMURA RS: Crista neglecta in the cat and human. Ann Otol Rhinol Laryngol *79*:105, 1970.

MONTGOMERY WW: *Surgery of the Upper Respiratory System.* Volume 1, 1st ed. Philadelphia, Lea & Febiger, 1971.

MORETTI, JA: Highly placed jugular bulb and conductive deafness. Secondary to sinusojugular hypoplasia. Arch Otolaryngol *102*:430, 1976.

MORTON LT: *A Medical Bibliography* (Garrison and Morton). An annotated check-list of texts illustrating the history of medicine. 4th ed. London, Gower Publishing Company, 1983.

MULLIGAN RM: Chemodectoma in the dog. Am J Pathol 26:680, 1950.

MYERSON MC, RUBIN H, GILBERT JG: Anatomic studies of the petrous portion of the temporal bone. Arch Otolaryngol 20:195, 1934.

NABEYA D: A study in the comparative anatomy of the blood-vascular system of the internal ear in Mammalia and in Homo (Japanese). Acta Sch Med Univ Imperiales Kioto 6:1, 1923a.

NABEYA D: The blood vessels of the middle ear, in relation to the development of the small ear bones and their muscles. (A preliminary report). Folia Anat Japon 1:243, 1923b.

NAGER GT, NAGER M: The arteries of the human middle ear, with particular regard to the blood supply of the auditory ossicles. Ann Otol Rhinol Laryngol 62:923, 1953.

NOVIKOFF AB, ESSNER E: Pathological changes in cytoplasmic organelles. Fed Proc Suppl 21:1130, 1962.

OGAWA A, SANDO I: Spatial occupancy of vessels and facial nerve in the facial canal. Ann Otol Rhinol Laryngol 91:14, 1982.

OGURA Y, CLEMIS JD: A study of the gross anatomy of the human vestibular aqueduct. Ann Otol Rhinol Laryngol 80:813, 1971.

OKANO Y, MYERS EN: Herniation of the singular nerve into the round window niche. Arch Otolaryngol 102:478, 1976.

OKANO Y, MYERS EN, DICKSON DR: Microfissure between the round window niche and posterior canal ampulla. Ann Otol Rhinol Laryngol 86:49, 1977.

OKANO Y, SANDO I, MYERS EN: Crista neglecta in man. Ann Otol Rhinol Laryngol 87:306, 1978.

OKANO Y, SANDO I, MYERS EN: Branch of the singular nerve (posterior ampullary nerve) in the otic capsule. Ann Otol Rhinol Laryngol 89:13, 1980.

OMBREDANNE M: Absence congénitale de fenêtre ronde dans certaines aplasies mineures. Ann Otolaryngol Chir Cervicofac 85:369, 1968.

O'RAHILLY R: The early development of the otic vesicle in staged human embryos. J Embryol Exp Morphol 11:741, 1963.

ORZALESI F, PELLEGRINI E: Sui rapporti fra i nervi intermedio e vestibolare e sulla struttura del ganglio e del nervo vestibolare nell'uomó. Arch Ital Anat Embriol 31:105, 1933.

OSTMANN P: Die Würdigung des Fettpolsters der lateralen Tubenwand. Ein Beitrag zur Frage der Autophonie. Arch Ohrenheilk 34:170, 1893.

OVERTON SB, RITTER FN: A high placed jugular bulb in the middle ear. A clinical and temporal bone study. Laryngoscope 83:1986, 1973.

PALVA T: Cochlear aqueduct in infants. Acta Otolaryngol (Stockh) 70:83, 1970.

PALVA T, DAMMERT K: Human cochlear aqueduct. Acta Otolaryngol (Stockh) Suppl 246:1, 1969.

PARISIER SC: The middle cranial fossa approach to the internal auditory canal—an anatomical study stressing critical distances between surgical landmarks. Laryngoscope Suppl 4, 87:1, 1977.

PEARSON AA: Developmental anatomy of the ear. Chapter 1 in *Otolaryngology*. Edited by GM English. Hagerstown, Harper & Row, 1984.

PÉREZ OLIVARES F, SCHUKNECHT HF: Width of the internal auditory canal. A histological study. Ann Otol Rhinol Laryngol 88:316, 1979.

PERLMAN HB: The saccule; observations on a differentiated reinforced area of the saccular wall in man. Arch Otolaryngol 32:678, 1940.

PETRAKIS NL, DOHERTY M, LEE RE, SMITH SC, PAGE NL: Demonstration and implications of lysozyme and immunoglobulins in human ear wax. Nature 229:119, 1971.

PLATZER W: Zur Anatomie der Eminentia pyramidalis und des M. stapedius. Monatschr Ohrenheilk Laryngorhinol 95:553, 1961.

POLITZER A: Ueber gestielte Gebilde im Mittelohre des menschlichen Gehörorganes. Wien Med Wchnschr, November 20, 1869.

POLITZER A: *Textbook of the Diseases of the Ear and Adjacent Organs. For Students and Practitioners.* Translated by O Dodd, edited by W Dalby. London, Bailliere, Tindall & Cox, 1894.

POLITZER A: *Geschichte der Ohrenheilkunde.* Volume 1. Stuttgart, F Enke, 1907.

POLITZER A: *History of Otology.* Volume I. English translation by S Milstein, C Portnoff, A Coleman. Phoenix, Columella Press, 1981.

PORTMANN G: Vertigo. Surgical treatment by opening the saccus endolymphaticus. Arch Otolaryngol 6:309, 1927.

PORTMANN M: A propos de la topographie des nerfs de l'oreille moyenne. Rev Laryngol 76:273, 1955a.

PORTMANN M: Quelques observations sur la systématisation des nerfs transpétreux. Rev Laryngol 76:281, 1955b.

PORTMANN M, STERKERS JM, CHARACHON R, CHOUARD C: *The Internal Auditory Meatus: Anatomy, pathology and surgery.* New York, Churchill Livingstone, 1975.

PROCTOR B: The development of the middle ear spaces and their surgical significance. J Laryngol Otol 78:631, 1964.

PROCTOR B: Embryology and anatomy of the eustachian tube. Arch Otolaryngol 86:503, 1967.

PROCTOR B: Alexander Prussak. Ann Otol Rhinol Laryngol 77:344, 1968.

PROCTOR B: Surgical anatomy of the posterior tympanum. Ann Otol Rhinol Laryngol 78:1026, 1969.

PROCTOR B: Anatomy of the eustachian tube. Arch Otolaryngol 97:2, 1973.

PROCTOR B: The petromastoid canal. Ann Otol Rhinol Laryngol 92:640, 1983.

PROCTOR B, NAGER GT: The facial canal: normal anatomy, variations and anomalies. Ann Otol Rhinol Laryngol Suppl 97, 91:33, 1982a.

PROCTOR B, NAGER GT: The facial canal: normal anatomy, variations and anomalies. Trans Am Otol Soc 70:49, 1982b.

PROCTOR B, NIELSEN E, PROCTOR C: Petrosquamosal suture and lamina. Otolaryngol Head Neck Surg 89:482, 1981.

PROOPS DW, HAWKE M, BERGER G, MACKAY A: The anterior process of the malleus. Abstr Seventh Midwinter Res Meet Assn Res Otolaryngol. Edited by DJ Lim. Columbus, Offset print, 1984.

PRUSSAK A: Zur Anatomie des menschlichen Trommelfells. Arch Ohrenheilk 3:255, 1867.

PYE A, HINCHCLIFFE R: Comparative anatomy of the ear. Chapter 13 in *Scientific Foundations of Otolaryngology.* Edited by R Hinchcliffe, D Harrison. London, William Heinemann Medical Books Publications, 1976.

RABL K: Über das Gebiet des Nervus facialis. Anat Anz (Jena) 2:219, 1887.

RAMADIER J: Les osteites petreuses profondes (petrosites). Otorhinolaryngol Int 17:816, 1933.

RASK-ANDERSEN H, BREDBERG G, STAHLE J: Structure and function of the endolymphatic duct. In *Meniere's Disease*. Edited by K-H Vosteen, H Schuknecht, CR Pfaltz, J Wersäll, RS Kimura, C Morgenstern, SK Juhn. New York, Thieme-Stratton Inc, 1981.

RASK-ANDERSEN H, STAHLE J, WILBRAND H: Human cochlear aqueduct and its accessory canals. Ann Otol Rhinol Laryngol Suppl 42, 86:1, 1977.

RASMUSSEN AT: Studies of the eighth cranial nerve of man. Laryngoscope 50:67, 1940.

RASMUSSEN GL: The olivary peduncle and other fiber projections of the superior olivary complex. J Comp Neurol 84:141, 1946.

RETZIUS G: Das Gehörorgan der Wirbeltiere. II. Das Gehörorgan der Reptilien, der Vögel, und der Säugetiere. Stockholm, Samson & Wallin, 1884.

RICHARDSON TL, ISHIYAMA E, KEELS EW: Submicroscopic studies of the round window membrane. Acta Otolaryngol (Stockh) 71:9, 1971.

RITTER FN, LAWRENCE M: A histological and experimental study of cochlear aqueduct patency in the adult human. Laryngoscope 75:1224, 1965.

ROGERS BD: Anatomy, embryology, and classification of auricular deformities. In *Symposium on Reconstruction of the Auricle*. Volume 10. Edited by RC Tanzer, MT Edgerton. St Louis, CV Mosby Co, 1974.

ROSEN S: Tympanic plexus. Anatomic study. Arch Otolaryngol 52:15, 1950.

ROSENWASSER H: Carotid body tumor of the middle ear and mastoid. Arch Otolaryngol 41:64, 1945.

SAINTE-MARIE G: A paraffin-embedding technique for studies employing immunofluorescence. J Histochem Cytochem 10:250, 1962.

SAITO H, RUBY RF, SCHUKNECHT HF: Course of the sensory component of the nervus intermedius in the temporal bone. Ann Otol Rhinol Laryngol 79:960, 1970.

SAITO R, IGARASHI M, ALFORD BR, GUILFORD FR: Anatomical measurement of the sinus tympani. Arch Otolaryngol 94:418, 1971.

SANDO I, DOYLE W, OKUNO H, TAKAHARA T, KITAJIRI M, COURY WJ III: How to remove, process, and study the temporal bone with the eustachian tube and its accessory structures: a method for histopathology study. Auris Nasus Larynx Suppl, in press.

SANDO I, EGAMI T, HARADA T: Course and contents of the paravestibular canaliculus. Ann Otol Rhinol Laryngol 89:147, 1980.

SCHACHERN PA, PAPARELLA MM, DUVALL AJ III, CHOO YB: The human round window membrane. Arch Otolaryngol 110:15, 1984.

SCHUKNECHT HF: *Stapedectomy*. Boston, Little, Brown & Co, 1971.

SCHUKNECHT HF: *Pathology of the Ear*. Cambridge, Harvard University Press, 1974.

SCHUKNECHT HF: Mondini dysplasia. A clinical and pathological study. Ann Otol Rhinol Laryngol Suppl 65, 89:1, 1980.

SCHUKNECHT HF, BELAL AA: The utriculo-endolymphatic valve: its functional significance. J Laryngol Otol 89:985, 1975.

SCHUKNECHT HF, SEIFI AE: Experimental observations on the fluid physiology of the inner ear. Ann Otol Rhinol Laryngol 72:687, 1963.

SENTURIA BH, Marcus MD, LUCENTE FE: *Diseases of the External Ear. An Otologic-dermatologic Manual*. New York, Grune & Stratton, 1980.

SHAMBAUGH GE: *Blood-vessels in the Labyrinth of the Ear*. Volume X, Dicennial Publication. Chicago, University of Chicago Press, 1903.

SHAMBAUGH GE: The distribution of blood-vessels in the labyrinth of the ear of the sheep and the calf. Arch Otol 34:71, 1905.

SHAMBAUGH G: On the structure and function of the epithelium in the sulcus spiralis externus. Arch Otolaryngol 37:538, 1908.

SHAMBAUGH GE JR: Facial nerve decompression and repair. In *Surgery of the Ear.* 2nd ed. Philadelphia, WB Saunders Co, 1967.

SHI S-R: Temporal bone findings in a case of otopalatodigital syndrome. Arch Otolaryngol *111*:119, 1985.

SHIMADA T, LIM D: Distribution of ciliated cells in the human middle ear: electron and light microscopic observations. Ann Otol Rhinol Laryngol *81*:203, 1972.

SHRAPNELL HJ: On the form and structure of membrana tympani. Lond M Gaz *10*:120, 1832.

SIEBENMANN F: *Die Korrosions-Anatomie des knochernen Labyrinthes des menschlichen Ohres.* Wiesbaden, JF Bergmann, 1890.

SIEBENMANN F: *Die Blutgefässe im Labyrinthe des menschlichen Ohres.* Wiesbaden, J Bergmann, 1894.

SILVERSTEIN H: Cochlear and vestibular gross and histologic anatomy (as seen from postauricular approach). Otolaryngol Head Neck Surg 92:207, 1984.

SMITH CA: Capillary areas of the cochlea in the guinea pig. Laryngoscope *61*:1073, 1951.

SMITH CA: The capillaries of the vestibular membranous labyrinth in the guinea pig. Laryngoscope *63*:87, 1953.

SMITH CA: Capillary areas of the membranous labyrinth. Ann Otol Rhinol Laryngol *63*:435, 1954.

SMITH CA: Microscopic structure of the utricle. Ann Otol Rhinol Laryngol *65*:450, 1956.

SMITH CA: Structure of the stria vascularis and the spiral prominence. Ann Otol Rhinol Laryngol *66*:521, 1957.

SOBOTTA J: *Atlas of Descriptive Human Anatomy.* Volume III, 7th English ed. Edited and translated by E Uhlenhuth. New York, Hafner Publishing Co, Inc, 1957.

SPECTOR GJ, GE X-X: Development of the hypotympanum in the human fetus and neonate. Ann Otol Rhinol Laryngol Suppl 88, 90:1, 1981.

SPECTOR GJ, LEE D, CARR C, DAVIS G, SCHNETTGOECKE V, STRAUSS M, RAUCHBACH E: Later stages of development of the periotic duct and its adjacent area in the human fetus. Laryngoscope Suppl 20, 90:1, 1980.

SPECTOR GJ, MAISEL RH, OGURA JH: Glomus tumors in the middle ear. I. An analysis of 46 patients. Laryngoscope *83*:1652, 1973.

SPOENDLIN H: The organization of the cochlear receptor. Adv Oto-rhinolaryngol *13*:1, 1966.

SPOENDLIN H, LICHTENSTEIGER W: The sympathetic nerve supply to the inner ear. Arch Klin Exp Ohr Nas Kehlkopfheilk *189*:346, 1967.

STAHLE J, WILBRAND H: The vestibular aqueduct in patients with Ménière's disease. A tomographic and clinical investigation. Acta Otolaryngol (Stockh) *78*:36, 1974a.

STAHLE J, WILBRAND H: The para-vestibular canaliculus. Can J Otolaryngol *3*:262, 1974b.

STEFFEN TN: Vascular anomalies of the middle ear. Laryngoscope *78*:171, 1968.

STREETER GL: On the development of the membranous labyrinth and the acoustic and facial nerves in the human embryo. Am J Anat 6:139, 1906.

STREETER GL: Development of the auricle in the human embryo. Contrib Embryol *14*:111, 1922.

SULTAN AA: Histoire de l'otologie. Chapitre XVII. Acta Otorhinolaryngol Belg Suppl IV, *35*:1141, 1981.

TANAKA K, SAKAI N, TERAYAMA Y: Organ of Corti in the human fetus. Scanning and transmission electronmicroscope studies. Ann Otol Rhinol Laryngol *88*:749, 1979.

TANDLER J: *Zur vergleichenden Anatomie der Kopfarterien bei den Mammalia.* Wien, C Gerold's Sohn, 1898.

TAYLOR GD: Evolution of the ear. Laryngoscope *79*:638, 1969.

THOMANDER L, ALDSKOGIUS H, GRANT G: Motor fiber organization in the intratemporal portion of the cat and rat facial nerve studied with the horseradish peroxidase technique. Abstr Uppsala Disert Fac Med No 404 iii, 1. Uppsala, Acta Universitatis Upsaliensis, 1981.

TOMASI TB JR: *The Immune System of Secretions.* Englewood Cliffs, NJ, Prentice-Hall, 1976.

TREMBLE GE: Pneumatization of the temporal bone. Arch Otolaryngol *19*:172, 1934.

TRÖLTSCH AF VON: Anatomische Beiträge zur Ohrenheilkunde. Virchow's Arch *17*:1, 1859.

TUMARKIN A: Evolution of the auditory conducting apparatus in terrestrial vertebrates. In *Hearing Mechanisms in Vertebrates.* Boston, Little, Brown & Co, 1968.

VALVASSORI GE, CLEMIS JD: The large vestibular aqueduct syndrome. Laryngoscope *88*:723, 1978.

VAN BERGEIJK WA: Evolution of the sense of hearing in vertebrates. Am Zoologist *6*:371, 1966.

VAN DE WATER TR, MADERSON PF, JASKOLL TF: The morphogenesis of the middle and external ear. Birth Defects *16*:147, 1980.

VAN DE WATER TR, RUBEN RJ: Organogenesis of the ear. Chapter 12 in *Scientific Foundations of Otolaryngology.* Edited by R Hinchcliffe, D Harrison. London, William Heinemann Medical Books Publication, 1976.

VIDIĆ B, YOUNG PA: Gross and microscopic observations on the communicating branch to the facial nerve to the lesser petrosal nerve. Anat Rec *158*:257, 1967.

WALTNER JG: Histogenesis of corpora amylacea of the cochlear aqueduct, the internal auditory meatus and the associated cranial nerves. Arch Otolaryngol *45*:619, 1947.

WALTNER JG: Barrier membrane of the cochlear aqueduct. Histologic studies on the patency of the cochlear aqueduct. Arch Otolaryngol *47*:656, 1948.

WERNER C: *Das Labyrinth.* Bau, Funktion und Krankheiten des Innenohres vom Standpunkt einer experimentellen und vergleichenden Pathologie. Leipzig, Verlag Georg Thieme, 1940.

WERSÄLL J: Studies on the structure and innervation of the sensory epithelium of the cristae ampullares in the guinea pig. A light and electron microscopic investigation. Acta Otolaryngol (Stockh) Suppl *126*:1, 1956.

WEVER EG, LAWRENCE M: *Physiological Acoustics.* Princeton, Princeton University Press, 1954.

WIGAND ME, TRILLSCH K: Surgical anatomy of the sinus epitympani. Ann Otol Rhinol Laryngol *82*:378, 1973.

WILLIAMS HL: Latent or dormant disease in the pneumatic cell tracts of the temporal bone. Trans Am Acad Ophthalmol Otolaryngol 70:545, 1966.

WINSHIP T, KLOPP CT, JENKINS WH: Glomus-jugularis tumors. Cancer 1:441, 1948.

WOLFF D, BELLUCCI RJ: The human ossicular ligaments. Ann Otol Rhinol Laryngol 65:895, 1956.

WOLFF D, BELLUCCI RJ, EGGSTON AA: *Microscopic Anatomy of the Temporal Bone.* Baltimore, Williams & Wilkins, 1957.

WOLFF D, BELLUCCI RJ, EGGSTON AA: *Surgical and Microscopic Anatomy of the Temporal Bone.* New York, Hafner Publishing Company, 1971.

WOOD-JONES F, WEN I-C: The Development of the External Ear. J. Anat 68:525, 1934.

WRIGHT JLW, ETHOLM B: Anomalies of the middle-ear muscles. J Laryngol Otol 87:281, 1973.

WRIGHT JW JR, TAYLOR CC, McKAY DC: Variations in the course of the facial nerve as illustrated by tomography. Laryngoscope 77:717, 1967.

ZETTERGREN L, LINDSTROM J: Glomus tympanicum, its occurrence in man and its relation to middle ear tumors of carotid body type. Acta Pathol Microbiol Scand 28:157, 1951.

ZIEGELMAN EF: The cellular character of one hundred temporal bones: clinical and surgical significance. Ann Otol Rhinol Laryngol 44:3, 1935.

ZUCKERKANDL E: Zur Anatomie des Warzenfortsatzes. Monatschr Ohrenheilk 13:49, 1879.

Glossary

ACOUSTIC   *Greek:* akoustikos, sound or its perception.

AD   *Latin:* to or toward.

ADITUS   [*plural:* aditus; *possessive:* aditus] *Latin:* approach to, access.

ALDERMAN'S NERVE   The auricular branch of the vagus (Xth cranial nerve), so named because of the reflex coughing caused by mechanical stimulation of the skin of the external auditory canal. *Synonym:* Arnold's nerve.

AMPULLA   [*plural:* ampullae; *possessive:* ampullae] *Latin:* diminutive of amp(h)ora; little jar or jug. The normal dilated end of a semicircular canal or duct.

AN(N)ULUS   [*plural:* an(n)uluses or an(n)uli; *possessive:* an(n)uli] *Latin:* diminutive of anus; a ring-like structure.
   a. tympanicus, the fibrous annulus, the peripheral fibrous margin of the tympanic membrane. The term **a. fibrocartilagineus membranae tympani** is a misnomer, as this structure contains no cartilage.

ANTE   *Latin:* in front of or before.

ANTERIOR VERTICAL CANAL   The superior semicircular canal.

ANTRUM   [*plural:* antra; *possessive:* antri] *Latin:* cave.
   a. mastoideum, mastoid antrum.

APERTURA   [*plural:* aperturae; *possessive:* aperturae] *Latin:* the past participle of aperire, to open; an orifice, hole, or other opening.
   a. tympanica canaliculi chordae tympani, the aperture through which the chorda tympani nerve gains access to the middle ear.

AQU(A)EDUCTUS   [*plural:* aqu(a)eductus; *possessive:* aqu(a)eductus] *Latin:* combination of aqua (water) and ductus (duct); a conduit or a channel for fluid.
   a. of Cotugno, canal for the inferior cochlear vein. *Synonyms:* canal of Cotugno, first accessory canal of Siebenmann. **a. fallopii,** canal for the facial nerve. *Synonyms:* aqueduct of Fallopius; fallopian canal. **a. vestibuli,** the vestibular aqueduct.

ARNOLD, TUBAL BRANCH OF   Derivative of the tympanic plexus that ramifies in the anterolateral wall of the cartilage and mucosa of the eustachian tube.

ARNOLD'S NERVE   The auricular branch of the vagus (Xth cranial nerve). *Synonym:* Alderman's nerve.

ARTICULATIO   [*plural:* articulationes; *possessive:* articulationis] *Latin:* articulatus, past participle of articulare, to divide into joints. A joint between two bones.

AUDITORY TUBE   The eustachian tube. *Synonym:* pharyngotympanic tube.

AURICLE OR AURICULA   [*plural:* auricles or auriculae; *possessive:* auriculae] *Latin:* auricula, diminutive of auris; the external part of the ear, the pinna.

AURICULAR BRANCH OF THE VAGUS NERVE   *Synonyms:* Arnold's nerve, Alderman's nerve.

AURIS   [*plural:* aures; *possessive:* auris] *Latin:* ear.
   a. externa, the external ear. **a. interna,** the inner ear. **a. media,** the middle ear.

BASILAR PAPILLA   The organ of Corti. *Synonyms:* papilla of Huschke, spiral organ.

BASIS   [*plural:* basis; *possessive:* basis] *Latin:* pedestal or base.
   b. stapedis, the footplate of the stapes.

BAST, UTRICULO-ENDOLYMPHATIC VALVE OF   The utriculo-endolymphatic valve.

BECHTEREW, GANGLION OF   Ganglion in the vestibule for fibers going to the basal end of the organ of Corti.

BECHTEREW, NUCLEUS OF   Superior vestibular nucleus.

BILL'S BAR   Vertical crest of the fundus of the internal auditory canal used as an anatomic landmark during translabyrinthine surgery. Named for William House.

BLUE MANTLES OF MANASSE   Uniform, basophilic-staining bone deposit, particularly in the perivascular resorption spaces, commonly seen with otosclerosis.

BOCK, PHARYNGEAL NERVE OF   The pharyngeal branch of the sphenopalatine nerve. *Synonym:* rami pharyngei nervi vagi.

BOETTCHER (BÖTTCHER) CELLS   Cells that form a layer located between the basilar membrane and the outer sulcus cells.

BRANCHIAL ARCH CARTILAGE, FIRST   *Synonyms:* mandibular cartilage, Meckel's cartilage.

BRANCHIAL ARCH CARTILAGE, SECOND   *Synonyms:* hyoid cartilage, Reichert's cartilage.

BRESCHET'S HIATUS   *Synonyms:* helicotrema, Scarpa's hiatus.

CAECUM   [*plural:* caeca; *possessive:* caeci] *Latin:* blind pouch.
   c. cupulare, the blind, pouch-like, apical end of the cochlear duct just beyond the hamulus of the spiral lamina. **c. vestibulare,** the cul-de-sac basal end of the cochlear duct that occupies the cochlear recess of the vestibule.

CAJAL, INTERSTITIAL NUCLEUS OF   Nucleus of the medial longitudinal fasciculus.

CANALICULI PERFORANTES OF SCHUKNECHT   Tiny openings in the tympanic shelf of the osseous spiral lamina that connect the scala tympani with the intercellular fluid spaces within and surrounding the organ of Corti. *Synonym:* perilymph canaliculi.

CANALICULUS   [*plural:* canaliculi; *possessive:* canaliculi] *Latin:* diminutive of canalis; a conduit or channel.
   c. cochleae, the cochlear aqueduct. **c. tympanicus** (superior), the innominate canal for the lesser superficial petrosal nerve. **c. tympanicus** (inferior), the canal for Jacobson's nerve. **c. perforantes,** small open-

ings in the tympanic shelf of the osseous spiral lamina. **subarcuate c.,** petromastoid canal. *Synonym:* antrocerebellar canal of Chatellier.

CANALIS [*plural:* canales; *possessive:* canalis] *Latin:* channel.

c. mastoideus, a channel from the lateral wall of the jugular fossa carrying Arnold's nerve to the tympanomastoid fissure. **c. semicirculares ossei,** the bony semicircular canals. **c. spiralis modioli** (**c. spiralis cochleae**), Rosenthal's canal. *Synonym:* spiral canal of the modiolus.

CAPITULUM [*plural:* capitula; *possessive:* capituli] *Latin:* diminutive of caput (head).

c. mallei, the head of the malleus. **c. stapedis,** the head of the stapes.

CAUDA [*plural:* caudae; *possessive:* caudae] *Latin:* tail.

c. helicis, the most inferior portion of the helix of the cartilage of the pinna.

CAVUM [*plural:* cava; *possessive:* cavi] *Latin:* hole or cavity.

c. conchae, the inferior depression of the concha of the auricle that leads into the external auditory canal. **c. tympani,** the tympanic cavity.

CELLULA [*plural:* cellulae; *possessive:* cellulae] *Latin:* diminutive of cella; a small chamber, a cell.

c. mastoideae, the aerated honeycomb of the mastoid bone. **c. tympanicae,** the tympanic air cells.

CERUMEN *Latin:* cera (wax).

CHATELLIER, ANTROCEREBELLAR CANAL OF The petromastoid canal. *Synonym:* subarcuate canaliculus.

CHORDA [*plural:* chordae; *possessive:* chordae] *Latin:* cord or sinew.

c. tympani, a sensory branch of the facial nerve that stretches across the middle ear.

CITELLI, SINODURAL ANGLE OF The sinodural angle.

CLAUDIUS' CELLS Those supporting cells of the organ of Corti that line the outer spiral sulcus.

COCHLEA [*plural:* cochleae; *possessive:* cochleae] *Latin:* snail shell. The bony configuration of the organ of hearing.

COCHLEARE [*plural:* cochleares; *possessive:* cochlearis] *Latin:* spoon.

As cochleariformis: **processus c.,** the bony projection that cradles the tendon of the tensor tympani muscle as it extends to the neck of malleus.

COLLUM [*plural:* colla; *possessive:* colli] *Latin:* neck.

c. mallei, the neck of the malleus.

COLUMELLA [*plural:* columellae; *possessive:* columellae] *Latin:* small column.

c. cochleae, the modiolus.

COMMON CARDINAL VEINS The ducts of Cuvier.

CONCHA [*plural:* conchae; *possessive:* conchae] *Latin:* a shell-like structure.

c. auriculae, the deepest depression of the auricular cartilage.

CONDYLOID *Greek:* kondylos; a rounded articulatory prominence at the end of the bone, as in the condyloid process of the mandible. The anterior condyloid foramen refers to the tunnel that transmits the XIIth cranial nerve in the condyloid process of the occipital bone.

CORTI, HAIR CELLS OF Outer hair cells of the organ of Corti.

CORTI, MEMBRANE OF Tectorial membrane.

CORTI, ORGAN OF *Synonyms:* basilar papilla, papilla of Huschke, spiral organ.

CORTI, PILLARS OF Pillar cells. *Synonym:* pillars of Corti's organ.

CORTI, TUNNEL OF Triangular channel, also known as the inner tunnel, which is formed by the articulation of the heads of the inner and outer pillar cells.

CORTILYMPH Name given by Engström to his proposed "third lymph" of the inner ear. This fluid theoretically is found in the tunnel of Corti, the spaces of Nuel, the outer tunnel, and the spaces around the hair cells. This fluid is now believed to be perilymph, which reaches these spaces by penetrating the osseous spiral lamina through channels known as the canaliculi perforantes of Schuknecht.

COTUGNO, CANAL OF Canal for the inferior cochlear vein (vein at the cochlear aqueduct). *Synonym:* aqueduct of Cotugno; first accessory canal of Siebenmann.

COTUGNO, FLUID OF Name originally given to perilymph. Breschet in 1836 adopted the name perilymph and used the term endolymph to describe Scarpa's fluid.

CRIBROSE *Latin:* cribrum (sieve); used in the form cribrose or cribrosa.
   macula c. inferior, the small cribrose area deep in the singular canal that transmits the fibers of the posterior ampullary nerve. **macula c. media,** the perforated area at the posteromedial aspect of the fundus of the internal auditory canal that transmits the fibers of the saccular nerve. **macula c. superior,** the perforated area at the posterosuperior aspect of the fundus of the internal auditory canal above the falciform (transverse) crest that transmits the fibers of the utricular and superior ampullary nerves. *Synonym:* Mike's dot. **c. tractus spiralis,** the one-and-one-half-turn spiral perforated area in the anteroinferior part of the fundus of the internal auditory canal for transmission of the cochlear nerve fibers.

CRISTA [*plural:* cristae; *possessive:* cristae] *Latin:* crest.
   c. falciformis, the transverse crest of the internal auditory canal. **c. stapedis,** an intercrural ridge occasionally found on the tympanic aspect of the footplate of the stapes. **c. vestibuli,** the vertical crest that separates the spherical recess housing the saccule from the elliptical recess housing the utricle. **c. ampullaris,** the neuroepithelial crest in an ampulla of a semicircular canal.

CRUS [*plural:* crura; *possessive:* cruris] *Latin:* leg.
   c. anterius, the anterior leg of the stapes. **c. breve,** the short process of the incus. **c. commune,** the common duct formed by the superior and posterior canals as their nonampullated ends enter the vestibule. **c. curvilineum,** the posterior leg of the stapes. **c. helicis,** the oblique ridge of the auricular cartilage that divides the concha into a superior cymba conchae and an inferior cavum conchae. **c. longum,** the long process of the incus. **c. posterius,** the posterior leg of the stapes. **c. rectilineum,** the anterior leg of the stapes.
   Plural: **c. anthelicis,** divides the superior division of the anthelix into two ridges between which is a shallow concavity named the triangular fossa.

CUL-DE-SAC *Latin:* culus (bottom); *French:* blind alley, bottom of the sac. A sac-like cavity or tube that is open only at one end.

CUPULA [*plural:* cupulae; *possessive:* cupulae] *Latin:* the diminutive of cupa; a tub or vat.
   c. cristae ampullaris, the gelatinous cap of the crista of the ampulla of the semicircular duct. **c. cochleae,** the termination of the cochlear duct at the helicotrema just distal to the hamulus of the spiral lamina.

CUVIER, DUCTS OF common cardinal veins.

CYMBA [*plural:* cymbae; *possessive:* cymbae] *Latin:* a small boat.

c. conchae, the concave depression of the concha that lies superior to the crus of the helix.

DEITERS' CELLS Supporting cells of the outer hair cells. *Synonyms:* outer phalangeal cells; sustentacular cells.

DEITERS' NUCLEUS Lateral vestibular nucleus.

DORELLO, CANAL OF Channel in the dura between the petrous tip and the sphenoid bone through which the abducens nerve and inferior petrosal sinus enter the cavernous sinus.

DUCTUS [plural: ductus; possessive: ductus] *Latin:* a drawing or row. **d. cochlearis,** the cochlear duct (scala media). **d. endolymphaticus,** endolymphatic duct. *Synonym:* otic duct. **d. perilymphatici,** the periotic duct (within the cochlear aqueduct). **d. reuniens,** the duct that establishes a communication between the saccule and the cochlear duct. *Synonym:* Reichert's canal. **d. semicirculares,** the membranous semicircular canals. **d. utriculosaccularis,** an alternate name for the utricular duct.

DURA MATER *Latin:* dura (hard) and mater (mother). The tough, fibrous layer enveloping the leptomeninges, the brain, and the spinal cord.

EMINENTIA [*plural:* eminentiae; *possessive:* eminentiae] *Latin:* prominence.

e. arcuata, the arcuate eminence, which is the bulge of the superior semicircular canal located in the floor of the middle cranial fossa. **e. conchae,** the bulge on the medial aspect of the auricle that corresponds to the cavum conchae. **e. fossae triangularis,** the bulge on the medial aspect of the auricle that corresponds to the triangular fossa. **e. pyramidalis,** the pyramidal eminence from which the tendon of the stapedius muscle emerges. **e. scaphae,** the medially located bulge of the auricle created by the scapha of the concha.

ENDOLYMPH *Greek:* endon (within). The intramembranous inner ear fluid. *Synonyms:* Scarpa's fluid; otic fluid.

ENDOLYMPHATIC DUCT *Synonym:* otic duct.

EPITYMPANUM *Greek:* epi-, prefix meaning upon; therefore. That portion of the middle ear cavity that lies above a horizontal plane drawn through the superior aspect of the tympanic annulus.

EUSTACHIAN TUBE *Synonyms:* auditory tube, pharyngotympanic tube.

FACIAL RECESS (SINUS) *Synonyms:* posterior recess, suprapyramidal recess.

FALLOPIAN CANAL Canal for the facial nerve. *Synonyms:* aqueduct of Fallopius, aqu(a)eductus Fallopii.

FENESTRA [*plural:* fenestrae; *possessive:* fenestrae] *Latin:* window or opening.

f. cochleae, the round window. **f. rotunda,** the round window. **f. vestibuli,** the oval window.

FISSULA [*plural:* fissulae; *possessive:* fissulae] *Latin:* fissus, the past participle of findo, findere; a cleavage or splitting.

f. ante fenestram, the evagination of the perilymphatic space immediately anterior to the oval window.

FISSURA [*plural:* fissurae; *possessive:* fissurae] *Latin:* from fissus, the past participle form of findere; to split or cleave.

f. antitragohelicina, the deep groove in the auricular cartilage that separates the tail of the helix from the antitragus.

FISTULA [*plural:* fistulae; *possessive:* fistulae] *Latin:* abnormal passage or communication, ulcer.

FOLIANUS, PROCESSUS The anterior process of the malleus. *Synonym:* processus gracilis mallei.

FORAMEN [*plural:* foramina; *possessive:* foraminis] *Latin:* a hole or opening.

> jugular f., the opening at the base of the skull for the internal jugular vein. f. magnum, the passageway at the base of the skull for the spinal cord. f. mastoideum, opening posterior to the mastoid process for the mastoid emissary vein and an artery. f. ovale, the passageway that transmits the third (mandibular) division of the trigeminal (Vth cranial) nerve. f. rotundum, the opening that transmits the second (maxillary) division of the trigeminal nerve. f. singulare, the orifice of the singular canal for the posterior ampullary nerve located in the posteroinferior part of the internal auditory canal. *Synonyms:* foramen singular of Morgagni; solitary canal; singular canal.

FOSSA [*plural:* fossae; *possessive:* fossae] *Latin:* ditch or trench.

> f. incudis, the notch in the epitympanum that houses the short process of the incus. jugular f., the depression on the inferior aspect of the temporal bone that houses the jugular bulb. mandibular f., the depression, also known as the glenoid fossa, that accommodates the temporomandibular joint. f. mastoidea, the small depression immediately posterior to the suprameatal spine of Henle, medial to which lies the mastoid antrum. f. triangularis, the concavity between the crura of the anthelix.

FOSSULA [*plural:* fossulae; *possessive:* fossulae] *Latin:* diminutive of fossa, a ditch.

> f. fenestrae cochleae (f. cochlear fenestra), the round window niche. f. fenestrae vestibuli (f. vestibular fenestra), the oval window niche. f. post fenestram, the extension of the perilymphatic labyrinth posterior to the oval window. f. rotunda, the round window niche. f. subarcuata, subarcuate fossa.

FOVEA [*plural:* foveae; *possessive:* foveae] *Latin:* small pit.

> f. saccus endolymphaticus, the shallow depression on the posterior wall of the petrous bone (foveate fossa) that accommodates the intradural portion of the endolymphatic sac.

GANGLION [*plural:* ganglia (or ganglions)] *Greek:* a cyst-like tumor, a clustering of neurons generally outside the central nervous system.

> Corti's g., the acoustic ganglion. gasserian g., *Synonyms:* semilunar ganglion; trigeminal ganglion. g. geniculi, the geniculate ganglion of the facial nerve. Meckel's g., sphenopalatine ganglion. Scarpa's g., the vestibular ganglion. g. spirale cochleae, g. spirale nervi cochleae, g. spirale partis cochlearis nervi octavi, the spiral ganglion of the cochlear nerve.

GENICULUM [*plural:* genicula; *possessive:* geniculi] *Latin:* diminutive of genu; knee.

> g. nervus facialis, the sharp bend in the course of the facial nerve at the geniculate ganglion where the labyrinthine segment ends and the tympanic segment begins.

GERLACH, TUBAL TONSIL OF Lymphatic follicles in and about the pharyngeal aspect of the auditory tube described by Gerlach.

GLANDULAE [*plural:* glandulae; *possessive:* glandulae] *Latin:* glandula; a glandular swelling.

> g. mucosae, the mucous glands in the cartilaginous portion of the eustachian tube.

GLASERIAN FISSURE Petrotympanic fissure (suture).

GLIAL-SCHWANN SHEATH JUNCTION *Synonym:* Obersteiner-Redlich zone.

GRACILIS, PROCESSUS The anterior process of the malleus. *Synonyms:*

processus gracilis mallei, processus Folianus.

GRADENIGO'S SYNDROME Symptom complex consisting of abducens palsy, retro-orbital facial pain, and suppurative disease of the middle ear indicative of involvement of the abducens and trigeminal nerves in petrous apicitis.

GRENZSCHEIDEN *German:* thin, basophilic staining membranes that normally line the inner surfaces of the bony lacunae and canaliculi, as well as the walls of the vascular channels of the temporal bone.

GRUBER'S LIGAMENT Petroclinoid ligament.

HABENULA [*plural:* habenulae; *possessive:* habenulae] *Latin:* diminutive of habena; strip or rein.

   h. arcuata, the inner portion of the cochlear basilar membrane. **h. perforata,** foramina nervosa limbus laminae spiralis, the openings in the tympanic lip of the limbus permitting passage of the cochlear nerve fibers.

HALLER, PLEXUS OF Plexus formed chiefly by fibers from branches of the vagus nerve with a contribution of fibers from the glossopharyngeal nerve and sympathetic trunks; this plexus supplies motor, general sensory, and sympathetic innervation to the muscles and mucosa of the pharynx and soft palate, save for the tensor veli palatini muscle. *Synonym:* pharyngeal plexus.

HAMULUS [*plural:* hamuli; *possessive:* hamuli] *Latin:* little hook.

   h. cochleae, h. laminae spiralis, the hooked apical end of the osseous spiral lamina. **h. pterygoideus,** a hook-like process on the inferior extremity of the medial pterygoid plate of the sphenoid bone, around which the tendon of the tensor veli palatini muscle passes.

HAVERSIAN SYSTEM Consists of a haversian canal and its concentrically arranged lamellae, comprising the basic unit of structure (osteon) of compact bone. A haversian system is directed primarily in the long axis of the bone.

HELD, RANDFASERNETZ OF *Synonyms:* Randfasernetz, Randfadennetz.

HELICOTREMA *Greek:* helico, form of helix (snail or coil) and trema (hole). The passage whereby the scala tympani communicates with the scala vestibuli at the apex of the cochlea. *Synonyms:* Breschet's hiatus; Scarpa's hiatus.

HELIX *Greek:* coil. The most peripheral arc of the free margin of the auricle.

HENLE'S SUPRAMEATAL SPINE Small spine at the posterosuperior margin of the external auditory canal.

HENSEN'S CELLS Tall supporting cells located in the organ of Corti external to the outer hair cells.

HENSEN'S STRIPE In histologic sections a basophilically staining band at the middle of the undersurface of the tectorial membrane. In its normal position, this stripe is located at and attached to the border cells just internal to the inner hair cells.

HIATUS [*plural:* hiatus; *possessive:* hiatus] *Latin:* an opening.

   h. canalis facialis, the dehiscence in the middle cranial fossa that transmits the greater superficial petrosal nerve, occasionally leaving the geniculate ganglion open at the floor of the middle cranial fossa.

HILLOCKS OF HIS Six developmental hillocks of the auricle that are derived from the first and second branchial arches.

HITSELBERGER'S SIGN Anesthesia of the posterior wall of the external auditory canal innervated by a sensory branch of the facial nerve.

HORIZONTAL CANAL The lateral semicircular canal.

HOWSHIP'S LACUNAE Excavations produced by osteoclastic erosion of bone.

HUGUIER, CANAL OF Channel beginning in the petrotympanic fissure through which the chorda tympani nerve passes as it exits the tympanic cavity anteriorly. *Synonym:* iter chordae anterius.

HUSCHKE, FORAMEN OF The lower of the two openings created by the partitioning of the tympanic annulus in the development of the tympanic ring; it is usually closed by early childhood.

HUSCHKE, PAPILLA OF The organ of Corti. *Synonyms:* basilar papilla, spiral organ.

HUSCHKE, STRIA VASCULARIS OF *Synonym:* stria vascularis.

HUSCHKE'S TEETH Tall cells covering the limbus.

HYOID CARTILAGE The second branchial arch cartilage. *Synonym:* Reichert's cartilage.

HYRTL'S FISSURE Extends from the hypotympanum just inferior to the round window niche to the posterior cranial fossa paralleling the cochlear aqueduct. (We have been unable to find Hyrtl's description of this fissure.) *Synonym:* tympanomeningeal hiatus.

INCISURA [*plural:* incisurae; *possessive:* incisurae] *Latin:* incisum, the past participal of incidere; to cut into or to cut open.

    i. anterior, the concavity that separates the crus of the helix from the tragus of the auricle. **i. intertragica,** the depression dividing the tragus from the antitragus. **i. mastoidea,** the digastric groove. **i. Rivini,** notch of Rivinus. *Synonym:* incisura tympanica. **i. tympanica.** *Synonyms:* incisura rivini; notch of Rivinus.

    plural: **i. cartilaginis meatus acustici externi,** the two fissures located in the anterior wall of the fibrocartilaginous part of the external auditory canal. *Synonym:* Santorini's fissures.

INCUS [*plural:* incudes; *possessive:* incudis] *Latin:* anvil. The middle ossicle in the sound transmission mechanism, so named because of its resemblance to an anvil.

INFERIOR COCHLEAR VEIN Vein at the cochlear aqueduct. *Synonym:* vena aquaeductus cochleae.

INFRAPYRAMIDAL RECESS The sinus tympani.

INTERHYAL(E) *Latin:* inter (between); *Greek:* hyoeides (U-shaped). During embryonic growth, a small shaft of bone that facilitates the articulation of the cornu of the hyoid with Meckel's cartilage, connecting the hyomandibular and the remainder of the hyoid in some vertebrates.

INTERNAL AUDITORY ARTERY Labyrinthine artery.

ISTHMUS [*plural:* isthmi; *possessive:* isthmi] *Latin:* derived from the Greek isthmos, narrow passage.

ITER [*plural:* itineres; *possessive:* itineris] *Latin:* a walk or a way.

    i. chordae anterius, the opening by which the chorda tympani nerve leaves the middle ear cavity. *Synonym:* canal of Huguier. **i. chordae posterius,** the opening by which the chorda tympani nerve gains access to the middle ear cavity.

JACOBSON'S NERVE Tympanic branch of the glossopharyngeal (IXth cranial) nerve. *Synonym:* tympanic nerve.

KOERNER'S (KÖRNER'S) FLAP Surgically created, laterally based, pedicled flap of skin of the posterior wall of the external auditory canal.

KOERNER'S (KÖRNER'S) SEPTUM The bony partition dividing the mastoid into a lateral squamous and medial petrous portions. *Synonym:* petrosquamosal septum.

LABYRINTHINE ARTERY *Synonym:* internal auditory artery.

LABYRINTHUS [*plural:* labyrinthi; *possessive:* labyrinthi] *Latin:* a maze or labyrinth.

> **l. membranaceus,** the membranous labyrinth of the inner ear. **l. osseus,** the bony labyrinth.

LACUNA [*plural:* lacunae; *possessive:* lacunae] *Latin:* pool, a small pit or hollow cavity.

LAMINA [*plural:* laminae; *possessive:* laminae] *Latin:* a thin plate.

> **l. basilaris,** the basilar membrane of the cochlea. **l. lateralis,** the lateral plate of cartilage of the eustachian tube. **l. medialis,** the medial plate of cartilage of the eustachian tube. **l. membranacea,** the band of connective tissue that defines the cartilaginous eustachian tube inferiorly and laterally. **l. spiralis ossea,** the osseous spiral lamina, the spiral projection that winds about the modiolus to end in the apex of the cochlea at the hamulus.

LATERAL SEMICIRCULAR CANAL *Synonym:* horizontal canal.

LATERAL VESTIBULAR NUCLEUS *Synonym:* Deiters' nucleus.

LEIDY, SCUTUM OF Bony lamina of the squama that comprises the lateral wall of the epitympanic recess. *Synonym:* lateral epitympanic bony wall.

LENTICULAR PROCESS OF THE INCUS *Synonyms:* os orbiculare, Sylvian apophysis.

LEVATOR [*plural:* levatores; *possessive:* levatoris] *Latin:* levare; to raise or lift.

> **l. veli palatini,** the muscle that, in conjunction with the tensor veli palatini, opens the eustachian tube at its pharyngeal orifice. *Synonym:* retrotubal muscle of Sebileau.

LIGAMENTUM [*plural:* ligamenta; *possessive:* ligamenti] *Latin:* a bandage or bond.

> **l. anulare stapedis,** the annular ligament of the stapes that anchors the footplate in the oval window. **l. auriculare anterius,** the anterior extrinsic ligament of the auricle. **l. auriculare posterius,** the posterior extrinsic ligament of the auricle. **l. auriculare superius,** the superior extrinsic ligament of the auricle. **l. incudis posterius,** the ligament that seats the short process of the incus in the incudal fossa to form the posterior axis of ossicular rotation. **l. mallei anterius,** the anterior ligament of the malleus that accompanies the anterior malleal process to form the anterior axis of ossicular rotation. This ligament must be differentiated from the anterior suspensory ligament of the malleus, which lies at a more superior level and tethers the head of the malleus to the anterior wall of the epitympanum. **l. mallei laterale,** the suspensory ligament that attaches the neck of the malleus to the margins of the tympanic notch. **l. mallei superius,** the suspensory ligament that connects the head of the malleus to the tegmen of the epitympanum. **l. spirale cochleae,** the thickened periosteum of the outer wall of the bony cochlea that acts as the outer supporting wall for the cochlear duct (spiral ligament).

LIMBUS [*plural:* limbi; *possessive:* limbi] *Latin:* border or fringe.

> **l. laminae spiralis osseae,** the fibroepithelial mound to which the tectorial and Reissner's membranes attach. **l. membranae tympani,** the thickened rim of the tympanic membrane.

LOBULUS [*plural:* lobuli; *possessive:* lobuli] *Latin:* diminutive of lobus; lobe.

> **l. auriculae,** the lobule of the auricle.

LUCAS, GROOVE OF Groove in the spina angularis of the sphenoid bone for the chorda tympani nerve.

LUSCHKA'S TONSIL *Synonyms:* nasopharyngeal lymphoid mass; pharyngeal tonsil.

LYMPHA [*plural:* lymphae; *possessive:* lymphae] *Latin:* water.

MACEWEN'S TRIANGLE Triangle formed at the lateral-most surface of the temporal bone by the posterior extension of the upper border of the root of the zygoma (the temporal line), the posterior wall of the external canal, and a line that connects the two; this triangle is lateral to the mastoid antrum. *Synonym:* suprameatal triangle.

MACULA [*plural:* maculae; *possessive:* maculae] *Latin:* spot or mark.
　　m. acustica sacculi, the sense organ of the saccule. **m. acustica utriculi,** the sense organ of the utricle. **m. cribrosa inferior,** the perforated area penetrated by fibers of the posterior ampullary nerve. **m. cribrosa media,** the perforated area of the spherical recess through which nerve fibers pass to the macula of the saccule. **m. cribrosa superior,** the perforated area of the elliptical recess through which nerve fibers pass to the utricle and ampullae of the superior and lateral canals. *Synonym:* Mike's dot. **m. sacculi,** the sense organ of the saccule. **m. utriculi,** the sense organ of the utricle.

MALLEUS [*plural:* mallei; *possessive:* mallei] *Latin:* hammer or mallet. The most lateral of the ossicles.

MALLEUS, ANTERIOR PROCESS OF *Synonyms:* processus Folianus, processus gracilis mallei.

MANASSE, BLUE MANTLES OF *Synonym:* blue mantles.

MANDIBULAR CARTILAGE *Synonyms:* first branchial arch cartilage, Meckel's cartilage.

MANUBRIUM [*plural:* manubria; *possessive:* manubrii] *Latin:* handle.
　　m. mallei, the descending shaft of the malleus.

MEATUS [*plural:* meatus, meatuses; *possessive:* meatus] *Latin:* a passage.
　　m. acusticus externus, the external auditory canal. **m. acusticus externus cartilagineus,** the fibrocartilaginous portion of the external auditory canal. **m. acusticus externus osseus,** the bony portion of the external auditory canal. **m. acusticus internus,** the internal auditory canal.

MECKEL'S CARTILAGE First branchial arch cartilage. *Synonym:* mandibular cartilage.

MECKEL'S GANGLION *Synonym:* sphenopalatine ganglion.

MEMBRANA [*plural:* membranae; *possessive:* membranae] *Latin:* a thin film or membrane.
　　m. obturatoria stapedis, the veil of mucous membrane that occasionally bridges the obturator foramen. **m. tympani,** the tympanic membrane. **m. tympani secundaria,** the round window membrane. **m. vestibularis,** Reissner's membrane. *Synonym:* vestibular membrane.

MIKE'S DOT Macula cribrosa superior that transmits nerve fibers to the utricle and ampullae of the superior and lateral semicircular canals. It is used as a landmark for the lateral end of the internal auditory canal in translabyrinthine surgery. Named for Michael Glasscock.

MODIOLUS [*plural:* modioli; *possessive:* modioli] *Latin:* hub of a wheel. The tapered pillar that constitutes the central support of the cochlea. *Synonym:* columella cochleae.

MORGAGNI, FORAMEN SINGULAR OF Foramen for the posterior ampullary nerve. *Synonyms:* foramen singulare; singular canal; solitary canal.

MORGAGNI, SINUS OF Gap between the upper border of the superior pharyngeal constrictor muscle and the base of the skull that transmits the levator veli palatini muscle and the eustachian tube.

MORIAT, GANGLION OF Ganglion cells located medially in the perimysium of the tensor tympani muscle.

NASOPHARYNGEAL LYMPHOID MASS *Synonyms:* Luschka's tonsil, pharyngeal tonsil.

NERVUS [*plural:* nervi; *possessive:* nervi] *Latin:* string or wire.
> **n. acusticus,** the VIIIth cranial nerve, both cochlear and vestibular divisions. **n. ampullaris canalis lateralis,** the nerve fibers supplying the ampulla of the lateral canal. **n. ampullaris canalis posterior,** the nerve fibers supplying the ampulla of the posterior canal. **n. ampullaris canalis superior,** the nerve fibers supplying the ampulla of the superior canal. **n. cochleae,** the cochlear nerve. **n. facialis,** the VIIth cranial nerve. **n. intermedius,** the nerve of Wrisberg. **n. petrosus superficialis major,** the greater superficial petrosal nerve. **n. saccularis,** the saccular nerve. **n. stapedius,** the nerve to the stapedius muscle. **n. tensoris tympani,** the nerve to the tensor tympani muscle. **n. utricularis,** the utricular nerve. **n. vestibularis,** the vestibular nerve (with either **inferioris** or **superioris**). **n. vestibulocochlearis,** the VIIIth cranial nerve.

NODULUS [*plural:* noduli; *possessive:* noduli] *Latin:* diminutive of nodus; a knob. A small knot, or irregular rounded lump.
> **n. lymphatici tubarii,** the lymphatic tissue of the eustachian tube.

NUCLEUS, LATERAL VESTIBULAR *Synonym:* Deiters' nucleus.

NUCLEUS OF THE MEDIAL LONGITUDINAL FASCICULUS *Synonym:* interstitial nucleus of Cajal.

NUEL, SPACES OF Spaces between the processes of the phalangeal cells in the organ of Corti.

OBERSTEINER-REDLICH ZONE Transition zone between peripheral myelin and central oligodendrital myelin of the cranial nerves. *Synonym:* glial-Schwann sheath junction.

OLIVOCOCHLEAR BUNDLE Efferent nerve fibers passing from neurons in the region of the olive to the cochlea. *Synonym:* Rasmussen's bundle.

OORT'S ANASTOMOSIS Anastomosis between the saccular branch of the inferior vestibular nerve and the cochlear nerve. Part of the olivocochlear (Rasmussen's) bundle. *Synonym:* vestibulocochlear anastomosis.

ORGANUM [*plural:* organa; *possessive:* organi] *Latin:* instrument or organ.
> **o. spirale,** the organ of Corti. *Synonyms:* basilar papilla; papilla of Huschke; spiral organ. **o. vestibulocochleare,** the statoacoustic organ (embryologic connotation).

OS ORBICULARE *Synonyms:* lenticular process of the incus, Sylvian apophysis.

OSTIUM [*plural:* ostia; *possessive:* ostii] *Latin:* an opening.
> **o. pharyngeum tubae auditivae,** the pharyngeal opening of the eustachian tube. **o. tympanicum tubae auditivae,** the tympanic orifice of the eustachian tube.

OSTMANN, LATERAL FAT PAD (BODY) OF Body of adipose tissue interspersed between the lateral aspect of the fibrocartilaginous eustachian tube and the tensor veli palatini muscle (Ostmann, 1893).

OTIC DUCT The endolymphatic duct.

OTOCONIA *Greek:* ous, ot- (ear); konis (dust). The calcium carbonate crystals of the otolithic organs.

OUTER HAIR CELLS OF THE ORGAN OF CORTI *Synonym:* hair cells of Corti.

PAPILLA, BASILAR The organ of Corti. *Synonyms:* papilla of Huschke, spiral organ.

PAPILLA OF HUSCHKE The organ of Corti. *Synonyms:* basilar papilla, spiral organ.

PARIES [*plural:* parietes; *possessive:* parietis] *Latin:* wall (of a house).
p. caroticus, the carotid (anterior) wall of the middle ear. **p. jugularis,** the jugular (inferior) wall of the middle ear. **p. labyrinthicus,** the labyrinthine (medial) wall of the middle ear. **p. mastoideus,** the mastoid (posterior) wall of the middle ear. **p. membranaceus,** the membranous (lateral) wall of the middle ear. **p. tegmentalis,** the roof of the middle ear. **p. vestibularis ductus cochlearis,** the membrane that separates the scala media from the scala vestibuli. *Synonyms:* membrana vestibularis; Reissner's membrane; vestibular membrane.

PARS [*plural:* partes; *possessive:* partis] *Latin:* part or portion.
p. cartilaginae tubae auditivae, the cartilaginous portion of the eustachian tube. **p. flaccida,** the flaccid portion of the tympanic membrane located superior to the lateral process of the malleus. *Synonym:* Shrapnell's membrane. **p. mastoideae,** the mastoid part of the temporal bone. **p. petrosa,** the petrous portion of the temporal bone. **p. propria,** the middle (fibrous) layer of the tympanic membrane. **p. squamosa,** the squamous portion of the temporal bone. **p. tensa,** the tense vibrating part of the tympanic membrane. **p. tympanica,** the tympanic portion of the temporal bone.

PERILYMPH *Greek:* peri (around). The inner ear fluid between the bony and membranous labyrinths. *Synonym:* fluid of Cotugno.

PERILYMPH CANALICULI *Synonym:* canaliculi perforantes of Schuknecht.

PERILYMPHATIC DUCT *Synonym:* periotic duct.

PERIOTIC DUCT Membranous tube within the cochlear aqueduct. *Synonym:* perilymphatic duct.

PETROCLINOID LIGAMENT *Synonym:* Gruber's ligament.

PETROMASTOID CANAL *Synonyms:* antrocerebellar canal of Chatellier, subarcuate canaliculus.

PETROSQUAMOSAL FISSURE (SUTURE) Narrow hiatus extending from the floor of the middle cranial fossa that corresponds to the union of the petrous and squamous portions of the temporal bone.

PETROSQUAMOSAL SEPTUM *Synonym:* Koerner's (Körner's) septum.

PETROTYMPANIC FISSURE (suture) Glaserian fissure.

PETROUS *Latin:* rock-like.
p. pyramid, the petrous portion of the temporal bone.

PHALANGEAL CELLS, OUTER *Synonyms:* Deiters' cells, sustentacular cells.

PHARYNGEAL NERVE OF BOCK Pharyngeal branch of the sphenopalatine nerve that supplies the superior wall of the pharyngeal orifice of the eustachian tube. *Synonym:* rami pharyngei nervi vagi.

PHARYNGEAL PLEXUS *Synonym:* plexus of Haller.

PHARYNGEAL RECESS *Synonym:* fossa of Rosenmüller.

PHARYNGEAL TONSIL *Synonyms:* Luschka's tonsil, nasopharyngeal lymphoid mass.

PHARYNGOTYMPANIC TUBE *Synonyms:* auditory tube, eustachian tube.

PILLAR CELLS Supporting cells of the organ of Corti occurring in inner and outer rows to form the inner tunnel (Corti's tunnel). *Synonyms:* pillars of Corti, pillars of Corti's organ.

PINNA [*plural:* pinnae; *possessive:* pinnae] *Latin:* a feather or fin. The external part of the ear, the auricle.

PLEXUS [*plural:* plexus; *possessive:* plexus] *Latin:* past participle of plectere, to plait or braid; a network.

p. tympanicus, the tympanic plexus of nerves on the promontory of the middle ear.

PLICA [*plural:* plicae; *possessive:* plicae] *Latin:* plicare, to fold; a fold.
p. incudis, the variably present fold of mucosa that extends from the body and short crus of the incus to the tegmen of the tympanic cavity. **p. mallearis anterior,** the variably present membranous fold that extends from the tympanic membrane to cover the anterior process and anterior ligament of the malleus as well as the adjacent chorda tympani nerve. **p. mallearis posterior,** the variably present membrane that extends between the posterior wall of the tympanic cavity and the manubrium of the malleus to surround the lateral ligament of the malleus and the posterior aspect of the chorda tympani nerve. **p. stapedis,** the variably present membranous fold that extends from the posterior wall of the middle ear to surround the stapes.

PONTICULUS [*plural:* ponticuli; *possessive:* ponticuli] *Latin:* diminutive of bridge. The bony bridge that extends from the posterior wall of the middle ear near the base of the pyramidal eminence to the promontory and forms the superior limit of the sinus tympani.

POST *Latin:* behind.

POSTERIOR RECESS Facial recess (sinus). *Synonym:* suprapyramidal recess.

POSTERIOR VERTICAL CANAL *Synonym:* posterior semicircular canal.

PROCESSUS [*plural:* processus; *possessive:* processus] *Latin:* an advance.
p. anterior. *Synonyms:* anterior process of the malleus; processus Folianus; processus gracilis mallei. **p. cochleariformis,** the cochleariform process. **p. lateralis mallei,** the lateral process of the malleus. **p. lenticularis.** *Synonyms:* lenticular process of the incus; os orbiculare; Sylvian apophysis.

PROMINENTIA [*plural:* prominentiae; *possessive:* prominentiae] *Latin:* prominens, a projection or headland.
p. canalis facialis, the bulge of the facial nerve canal as it courses in its tympanic segment. **p. canalis semicircularis lateralis,** the bulge of the lateral semicircular canal on the medial aspect of the tympanic cavity and mastoid antrum. **p. mallearis,** the lateral process of the malleus. **p. styloidea,** an eminence on the floor of the tympanic cavity that represents the root of the styloid process.

PRUSSAK'S SPACE Superior recess of the tympanic membrane. The superior tympanic recess is limited by the pars flaccida, the lateral malleal ligament, and the anterior and posterior malleal folds. *Synonyms:* Prussak's pouch; superior tympanic recess.

RAMI PHARYNGEI NERVI VAGI The pharyngeal branch of the sphenopalatine nerve. *Synonym:* pharyngeal nerve of Bock.

RANDFASERNETZ OF HELD Refers to the portion of the tectorial membrane that blankets the organ of Corti on the "slope of Hensen's cells" and additionally an outer sheet that passes as far as the base of Hensen's cells. In some specimens this sheet seems to cross the outer sulcus and to extend to the spiral prominence (Lawrence, 1981). *Synonym:* Randfadennetz (Kolmer, 1927).

RASMUSSEN'S BUNDLE The olivocochlear bundle.

RECESSUS [*plural:* recessus; *possessive:* recessus] *Latin:* a secluded spot or inner room.
r. cochlearis, the concavity delimited by two limbs of the vestibular crest that houses the blind end (vestibular cecum) of the cochlear duct. **r. ellipticus,** the recess of the posterior and superior aspects of the medial wall of the vestibule that houses the utricle. **r. membranae tympani superior,** Prussak's pouch. *Synonyms:* Prussak's space; supe-

rior tympanic recess. **r. membranae tympani anterior** or **posterior,** the anterior and posterior pouches of von Tröltsch (Troeltsch). **r. sphericus,** the round depression on the medial wall of the vestibule that houses the saccular macula.

REICHERT'S BAR   Cartilaginous and osseous remnant of Reichert's cartilage that persists at least until early infancy; located posteromedial to the facial nerve.

REICHERT'S CANAL   The ductus reuniens.

REICHERT'S CARTILAGE   Second branchial arch cartilage. *Synonym:* hyoid cartilage.

REISSNER'S MEMBRANE   Vestibular membrane that forms the anterior wall of the cochlear duct, bridging the space from the anterior edge of the spiral ligament to the inner margin of the limbus. Named by Kölliker (1861). *Synonyms:* membrana vestibularis; paries vestibularis ductus cochlearis.

RETICULUM   [*plural:* reticula; *possessive:* reticuli] *Latin:* diminutive of rete, net.

RIVINUS, NOTCH OF   Superior deficiency in the tympanic ring that acts as the superior attachment of the pars flaccida of the tympanic membrane. *Synonyms:* incisura rivini; tympanic incisura.

ROSENMÜLLER, FOSSA OF   Recess in the nasopharynx located posterior to the torus tubarius, the prominence of the eustachian tube. *Synonym:* pharyngeal recess.

ROSENTHAL'S CANAL   Canal in the modiolus for the spiral ganglion. *Synonyms:* canalis spiralis cochleae; canalis spiralis modioli; spiral canal of the modiolus.

RÜDINGER'S SAFETY TUBE   A small potential space seen superiorly on transverse section of the cartilaginous portion of the eustachian tube. *Synonyms:* security canal of Rüdinger; Sicherheitsrohr.

SACCULUS   [*plural:* sacculi; *possessive:* sacculi] *Latin:* diminutive of saccus, a bag or pouch. The saccule.

SACCUS   [*plural:* sacci; *possessive:* sacci] *Latin:* bag.
   s. endolymphaticus, the endolymphatic sac.

SALPINGOPALATINE FOLD OF TORTUAL   Extension of the anterior lip of the eustachian tube onto the lateral wall of the nasopharynx.

SCALA   [*plural:* scalae; *possessive:* scalae] *Latin:* staircase.
   s. media, the middle compartment of the cochlea (cochlear duct). **s. tympani,** the perilymphatic compartment of the cochlea located posterior to the scala media. **s. vestibuli,** the perilymphatic compartment of the cochlea anterior to the scala media.

SCAPHA   [*plural:* scaphae; *possessive:* scaphae] *Latin:* a small boat. The scaphoid fossa of the auricle. *Synonym:* fossa helicis.

SCARPA'S FLUID   Breschet (1836) renamed it endolymph. *Synonym:* otic fluid.

SCARPA'S GANGLION   Peripheral ganglion of the vestibular nerve.

SCARPA'S HIATUS   The helicotrema. *Synonym:* Breschet's hiatus.

SCHUKNECHT, CANALICULI PERFORANTES OF   *Synonyms:* perilymph canaliculi, canaliculi perforantes.

SCUTUM   [*plural:* scuta; *possessive:* scuti] *Latin:* shield. The part of the squamous portion of the temporal bone that forms the lateral wall of the epitympanic recess.

SEBILEAU, RETROTUBAL MUSCLE OF   *Synonym:* levator veli palatini.

SECURITY CANAL OF RÜDINGER   *Synonyms:* Rüdinger's safety tube, Sicherheitsrohr.

SEMILUNAR GANGLION *Synonyms:* trigeminal ganglion, gasserian ganglion.

SEPTUM [*plural:* septa; *possessive:* septi] *Latin:* a partition or barrier.
 mucosal s., any of the multiple mucosal folds that subdivide the tympanic cavity. **s. canalis musculotubarii,** the superiorly located septum in the osseous portion of the eustachian tube that separates its lumen from the tensor tympani muscle.

SHAMBAUGH, GLANDS OF The modified epithelium along the outer wall of the cochlear duct in the region of the stria vascularis which, in fetal development, resembles a glandular epithelium.

SHRAPNELL'S MEMBRANE Pars flaccida of the tympanic membrane.

SICHERHEITSROHR *Synonyms:* Rüdinger's safety tube, security canal of Rüdinger.

SIEBENMANN, FIRST ACCESSORY CANAL OF *Synonyms:* aqueduct of Cotugno, canal of Cotugno.

SINGULAR CANAL Canal for the posterior ampullary nerve. *Synonyms:* foramen singulare; foramen singular of Morgagni; solitary canal.

SINODURAL ANGLE OF CITELLI Angle between the middle cranial fossa superiorly and the posterior cranial fossa and sigmoid sinus posteriorly. It marks the position of the superior petrosal sinus at the juncture of the dura of the middle and posterior cranial fossae. *Synonym:* sinodural angle.

SINUS [*plural:* sinus; *possessive:* sinus] *Latin:* a hollow or valley.
 facial s., the facial recess. *Synonyms:* posterior recess; suprapyramidal recess. **s. posterior,** a depression between the posterior iter of the chorda tympani nerve and the pyramidal eminence. **s. tympani (tympanic s.),** the depression located in the medial wall of the middle ear, posterior to the round and oval windows, medial to the facial nerve, and bounded by the ponticulus superiorly and the subiculum inferiorly. *Synonym:* infrapyramidal recess.

SOLITARY CANAL *Synonyms:* foramen singulare, foramen singular of Morgagni, singular canal.

SPHENOPALATINE GANGLION *Synonym:* Meckel's ganglion.

SPINA [*plural:* spinae; *possessive:* spinae] *Latin:* thorn or spine.
 s. helicis, a small projection of cartilage that extends anteriorly from the crus of the helix of the ear. **s. tympanica major,** the anterior spine of the bony tympanic ring at the notch of Rivinus. **s. tympanica minor,** the posterior spine of the bony tympanic ring at the notch of Rivinus.

SPIRAL CANAL OF THE MODIOLUS Rosenthal's canal. *Synonym:* canalis spiralis cochleae.

SPIRAL ORGAN The organ of Corti. *Synonyms:* basilar papilla, papilla of Huschke.

SQUAMA [*plural:* squamae; *possessive:* squamae] *Latin:* a scale or plate-like structure. The portion of the temporal bone that partially forms the lateral bony wall of the middle cranial fossa and part of the mastoid.

STRATUM [*plural:* strata; *possessive:* strati] *Latin:* a covering or a pavement, a sheet-like mass of nearly uniform thickness.
 s. cutaneum, the epidermal (outer) layer of the tympanic membrane. **s. mucosum,** the mucosal (inner) layer of the tympanic membrane. **s. radiatum,** the fibrous (middle) layer of the tympanic membrane.

STRIA [*plural:* striae; *possessive:* striae] *Latin:* channel or groove.
 s. mallearis, the pale white streak seen upon otoscopic visualization of the tympanic membrane that represents the manubrium of the malleus. **s. vascularis,** the highly specialized and vascularized spiral struc-

ture located on the internal surface of the spiral ligament between the attachment of Reissner's membrane and the spiral prominence. *Synonym:* stria vascularis of Huschke.

SUBARCUATE CANALICULUS *Synonyms:* antrocerebellar canal of Chatellier, petromastoid canal.

SUBICULUM [*plural:* subicula; *possessive:* subiculi] *Latin:* diminutive of subex, a support or underlayer.

    s. promontorii, the ridge of bone inferior and posterior to the round window that defines the inferior limit of the sinus tympani.

SULCUS [*plural:* sulci; *possessive:* sulci] *Latin:* sulcus, a groove or furrow.

    s. anthelicis transversus, the depression on the medial aspect of the auricle corresponding to the anthelix. **s. auriculae posterior,** the depression that separates the antitragus from the anthelix. **s. cruris helicis,** the depression of the medial aspect of the auricle corresponding to the crus of the helix. **s. tympanicus,** the groove in the tympanic bone to which the tympanic membrane is attached.

SUPERIOR SEMICIRCULAR CANAL *Synonym:* anterior vertical canal.

SUPERIOR TYMPANIC RECESS *Synonyms:* Prussak's pouch, Prussak's space.

SUPERIOR VESTIBULAR NUCLEUS *Synonym:* nucleus of Bechterew.

SUPRAMEATAL SPINE *Synonym:* Henle's suprameatal spine.

SUPRAMEATAL TRIANGLE *Synonym:* Macewen's triangle.

SUPRAPYRAMIDAL RECESS Facial recess (sinus). *Synonym:* posterior recess.

SUSTENTACULAR CELLS Deiters' cells. *Synonym:* outer phalangeal cells.

SYLVIAN APOPHYSIS Lenticular process of the incus. *Synonyms:* os orbiculare; processus lenticularis.

SYNDESMOSIS [*plural:* syndesmoses; *possessive:* syndesmosis] *Latin:* from the Greek syndesmos, ligament.

    s. tympanostapedia, the stapediovestibular articulation.

TECTORIAL MEMBRANE *Synonym:* membrane of Corti.

TEGMEN [*plural:* tegmines; *possessive:* tegminis] *Latin:* a roof or cover.

    t. mastoideum, the roof of the mastoid. **t. tympani,** the roof of the middle ear cavity.

TENSOR *Latin:* tensio, tendere, to stretch.

    t. tympani, the middle ear muscle that forms a tendinous attachment to the malleus.

TENTORIUM [*plural:* tentoria; *possessive:* tentorii] *Latin:* a tent.

    t. cerebelli, the layer of dura mater that serves as a roof for the cerebellum and also acts as a support for the occipital lobes. It encloses the transverse venous sinus posteriorly.

TORTUAL, SALPINGOPALATINE FOLD OF Extension of the anterior lip of the eustachian tube onto the lateral wall of the nasopharynx.

TRACTUS [*plural:* tractus; *possessive:* tractus] *Latin:* a trail.

    t. tegmentalis centralis, that area of the medial wall of the vestibule through which nerves pass to the cochlea of the inner ear. *Synonym:* tractus spiralis foraminosus.

TRAGUS [*plural:* tragi; *possessive:* tragi] *Latin:* from the Greek tragos, goat (apparently from the resemblance of the hairs of the tragus to a goat's beard). The singular form is used to refer to that projection of cartilage that is located at the anterior aspect of the external auditory meatus. The plural form is used to refer to the hairs of the auricle, especially those on the tragus.

TRAUTMANN'S TRIANGLE Area of the mastoid bounded posteriorly by the lateral venous sinus, superiorly by the tegmen and superior petrosal sinus, and anteriorly by the bony labyrinth.

TRIGEMINAL GANGLION   *Synonyms:* semilunar ganglion, gasserian ganglion.

TUBA   [*plural:* tubae; *possessive:* tubae] *Latin:* Roman war trumpet.
   t. auditiva, the eustachian tube. *Synonyms:* auditory tube; pharyngotympanic tube.

TUBERCULUM   [*plural:* tubercula; *possessive:* tuberculi] *Latin:* diminutive of tuber, a lump or swelling.
   t. auriculae, the Darwinian tubercle, a variably present protrusion on the posterosuperior aspect of the free margin of the helix of the auricle representing the homolog for the tip of the auricle of lower mammals.
   t. supratragicum, a small protrusion of the anterior aspect of the auricle just superior to the tragus.

TUNICA   [*plural:* tunicae; *possessive:* tunicae] *Latin:* a sheath or tunic.
   t. mucosa, the mucous membrane lining of the eustachian tube. **t. mucosa cavi tympani,** the mucous membrane lining of the tympanic cavity.

TYMPANIC INCISURA   The notch of Rivinus.

TYMPANIC NERVE   The tympanic branch of the glossopharyngeal nerve. *Synonym:* Jacobson's nerve.

TYMPANOMASTOID FISSURE   The fissure at the posteroinferior aspect of the lateral bony external auditory canal, separating the mastoid and tympanic portions of the temporal bone and transmitting the auricular branch of the vagus (Arnold's nerve).

TYMPANOMENINGEAL HIATUS   Hyrtl's fissure.

TYMPANUM   [*plural:* tympana; *possessive:* tympani] *Latin:* a drum. The middle ear cavity, which somewhat resembles a drum in structure.

UMBO   [*plural:* umbones; *possessive:* umbonis] *Latin:* the center of a shield. The central region of the tympanic membrane marking the location of the tip of the manubrium.
   u. membranae tympani, the umbo.

UTRICULO-ENDOLYMPHATIC VALVE OF BAST   Valve characterized as a thickened portion of the utricular wall that is located at the inferior part of the utricle and marks the beginning of the utricular duct. *Synonym:* utriculo-endolymphatic valve.

UTRICULUS   [*plural:* utriculi; *possessive:* utriculi] *Latin:* diminutive of uter, a leather bag or bottle. The funnel-shaped sense organ of the vestibular part of the membranous labyrinth. *Synonym:* utricle.

VAGINA   [*plural:* vaginae; *possessive:* vaginae] *Latin:* a sheath or scabbard.
   v. processus styloidei, the sheath extending from the temporal bone that surrounds the superior-most portion of the styloid process.

VAS   [*plural:* vasa; *possessive:* vasis] *Latin:* vessel or receptacle.
   v. spirale, the vessel located just posterior to the inner tunnel of the organ of Corti on the scala tympani side of the basilar membrane.

VEIN AT THE COCHLEAR AQUEDUCT   The inferior cochlear vein. *Synonym:* vena aquaeductus cochleae.

VENA AQUAEDUCTUS COCHLEAE   The inferior cochlear vein. *Synonym:* vein at the cochlear aqueduct.

VERTICAL CANAL, ANTERIOR   The superior semicircular canal.

VESTIBULAR MEMBRANE   Reissner's membrane. *Synonym:* membrana vestibularis.

VESTIBULOCOCHLEAR ANASTOMOSIS   *Synonym:* Oort's anastomosis.

VESTIBULUM   [*plural:* vestibula; *possessive:* vestibuli] *Latin:* a courtyard or entrance to a court. The vestibule of the inner ear.

VOIT'S ANASTOMOSIS   A small nerve branch that leaves the superior division of the vestibular nerve to innervate part of the saccule.

VOLKMANN'S CANALS   Channels, other than haversian canals, for the passage of blood vessels through bone.

VON TRÖLTSCH (TROELTSCH), ANTERIOR POUCH OF   Anterior recess of the tympanic membrane.

VON TRÖLTSCH (TROELTSCH), POSTERIOR POUCH OF   Posterior recess of the tympanic membrane.

VON TRÖLTSCH (TROELTSCH), SALPINGOPHARYNGEAL FASCIA OF   Aponeurosis of the eustachian tube. The continuation of the sheath of the tensor veli palatini muscle toward the pharyngeal opening of the eustachian tube, this sheath is attached to the inferior and external edge of the tubal cartilage.

WEBER-LEIL, FASCIA OF   Fascia on the external surface of the tensor palatini muscle.

WRISBERG, ANASTOMOSIS OF   Anastomotic branch between the facial nerve and the nervus intermedius.

WRISBERG, NERVE OF   The nervus intermedius.

ZAUFAL, SALPINGOPHARYNGEAL FOLD OF   Continuation of the posterior lip of the eustachian tube onto the lateral pharyngeal wall.

ZINN, ZONA COCHLEAE OF   Membranous part of the spiral lamina.

ZONA   [*plural:* zonae; *possessive:* zonae] *Latin:* a zone.

   z. arcuata, the inner one third of the basilar membrane (the pars tecta).

   z. pectinata, the outer two thirds of the basilar membrane (the pars pectinata).

ZUCKERKANDL, PHARYNGOTUBAL LIGAMENT OF   Elastic fibers between the pharyngopalatini and salpingopharyngeal (pharyngotubal) muscles.

Historical Bibliography of Ear Anatomy

The following historical bibliography of ear anatomy represents information culled from a variety of primary and secondary sources. The secondary sources to which the interested reader is referred, and which we found particularly helpful in locating more detailed information, include writings by Politzer (1907, English translation by Milstein et al., 1981), Garrison (1929), Dobson (1962), Sultan (1981), and Morton (1983).

The historical persons cited have been selected on the basis of their significant contribution to the understanding of the anatomy of the ear. Inevitably in such an arbitrary listing there are omissions; we apologize for any particularly egregious oversights.

We acknowledge the kind assistance of Mr. Charles Snyder, former director of the Lucian Howe Library of the Massachusetts Eye and Ear Infirmary.

ALCMAEON, GREECE (circa 500 B.C.)
Quoted by Politzer in *Geschichte der Ohrenheilkunde* (Vol 1, Stuttgart, F Enke, 1907) and *History of Otology* (English translation by S Milstein, C Portnoff, and A Coleman, Phoenix, Columella Press, 1981).

According to Aristotle (as mentioned by Plutarch in *De Placitis Philosophorum*. Paris, v. Dübner, 1841), Alcmaeon made the observation that goats breathe through their ears. However, Politzer (1981) does not feel that the assumption that Alcmaeon knew of or discovered the eustachian tube, as credited by many authors, is warranted.

EMPEDOCLES, GREECE (circa 495–435 B.C.)
As detailed by Plutarch (*De Placitis Philosophorum*. Paris, v. Dübner, 1841) and quoted by Politzer (1907, English translation by Milstein et al., 1981), this Greek philosopher discovered a "snail-shaped cartilage" in the ear. This discovery is remarkable in that his knowledge of the ear was limited to the tympanic membrane and tympanic cavity. He also was aware of the fact that vibrations in air produce sound, and he felt that the "snail-shaped cartilage" produced a tone similar to that of a bell when set in motion by air currents.

HIPPOCRATES, GREECE (460–377 B.C.)
De Carnibus. In *Hippocrates' Works*. Edited by Littrés. Paris, 1839–1861.

According to Politzer, Hippocrates was the first to emphasize the fact that the tympanic membrane was an integral part of the organ of hearing. He described the symptoms of acute otitis media, chronic suppurative otitis media, and otitic meningitis. Hippocrates was well aware of the consequences of auricular hematoma and fractures of the cartilage of the auricle. He also included injury to the skull as a potential cause of deafness.

ARISTOTLE, GREECE (384–322 B.C.)
De Animalibus Historiae Libra I. St v Stein, Lit d Anat u Physiolog, 1890.

Aristotle knew only of the existence of the external auditory canal and the auricle in the human, although some of his writings suggest that he had seen the eustachian tube and cochlea in the course of animal dissection. He assumed the existence of an inner "air" ("aer innatus" or "aer implantus"), separated from the external ear, which he felt was the conductor of sound within the ear. This theory dominated the thoughts of subsequent investigators for many centuries.

GALEN, GREECE (130–200 A.D.)
Comment de Placit. Hippocrat et Plat, Lib VI.
De Nervorum Dissectione. Hippocrat et Plat, Lib VI.
De usu Partium. Hippocrat et Plat, Lib VIII.

In the first listed work, Galen credits Erasistratus (circa 310–250 B.C.) with accurate knowledge of the auditory nerve. In the second work Galen realized that the acoustic and facial nerves are separate branches of the "Vth cranial nerve" as numbered by Galen's teacher, Marinus. Apparently he was overwhelmed by the complexity of the numerous apertures and canals of the dissected temporal bone, and likened them to a labyrinth. In the third work, Galen included the first description of the course of the facial nerve. He indicated that it entered the foramen caecum (the internal auditory canal) and traveled in a tortuous bony canal to exit at the end of the styloid canal.

JACOPO BERENGARIO DA CARPI, ITALY (1470–1550)
Anatomi Carpi Isagogae breves perlucidae ac uberrimae in anatomiam humani corporis a communi medicorum academia usitatam, etc. Bonon, 1514.

In this work, Da Carpi describes the auditory ossicles, but does not claim to be the discoverer of them.

NICCOLÒ (NICOLAUS) MASSA, ITALY (1499–1569)
Anatomiae Liber Introductorius. Venetiis, F Bindoni ac M Pasini, 1536.

Massa described a dissection technique for demonstrating the tympanic membrane and the auditory ossicles.

GUIDO GUIDI (VIDUS VIDIUS), ITALY AND FRANCE (1500–1569)
De Anatomica Corporis Humani. Lib VII. Venetiis, 1611 (Francof, 1611, 1626), 1645, 1677.

Guidi was the first to describe the vidian nerve and its stem of origin shared with the palatine nerve.

GIOVANNI FILIPPO INGRASSIA, SICILY (1510–1580)
In *Galeni Librum de Ossibus Dectissima et Exspectatissima Commentaria.*
Panormi, edited post mortem, 1603.

In 1546 Ingrassia, an osteologist, discovered the stapes. He also described the oval and round windows and the chorda tympani nerve. He was the first to note the sound-conductivity of the teeth.

ANDREAS VESALIUS, BELGIUM AND ITALY (1514–1564)
De Fabrica Humani Corporis. Lib VII, first edition. Ex Off Joann Oporin,
Basil, 1543.
Anatomicarum Gabrielis Falloppii observationum examen. Venetiis, 1564.

The 1543 work includes the first drawing of the malleus and incus and a demonstration of the organ of hearing in cross section. (The illustrator was Joh. Stephan von Calcar, a student of Titian.) The subsequent volume corrects many of the errors found in the 1543 edition. It also includes further details of the anatomy of the organ of hearing. Vesalius described for the first time the round window, oval window, and the promontory; he referred to the latter structure as the tuberculum inter fenestram.

MATTEO REALDO COLOMBO, ITALY (1516–1559)
De Re Anatomica. Lib XV. Venetiis, 1559.

Colombo was the first anatomist to remark upon the blood supply of the inner ear. He also first described the lenticular process of the incus.

GABRIELE FALLOPPIO (FALLOPPIUS, FALLOPPIA), ITALY (1523–1562)
Observationes Anatomicae. Venetiis, MA Ulmus, 1561.

This work is the most complete treatise of the so-called "Founder of the Italian School of Anatomy." He studied the embryologic development of the organ of hearing and determined that the components of the adult ear could be found at early stages of development. He also realized that, although in the fetus the tympanic ring is separated from the temporal bone, in later development these two structures fuse. His was the first clear description of the tympanic membrane and its inclination with respect to the horizontal plane. He described the tympanic cavity and was the first to name it the "tympanum." In 1561 he discovered the "canalis sive aqueductus," which houses the intratemporal part of the facial nerve. He recognized that the inner ear consists of two parts: the secunda cavitas, comprised of the semicircular canals and the vestibule, which he named the labyrinth, and the tertia cavitas, which he named the cochlea. His description of both the coiled tubular nature of the cochlea and of the vestibular labyrinth surpassed all preceding descriptions and was superior to many that followed. He also was the first to describe the spiral lamina and to detail the anatomy of the auricular muscles. He discovered and described the chorda tympani nerve, a finding that was recapitulated in the postmortem studies of Ingrassia.

BARTOLOMEO EUSTACHIO (BARTOLOMMEO EUSTACHI, EUSTACHIUS),
ITALY (1524–1574)
Epistula de auditus organis. In *Opuscula Anatomica.* Venetiis, 1563.
Tabulae anatomicae cl viri Bartholomaei Eustachii, quae a tenebris tandem vindicatas, et sanct. Dom Clementis IV, Pont max munificentia dono acceptas, praefatione notisque illustravit Jo Maria Lancisius, intimus cubicularius et archiater pontificis. Romae, 1714; in fol editio 1728.

Independently of Ingrassia and Colombo, Eustachio also discovered the stapes. He described the tensor tympani muscle precisely and was the first to establish that the chorda tympani is a nerve; he documented that it joined with the mandibular branch of the trigeminal nerve, i.e., the lingual nerve. He was the first to describe precisely the configuration of the eustachian tube, supposedly first described by Alcmaeon in 500 B.C. He is credited with the discovery of the modiolus and provided superior descriptions of the cochlear osseous spiral lamina.

HIERONYMUS MERCURIALIS (GERONIMO MERCURIALI), ITALY (1530–1606)
De compositione medicamentorum tractatus, tres libros complectens, eiusdem de oculorum et aurium affectionibus praelectiones seorsim. Francoforti, Apud J Wechelum, 1584.

Mercurialis recognized that deafness could be caused not only by pathologic processes in the organ of hearing, but also by diseases of the brain. His therapeutic treatise was the first clinical manual on diseases of the ear.

VOLCHER KOYTER (COITER, COEITER, KOITER), HOLLAND AND ITALY (1534–1600)
De auditus instrumento. In *Externarum et Internarum Principalium Corporis Humani Partium Tabulae Atque Anatomicae Exercitationes*, etc. Norimbergae, in off T Gerlatzeni, 1573.

This work was the first monograph on the organ of hearing. Koyter was a student of Falloppio and was one of the first scientists to publish a theory of hearing. This theory included the concept of an inner ear, "aer implantatus," implanted into the ear by the Maker.

FABRICIUS AB AQUAPENDENTE (GIROLAMO FABRIZIO), ITALY (1537–1619)
De Visione, Voce et Auditu. Venetiis, F Bolzettam, 1600.
De Formato Foetu. Venetiis, 1600.

This student of Falloppio did not add any new information of anatomic significance with regard to the ear. He did, however, present a theory of hearing that was similar to that of Koyter. He believed that the "aer implantatus" was the carrier of sound perception; however, he felt that the vestibule was the center for hearing and that the other canals functioned to diminish the amplitude and echo of sound.

SALOMON ALBERTI, GERMANY (1540–1600)
Historia Plerarumque Partium Humani Corporis, in Usum Tyronum Edita. Viteberg, 1585.

This work includes chapters that deal specifically with the organ of hearing. Alberti is credited by Morgagni with recognizing that the vestibule (the vestibulum) is a distinct part of the labyrinth.

CONSTANTIUS VAROLIUS (CONSTANZO VAROLIO), ITALY (1543–1575)
Anatomia, s De Resolutione Corporis Humani. Lib IV. Francof, 1591.

Varolius was the first to describe the stapedius muscle.

GIULIO CASSERIO (CASSERIUS PLACENTINUS), ITALY (1561–1616)
De Vocis Auditusque Organis Historia Anatomicae Tractatibus II. Explicata. Ferrariae, Victorius Baldinus, 1600–1601.
Pentaesthesion, H E de Quinque Sensibus Liber. Lib VI. Venetiis, 1609; Francofurti, 1610.
Tabulae Anatomicae LXXIX. Omnes novae nec ante hoc visae. Venetiis, 1627. Cum Supplementis Dan Bucretii. S.i. et a.f. Francof, 1632.

Casserio's major contribution to otology consisted of a careful comparative anatomic study of the organ of hearing. This student of Fabrizio discovered the incisurae in the cartilaginous part of the external auditory canal. He also was the first to describe otoliths in fish. Although the membrana fenestrae cochleae (round window membrane) had already been mentioned by Guido Guidi, Casserius was the first to describe this structure precisely. He used the term "canalis facialis" for the fallopian canal. Casserio noted that there were three semicircular canals, and distinguished three cochlear turns. Although the membranous portion of the spiral lamina (septum spirale) had been mentioned by Eustachio, Casserio defined it more clearly. He also studied the embryology of the human ear.

CLAUDE PERRAULT, FRANCE (1613–1688)
Observations sur l'Organe de l'Ouie, Mémoires de l'Ac de Paris. Vol I. Essais de Physique ou Recueil de Plusieurs Traitez Touchant les Choses Naturelles. Edit JB Caignard, Paris, T I, II, III, 1680; T IV, 1688. Oeuvres Diverses. Leiden, 1721.

Claude Perrault extended the work of Casserius in comparative anatomy. He was the first to describe the bony lip overhanging the round window.

CAECILIUS FOLIUS (FOLIO), ITALY (1615–1650)
Nova Auris Internae Delineatio. Venetiis, 1645.

Folius is credited with the discovery of the processus longus spinosus s. Folii (anterior process) of the malleus, although this structure was known to both Koyter (Proc. primus) and Casserio (Proc. anterior elatior et exilior). Jac. Ravius described it as seen in the newborn, hence the occasional term "processus Ravii." Folius is credited with describing the semicircular canals; he limited the number of their communications with the vestibule to five.

THOMAS WILLIS, ENGLAND (1622–1675)
Cerebri Anatome, Cui Accessit Nervorum Descriptio et Usus. London, 1664.
De Anima Brutorum quae hominis vitalis ac sensitiva est, exercitationes duae, etc. London, R Davis, 1672.

Willis was the first to observe the phenomenon in which certain individuals with a hearing loss hear better when noise is present. This phenomenon now carries the name paracusis Willisii. He discovered the helicotrema independently of Méry, and he was the first to ascribe properly the role of hearing to the cochlea.

LUDOVICUS BILS (JONKER LONGS DE BILS), HOLLAND (1624–1670)
Anatomisch Vertoon van het Gehoor. Brüghe, 1655.

Bils described the temporal bone as consisting of four parts delineated by sutures.

JOHANN HEINRICH GLASER, SWITZERLAND (1629–1675)
Tractatus posthumus de cerebro, in quo hujus non fabrica tantum, sed actiones omnes principes, sensus ac motus ex veterum et recentiorum placitis et observationibus perspicue ac methodice explicantur. Basileae, 1680.

Glaser is given credit for the discovery of the petrotympanic fissure which bears his name (Glaserian fissure). Politzer, however, was not able to find the pertinent passage in his main work referenced above.

FREDRIK RUYSCH, HOLLAND (1638–1731)
In resp ad Epist probl VIII. Thesauri anatomici decem. Amst, 1701–1716.

Ruysch was the first to ascribe a trilamellar structure to the tympanic membrane. He also provided evidence that contradicted the thesis of Rivinius, which suggested the presence of an opening in the normal tympanic membrane. Ruysch showed that the ossicles possess a periosteal covering.

NIELS STENSEN (NIKOLAUS STENO), DENMARK (1638–1682)
De glandulis oris et nuper observatis inde prodentibus vasi. Lugduni Batavorum, J Chouet, 1661.

Steno was the first to describe the ceruminous glands of the external auditory canal.

JEAN MÉRY, FRANCE (1645–1722)
Description Exacte de l'Oreille de l'Homme avec Explication Méchanique et Physique des Fonctions de l'âme Sensitive. Paris, 1677, 1681, 1687.

Méry was the first to describe the spine of the helix (the spina s. processus acutus helicis) and added further details to the description of the fissures in the cartilage of the external auditory canal first observed by Casserius. Méry also was the first to observe the synovial capsules of the ossicular articulations.

JOHANNES MUNNI(C)KS, THE NETHERLANDS (1652–1711)
De Re Anatomica liber. Utrecht, 1697.

Munniks was the first to describe the notch in the bone of the superior part of the tympanic annulus (now known as the notch of Rivinus).

JOSEPH GUICHARD DUVERNEY, FRANCE (1648–1730)
Traité de l'organe de l'ouie, contenant la structure, les usages et les maladies de toutes les parties de l'orielle. Paris, E Michallet, 1683.

Duverney is heralded as the founder of the French school of anatomy of the eighteenth century. His contributions to the field of otology are many, and among his impressive list of firsts are included: description of the posterior auricular ligament, illustration of the vascular and neural branches of the auricle, accurate description of the bony external auditory canal as originating from the tympanic annulus, illustration of the route of communication between the tympanic cavity and the cells of the mastoid process, description of the epitympanum, and relationship of the eustachian tube to the medial wall of the tympanic cavity. His "Traité" is the first treatise in which the anatomy and the pathology of the ear are presented in a coherent and analytic manner. His theory of hearing, which he developed with the physicist Mariotte (the Duverny-Mariotte theory of hearing), ascribed to the labyrinth a role in the perception of different tones. He believed that the vibrations of the tympanic membrane were transmitted to the labyrinth through the ossicular chain. This theory of hearing was later expanded upon and eventually accredited to Helmholtz.

AUGUSTUS QUIRINUS RIVINUS (RIVINIUS), GERMANY (1652–1723)

In 1689 the senior Rivinus believed that he had discovered an opening in the tympanic membrane in its normal state. He relayed this finding in 1691 in a letter to Anton Nuck, a Dutch anatomist. His son, Joh. Aug. Rivinus, reported the finding in "De Auditus Vitiis" Dissertatio (Lipsiae, 1717). Rivinus located his opening, which he thought also had a fibrous sphincter, near the head of the malleus in the tympanic membrane of sheep and calves. In today's terminology, the notch of Rivinus describes a deficiency in the superior aspect of the tympanic ring, where Shrapnell's membrane (pars flaccida) attaches to the petrous bone.

ANTONIO MARIA VALSALVA, ITALY (1666–1723)
Tractatus de Aure Humana. Bologna, Typ C Pisarii, 1704.

Valsalva was a pupil of Malpighi and was the teacher of Morgagni. He was well known for his method of inflating the middle ear, i.e. Valsalva's maneuver; he also was the first to present an anatomic preparation of the complete organ of hearing. He divided the ear into an external compartment, a middle compartment, and an internal compartment. Valsalva was the first to describe clearly a muscular dilator that widened the eustachian tube, and he named the auditory tube in Eustachius' honor. Valsalva used the term "labyrinth" to denote the entire inner ear; moreover, in 1707 he was the first to observe that the entire labyrinth was filled with a watery fluid. He named the scala vestibuli and the scala tympani. He noted ankylosis of the stapes to the margin of the oval window in an autopsy of a deaf person.

GIOVANNI DOMENICO SANTORINI, ITALY (1681–1737)
Observationes Anatomicae. Venetiis, 1724.

Santorini provided a more detailed description of the incisures of the external auditory canal (incisurae Santorini) previously described by Méry and Duverney. He noted that muscle fibers could occasionally be seen passing over the first (largest) incisura (Santorian muscle), and he first described the major and minor musculus helicis.

GIOVANNI BATTISTA MORGAGNI, ITALY (1682–1771)
Epistolae anatomicae. Appendix in *Valsalva's Tractatus de Aure Humana.* Venice, 1740.

Morgagni was a pupil of Valsalva and Malpighi. His research was incorporated into Valsalva's treatise as an appendix; it was an extension of Valsalva's research. He described the vestibular segment of the vestibular aqueduct, as well as the spherical recess (cavitas hemisphaerica) and the elliptical recess (cavitas semiovalis). He contradicted the teaching of Valsalva by showing for the first time that intracranial suppuration is the consequence of infection from the ear rather than conversely, as Valsalva had hypothesized.

JOHANN FRIEDRICH CASSEBOHM, GERMANY (1699–1743)
Tractatus Quatuor Anatomici de Aure Humana. Sumtibus Orphanotrophei, Halae Magdeburgi, 1734.
Tractatus quintus anatomicus de aure humana cui accedit tractatus sextus de aure monstri humani. Halae Magdeburgi, 1735.

Cassebohm made many original contributions to the field of otology. He was the first to mention the notch at the tip of the short process of the anvil (incus) and was the first to describe the concavity of the inner aspect of the stapedial crura. He antedated Cotugno in his awareness of the presence of two recesses within the vestibule. He was the first to describe in some detail the communication of the two scalae in the apex of the cochlea; he first noted the falciform crest dividing the internal auditory canal into the superior and inferior halves. Cassebohm also studied the ossification process of the otic capsule and located the beginning of this process in the periphery of the round window.

JOHANN GOTTFRIED ZINN, GERMANY (1727–1759)
Observationes quaedam botanicae et anatomicae de vasis subtilioribus oculi et cochleae auris internae. Goettingen, 1753.

Thorough microscopic examination enabled Zinn to provide the first precise description of the cochlear (osseous) spiral lamina. Zinn traced the path of the cochlear nerve, and described how it entered the cochlea as a spiral band. He also was the first to describe in clear detail the vasculature of the cochlea, especially that of the apex.

DOMENICO COTUGNO (COTTUNNI, COTUNNI, COTUGNI, COTUNNIUS), ITALY (1736–1822)
De aquaeductibus auris humani internae anatomica dissertatio. Ex typ Naples, Simoniana, 1761.

Although Pyl had recognized the existence of fluid within the labyrinth, Cotugno, a student of Morgagni, is often credited as one of the first to be aware of the importance of these fluids, both in an anatomic and a physiologic sense. He was the first to establish the fact that the labyrinth was filled completely by fluid and contained no air. He incorporated the knowledge of the presence of a labyrinthine fluid into a theory of hearing that established the foundation for modern theories of hearing and finally laid to rest Aristotle's ancient "aer innatus" concept of the physiology of hearing. Cotugno felt that the impact of sound waves precipitated movement of the stapes, which in turn set into motion the labyrinthine fluid in which the nerves were suspended. He discovered the vestibular aqueduct and traced it to its opening on the posterior aspect of the petrous pyramid. He also discovered the intradural sac of the vestibular aqueduct (endolymphatic sac), which he called "cavitas aquaeductus membranacea" and correctly identified it as a prolongation of the endolymphatic duct. Cotugno discovered the cochlear aqueduct, which he traced from the scala tympani orifice ("orificium superius") to its funnel-shaped terminus at the "orificium inferius." He believed that these two aqueducts drained off labyrinthine fluid after medial movement of the stapes.

ANTONIO SCARPA, ITALY (1747–1832)
De structura fenestrae rotundae auris et de tympanos secundario anatomicae observationes. Apud soc typog. Mutinae, 1772.

Anatomicarum annotatianum liber primus de nervorum gangliis et plexibus. Mutinae, 1779.

Disquisitiones anatomicae de auditu et olfactu. Ticini et Mediolani, 1789.

Scarpa, probably one of the greatest anatomists of all time, possessed superb dissection technique, and his "Disquisitiones" marks the end of the premicroscopic era of otologic research. He complemented the visualization of his dissections by using a magnifying glass and by means of injection. He contended that sound waves entered the cochlea by both the round and oval windows. He also believed that the round window membrane could function as a tympanic membrane. In support of this contention, he presented the finding that a vibrating instrument held between the teeth could still be heard even after the tympanic membrane, ossicular chain, and the entire external ear had been destroyed. His treatise "De structura" deals with the architecture of the round window and its membrane. Scarpa's description of the anatomy of the labyrinth far excelled that of his predecessors. He was the first to demonstrate the existence of the saccule in the spheric vestibular recess and the utricle in the elliptic vestibular recess; he discovered the existence of membranous canals within the bony semicircular canals. He recognized the utricle as the common reservoir of the semicircular ducts; moreover, he noted that, upon squeezing the utricle, fluid could be forced into the semicircular ducts, but not into the saccule. He expanded upon the knowledge of the labyrinthine fluid because, although Cotugno had been aware of the existence of perilymph, knowledge of the membranous labyrinth was a prerequisite for the discovery of endolymph. Scarpa identified endolymph in the vestibular system but was unaware of the cochlear duct.

THEODOR PYL, (?) (1749–1794)

Dissertatio medica de auditu in genere et de illo qui fit per os in specie. Gryphiswald, 1742.

Pyl antedated Cotugno in recognizing the existence of fluid in the labyrinth. His theory of hearing, presented in 1742, was the first to be founded totally on the presence of a fluid medium in the inner ear.

ADOLPH MURRAY, (?) (1751–1803)

Anatomische Bemerkungen über die Durchbohrung der Apophysis mastoidea als Heilmittel gegen verschiedene Arten von Taubheit. In *K Schwed Akad d Wissenschaft neuen Abhandlungen aus der Naturlehre,* 1789.

Abscessus auris interne observatio. Upsal, 1796.

Murray detailed the anatomy of the air cells of the mastoid process and described the communication of these cells with each other and with the tympanic cavity. He observed variability in the degree of pneumatization of the mastoid process.

SAMUEL THOMAS VON SOEMMERRING, WESTERN PRUSSIA, GERMANY (1755–1830)

De corporis humani fabrica. Traj ad Moen, 1794.

Icones organi auditus humani. Frankfurt, 1806.

Abbildungen des menschlichen Hörorgans. Frankfurt am Main, Varrentrapp u Wenner, 1806.

Von Soemmerring was the first to describe the superior suspensory ligament of the malleus. He also was the first to utilize a chemical preparation of the organ of hearing to further his anatomic studies. Dilute nitric acid softened the bony shell, which he then removed; in this way, he visualized the course of the nerves in the modiolus and also in the osseous spiral lamina.

FLORIANO CALDANI, ITALY (?)
Osservazioni sulla membrana del tympano e nuove ricerche sulla elettricita animale. Padua, 1799.

Caldani was first to note that the fibrous layers of the tympanic membrane were arranged in both a radial and a circular manner.

SIR ASTLEY PASTON COOPER, ENGLAND (1768–1841)
Further observations on the effects which take place from the destruction of the membrana tympani of the ear; with an account of an operation for the removal of a particular species of deafness. Phil Trans, **91**:435, 1801.
Dictionary of Practical Surgery. London, 1825.

Sir Astley was the first to employ paracentesis of the tympanic membrane (myringotomy) on a rational basis. This operation was first performed in 1760 by Eli, a wandering quack who used it for the relief of certain cases of deafness. In his 1801 publication, Sir Astley presents three cases of deafness associated with eustachian tube obstruction that were relieved by myringotomy. He reasoned that the perforated tympanic membrane provided a substitute for the blocked eustachian tube.

JEAN MARIE GASPARD ITARD, FRANCE (1775–1838)
Traité des Maladies de l'Oreille et de l'Audition. Vols 1 and 2. Paris, Méquignon Marvis, 1821.

This surgeon did much to establish the field of otology and wrote the first modern textbook describing diseases of the ear.

FRIEDRICH CHRISTIAN ROSENTHAL, GERMANY (1780–1829)
Ueber den Bau der Spindel im menschlichen Ohr. In *Meckels Archiv, Bd VIII*, 1823.

Rosenthal was the first to describe the "canalis spiralis modioli," which now bears his name (Rosenthal's canal). It houses the spiral ganglion.

JOHN HOWSHIP, ENGLAND (1781–1841)
On the natural and diseased state of the bones. London, 1820.

Howship, a victim himself of tibial osteomyelitis, was especially interested in bone disease. The excavation defects created in bone by osteoclastic activity are called Howship's lacunae.

JOHANN FRIEDRICH MECKEL, GERMANY (1781–1833)
Abhandlungen aus der vergleichenden und menschlichen Anatomie. Halle, 1805.

Johann Meckel originally described the cartilage of the first branchial arch.

LUDWIG LEVIN JACOBSON, DENMARK (1783–1843)
Supplementa ad otoiatriam. Supplementum primum de anastomosi ner-

vorum nova in aure detecta. Acta Reg Soc Med Havnien, *5:293,* 1818.

Jacobson described the tympanic branch of the glossopharyngeal nerve, its canal, and its plexus, all of which now bear his name.

GILBERT BRESCHET, FRANCE (1784–1845)
Études anatomiques et physiologiques sur l'organe de l'ouie et sur l'audition, dans l'homme et les animaux vertébrés. Presentés à l'académie royale des sciences, 27 Août 1832.
Recherches anatomiques et physiologiques sur l'organe de l'ouie des poissons. Paris, JP Baillière, 1838.

Breschet named the individual labyrinthine components according to a uniform and rational system. He was the first to use the term "helicotrema" to describe the communication of the scala tympani and scala vestibuli at the apex of the cochlea. He distinguished otoliths (ear stones), which are the large enamel-like stones in fish, from otoconia (ear dust), a term that describes the fine granules of higher animals. He documented the relationships of the scala tympani and the vestibule, and first used the terms "perilymph" and "endolymph" to denote Cotugno's and Scarpa's fluids, respectively. He accurately delineated the arteries of the spiral lamina as part of his description of the vascular arborizations within the labyrinth.

AUGUST ALBRECHT MECKEL, GERMANY AND SWITZERLAND (1790–1829)
Bemerkungen über die Hohle des knöchernen Labyrinthes (mit Abbildungen). Meckels Arch f Anat u Physiol, 1827.

August Meckel introduced the corrosion method of preparation of the bony labyrinth in the macerated temporal bone.

CARL ERNST VON BAER, RUSSIA (1792–1876)
Ueber Entwicklungsgeschichte der Thiere. Bd I, Königsberg, 1828–1834; Bd II, 1837.

Von Baer is often referred to as the "Father of the New Embryology" and was the first to study the embryologic development of the organ of hearing on a comparative basis.

MARTIN HEINRICH RATHKE, POLAND AND GERMANY (1793–1860)
Entwicklungsgeschichte der Menschen und der Thiere. Leipzig, 1832.

Rathke, in 1825, was the first to observe transverse fissures (gill slits), which he found present in the cervical region of pig embryos. He determined that the exterior part of the first gill slit became the external auditory canal in the course of embryologic development. Rathke is better known for Rathke's pouch, a diverticulum from the embryonic buccal cavity from which the anterior lobe of the pituitary is developed.

MARIE JEAN PIERRE FLOURENS, FRANCE (1794–1867)
Memoires présentés à l'academie royale des sciences, 27 Decembre 1824.
Recherches experimentales sur les propriétés et les fonctions du système nerveux dans les animaux vertébrés. Paris, Crevot, 1824.
Nouvelles experiences sur l'independance respective des fonctions cérébrales. Compt Rend T LII, 1861.

Through animal experimentation, Flourens demonstrated that lesions of the semicircular canals resulted in dysequilibrium and motor incoordination. His experiments provided the foundation for the modern physiology of the semicircular canals and vestibule. Although Friedrich Goltz (1834–1902) was the first to suspect that the semicircular canals were the organs of balance, Flourens' experiments showed that the cochlea was the sole organ for the perception of sound and that the vestibular and semicircular canal structures were not involved in sound perception.

EMIL HUSCHKE, GERMANY (1797–1858)
S Th Soemmerring, Lehr von den Eingeweiden und Sinnesorganen des menschlichen Körpers. Revised and concluded by Emil Huschke, Leipzig, 1844.

Huschke was the discoverer of the sensory papilla of the cochlea, which later came to bear Corti's name. Huschke also gave a clear description of the stria vascularis, the dentate zone of the cochlea, and the tall cells that cover the limbus (Huschke's teeth).

FRIEDRICH CORNELIUS, ESTONIA (1799–1848)
De membranae tympani usu. Dorpat, 1825.

Cornelius was the first to observe and illustrate the "internal fold of the tympanic membrane" and the "posterior pocket of the tympanic membrane," which it formed. Thus, he anticipated von Tröltsch after whom this posterior pouch is now named.

JOHANNES PETER MÜLLER, GERMANY (1801–1858)
Handbuch der Physiologie des Menschen. Koblenz, 1837.

This German physiologist was the first to recognize the differential acoustic properties of air and water and the logical necessity of a transformer mechanism to convert air vibrations to those of fluid.

KASPAR THEOBALD TOURTUAL, PRUSSIA (1802–1865)
Neuen Untersuchungen über den Bau des menschlichen Schlund- und Kehlkopfes mit vergleichend-anatomischen Bemerkungen. Leipzig, 1846.

Tourtual was the first to provide an accurate description of the origin and relationships of the tensor veli palatini muscle, with special attention to its relationship to the eustachian tube. His description of the fossa of Rosenmüller excelled that of its namesake. He also described the location and course of the fold that bears his name, the plica salpingopalatina.

FRIEDRICH ARNOLD, GERMANY AND SWITZERLAND (1803–1890)
Diss inaug med sist observationes nonnullas neurologicas de parte cephalica nervi sympathici in homine. Heidelberg, 1826.
Ueber den Ohrknoten. Eine anatomisch-physiologische Abhandlung. Heidelberg, 1828.
Ueber den Canalis tympanicus u mastoideus. Tiedemanns Ztschr f physiol, Bd IV, 1832.

Arnold published his discovery of the otic ganglion in his 1826 inaugural dissertation. He was the first to describe and name the nervus petrosus superficialis minor (lesser superficial petrosal nerve) and the nervus petrosus profundus minor (lesser deeper petrosal nerve). An additional contribution to the field of neuroanatomy was his discovery and description of the auricular branch of the vagus and the canaliculus mastoideus, which it transverses.

PIERRE CHARLES HUGUIER, FRANCE (1804–1874)
Bichats' Anatomie descriptive. Paris, 1834.

Huguier is well known for his description of the canal near the petrotympanic fissure that transmits the chorda tympani nerve (canal of Huguier). He also described the sinus tympani (cavité sous-pyramidale).

FRIEDRICH GUSTAV JACOB HENLE, GERMANY (1809–1885)
Allgemeine Anatomie. Leipzig, 1841.
Handbuch der systematische Anatomie des Menschen. Brunswick, 1855–1872.

Henle was the first to describe the processus auditorius of the temporal bone, otherwise known as the suprameatal spine of Henle.

JOSEPH HYRTL, HUNGARY AND AUSTRIA (1811–1894)
Vergleichend-anatomische Untersuchungen über das innere Gehörorgan des Menschen und der Säugethiere. Prague, Friedrich Ehrlich, 1845.
Ueber spontane Dehiszenz des Tegmen tympani u d Cellulae mastoideae. Wien, 1858.
Die Korrosionsanatomie u ihre Ergebnisse. Wien, 1873.

In the first of these publications, Hyrtl expanded the knowledge of the comparative anatomy of the organ of hearing, particularly with respect to the structure of the inner ear. In 1858, Hyrtl wrote a short paper pointing out the frequent occurrence of dehiscence of the tegmen tympani, which could not be explained by the changes of aging or infection; he noted that these openings most frequently could be found superior and posterior to the incudomalleal articulation. In the third of the listed works, Hyrtl describes the results of his work in corrosion anatomy combined with injection of the external auditory canal, the tympanic cavity, the mastoid air cell system, and the eustachian tube. This study laid the foundation for the elucidation of the topographic anatomy of these regions of the organ of hearing. We have studied Hyrtl's publications but have been unable to confirm that he ever described the fissure that bears his name, Hyrtl's or tympanomeningeal fissure.

KARL BOGISLAUS REICHERT, EAST PRUSSIA (1811–1883)
De embryonum arcubus sic dictis branchialibus. Berlin, 1836.
Ueber die Visceralbogen der Wirbelthiere. Berlin, Sittenfeld, 1837.

Reichert declared that the second (hyoid) visceral bar, which he first described, gave rise to the entire stapes. It is now known, however, that the footplate of the stapes (basis stapedis) derives from the otic capsule.

HENRY JOHN (JONES) SHRAPNELL, ENGLAND (1814–1834)
On the form and structure of the membrana tympani. Lond Med Gaz, *10:120*, 1832.

Shrapnell was the first to distinguish between the pars tensa and the pars flaccida (Shrapnell's membrane) of the tympanic membrane.

JOSEPH TOYNBEE, ENGLAND (1815–1866)
On the functions of the membrana tympani, the ossicles and muscles of the tympanum, and of the eustachian tube and their actions in different classes of animals. Abstr Papers Commun Roy Soc Lond, 6:217, 1850–1854.
On the structure of the membrana tympani in the human ear. Phil Trans, 1851, pp. 159–168.
The Diseases of the Ear: Their Nature, Diagnosis, and Treatment. London, J Churchill, 1860.

The tensor tympani muscle is known as Toynbee's muscle because of his investigations. Knowledge of the existence of this muscle dated back to the time of Eustachius (1524–1574). Bernhard Albinus (1697–1770), a surgeon and anatomist at Leyden University, is credited with the appellation of the tensor tympani muscle.

The third work is a medical classic written by this "Father of British Otology." In this text he delineates his method for removal of the temporal bone (of which he dissected 2000). He correlated the postmortem findings with symptoms manifested during life, thus being the first to correlate pathology with the clinical presentation of otologic disease.

RUDOLF ALBERT VON KÖLLIKER, SWEDEN (1817–1905)
Entwicklungsgeschichte des Menschen und der höhren Thiere. Leipzig, W Engelmann, 1861.

In 1861 Kölliker honored Reissner by being the first to call the vestibular membrane by Reissner's name.

FRIEDRICH MATTHIAS CLADIUS (CLAUDIUS), GERMANY (1822–1869)
Physiologische Bermerkung ueber das Gehörorgan. Kiel, 1858; Marburg, 1862.

Claudius is credited with the original description of the cells that line the outer spiral sulcus of the cochlear duct; these cells are known as the cells of Claudius.

ALFONSO MARCHESE CORTI, ITALY (1822–1888)
Recherches sur l'organe de l'ouie des mammifères. Z Wiss Zool, 3:109, 1851.

Corti gave a more detailed description of the structure of the auditory papilla first discovered by Huschke. Hence, many of its structures bear his name—the organ of Corti, the pillars of Corti, the tunnel of Corti, the outer hair cells of Corti, and the (tectorial) membrane of Corti.

ERNST REISSNER, LATVIA (1824–1878)
De auris internae formatione. Dorpati Livonorum, H Laakmann, 1851.

In 1851 Reissner proved conclusively that there was a special canal in the cochlea termed the "canalis cochlearis." Three years later he described the embryologic development of the otic vesicle and demonstrated how the vesicle was transformed into its three derivatives: (1) the recessus labyrinthi, which up to that time was called the aquaeductus vestibuli, and was incorrectly considered to be the aquaeductus cochlearis, (2) the vestibular region with the semicircular ducts, and (3) the scala media or cochlear duct. He described the vestibular membrane that bears his name.

MAXIMILIAN JOHANN SIGISMUND SCHULTZE, GERMANY (1825–1874)
Ueber die Endigungsweise der Hörnerven im Labyrinth. Arch f Anat Physiol u Wiss Med, 1858, p. 343.

Schultze was an important figure in the development of the science of histology. Among his monographs on the nerve endings of the sense organs is the description of the nerve endings of the labyrinth.

ANTON FRIEDRICH VON TRÖLTSCH (TROELTSCH), GERMANY (1829–1890)
Anatomische Beiträge zur Ohrenheilkunde. Virchows Arch, *17:1*, 1859.
Die Untersuchung des Gehörgangs und Trommelfells. Ihre Bedeutung. Kritik der bisherigen Untersuchungsmethoden und Angabe einer neuen. Dtsch Klinik, *12:113*, 1860.
Ein Fall von Anbohrung des Warzenfortsatzes bei Otitis interna mit Bemerkungen über diese Operation. Virchows Arch f Path Anat, *21:295*, 1861.
Die Krankheiten des Ohres, ihre Erkenntniss und Behandlung. Würzburg, Stahel, 1862.
Lehrbuch der Ohrenheilkunde, mit Einschluss der Anatomie des Ohres. 7th ed. Leipzig, FCW Vogel, 1881.

Von Tröltsch developed the first modern otoscope; he originated the modern radical mastoidectomy. The anterior and posterior malleal folds of the tympanic membrane, as well as the pouches they delimit, are named after von Tröltsch. He believed that sclerotic changes in the middle ear mucosa were responsible for stapes fixation and thus developed the term "otosclerosis."

ARTHUR BÖTTCHER (BOETTCHER), ESTONIA (1831–1889)
Observationes microscopicae de ratione qua nervus cochleae mammalium terminatur. Dorpat, 1856.
Ueber Entwickelung und Bau des Gehörlabyrinths nach Untersuchungen an Säugethieren. 1. Theil. 4°. E Blockmann u sohn, 1869.

In 1869, Böttcher was the first to use the term "cartilage islands" to refer to the globuli interossei of the temporal bone. His name is applied to the cells on the basilar membrane of the cochlea that lie medial and deep to the cells of Claudius as well as to the saccular duct connecting the saccule and utricle. He also studied the terminal endings of the cochlear nerve.

MORITZ FERDINAND TRAUTMANN, GERMANY (1832–1902)
Embolische Processe des Mittelohrs. Berlin, 1886.

Trautmann was the professor of aural surgery at Berlin University in the 1870s. His name is associated with the triangular area bounded by the superior petrosal sinus, the sigmoid sinus, and the bony labyrinth (Trautmann's triangle).

OTTO FRIEDRICH CARL DEITERS, GERMANY (1834–1863)
Untersuchungen über die Lamina spiralis membranacea. Bonn, 1860.

In 1860, Deiters was the first to describe the inner hair cells of the organ of Corti and their supporting cells. The outer phalangeal cells bear Deiters' name in honor of this discovery.

VIKTOR HENSEN, GERMANY (1835–1924)
Zur Morphologie der Schnecke des Menschen und der Säugthiere. Ztschr Wiss Zool, *13:481*, 1863.

In 1863, Hensen was the first to describe numerous structures of the inner ear, including: (1) the ductus reuniens (known as Hensen's canal), (2) a thickened band on the inferior surface of the tectorial membrane now known as Hensen's stripe, (3) the supporting cells radially outside the outer hair cells, which are now known as Hensen's cells, and (4) the hairs (stereocilia) of the hair cells. He was the first to demonstrate that the basilar membrane gradually widened from base to apex of the cochlea. He believed that alterations in the consistency of the protoplasm of the cells of the organ of Corti triggered off the nerve impulses. Moreover, he agreed with Claudius in believing that sound impulses entered the cochlea through the round window and that the scala tympani was stimulated through the basilar membrane.

ADAM POLITZER, HUNGARY AND AUSTRIA (1835–1920)
Ueber ein neues Heilverfahren gegen Schwerhörigkeit in Folge von Unwegsamkeit der Eustachischen Ohrtrompete. Wien Med Wschr, 13:84, 1863.
Die Beleuchtungsbilder des Trommelfells im gesunden und kranken Zustande. Wein, W Braumüller, 1865.
Lehrbuch der Ohrenheilkunde. Vols 1 and 2. Stuttgart, F Enke, 1878–1882.
On a peculiar affection of the labyrinthine capsule as a frequent cause of deafness. Trans 1st Panam Med Congr (1893), 1895.
Geschichte der Ohrenheilkunde. Stuttgart, F Enke, Vol 1, 1907; Vol 2, 1913.
History of Otology. English translation by S Milstein, C Portnoff, and A Coleman. Phoenix, Columella Press, 1981.

While Politzer made no contributions to new knowledge of anatomy, his contributions to otology were prolific.

In the first of the cited references, Politzer describes his method for achieving patency of the eustachian tube. The second is an atlas of colored illustrations of the tympanic membrane. The third is his textbook of otology, which for many years served as the preeminent source book on the subject. In the fourth, he described for the first time the clinical entity of otosclerosis as being distinct from chronic middle ear disease. The fifth reference is his classic two-volume history of otology, which recently (1981) was translated into English by Milstein et al.

GUSTAV MAGNUS RETZIUS, SWEDEN (1842–1919)
Das Gehörorgan der Wirbelthiere. Vols 1 and 2. Stockholm, Samson and Wallin, 1881–1884.
Die Endigungsweise des Gehörnerven. Biol Untersuch, 3:29, 1892.

Retzius was one of the foremost histologists of the recent past, and his diagrams of the organ of hearing in bony fish and vertebrates can scarcely be excelled, even in modern times. He felt that the hair cells were the ultimate receptors of the hearing organ and noted their innervation by auditory nerve fibers.

FRIEDRICH SIEBENMANN, SWITZERLAND (1852–1928)
Die Blutgefässe im Labyrinth des menschlichen Ohres nach eigenen Untersuchungen an Celloiden-Korrosionen und an Schnitten. Weisbaden, JF Bergmann, 1894.
Demonstration mikroscopischer und macroscopisher Präparate von Otospongiosis progressiva. Int Otol Congr Bost, 9:207, 1912.

Siebenmann used the corrosion method of preparation of the temporal bone in his anatomic studies. His name is eponymically associated with the channels traveling with the cochlear aqueduct (paravestibular canaliculi). He described the blood supply of the inner ear.

SANTIAGO RAMÓN Y CAJAL, SPAIN (1852–1934)
Manual de Anatomia Patologica General. Barcelona, 1890 (7th ed, Madrid, Moya, 1922).
This Nobel laureate studied and described the histology of the nervous system including the cochlear nuclei.

MAX BRÖDEL, U.S.A. (1870–1941)
Three Unpublished Drawings of the Anatomy of the Human Ear. Philadelphia, WB Saunders Co, 1946.
Brödel was a master artist who contributed elegant drawings of the anatomic structures of the human body, including the ear.

KENKICHI ASAI, JAPAN (1872–1945)
Die Blutgefässe des häutigen Labyrinthe der Ratte. Anat Hefte, 36:711, 1908.
Die Blutgefässe des häutigen Labyrinthe des Hundes. Anat Hefte, 36:369, 1908.
Asai described in detail the blood vessels of the inner ear.

ROBERT BÁRÁNY, AUSTRIA (1876–1936)
Ueber die vom Ohrlabyrinth ausgelöste Gegenrollung der Augen bei Normalhörenden. Arch Ohrenheilk, 68:1, 1906.
Untersuchungen über den vom Vestibularapparat des Ohres reflektorisch ausgelösten rhythmischen Nystagmus und seine Begleiterscheinungen. Mschr Ohrenheilk, 40:193, 1906; 41:477, 1907.
Bárány (Nobel laureate, 1914) made no important anatomic studies, but is remembered for developing and popularizing the caloric test as an indicator of vestibular function.

KARL WITTMAACK, GERMANY (1876–1972)
Über sekundäre Degeneration im inneren Ohre nach Akustikustammuerletzungen. Verh Dtsch Otol Ges, 20:289, 1911.
Die Ortho- und Pathobiologie des Labyrinthes. Stuttgart, Georg Thieme Verlag, 1956.
Wittmaack was a pathologist and researcher known for his detailed studies of human inner ear disease based on light microscopic studies.

THEODORE HIERONYMOUS BAST, U.S.A. (1890–1959)
With BJ Anson. *The Temporal Bone and the Ear.* Springfield, Charles C Thomas, 1949.
Bast contributed greatly to today's knowledge of the anatomy of the temporal bone, both adult and developmental. He is credited with the discovery of the utriculo-endolymphatic valve.

GOSTA DOHLMAN, SWEDEN (1890–1983)
The mechanism of secretion and absorption of endolymph in the vestibular apparatus. Acta Otolaryngol (Stockh), *59:275*, 1965.

Dohlman described the physiologic behavior of the cupula. He was a strong proponent of the theory that ruptures of the membranous labyrinth are responsible for the acute vertiginous episodes in Ménière's disease.

STACY RUFUS GUILD, U.S.A. (1890–1966)
A hitherto unrecognized structure, the glomus jugularis, in man. Anat Rec, Suppl 2, *79:28*, 1941.
The glomus jugulare, a non-chromaffin paraganglion in man. Ann Otol Rhinol Laryngol, *62:1045*, 1953.
A graphic reconstruction method for the study of the organ of Corti. Anat Rec, *22:141*, 1921.

Guild was the first to describe the normally occurring "glomus body" in the middle ear and first demonstrated the method of graphic reconstruction of the cochlea from serial histologic sections.

BARRY JOSEPH ANSON, U.S.A. (1894–1974)
With TH Bast. *The Temporal Bone and the Ear*. Springfield, Charles C Thomas, 1949.

Anson made numerous anatomic descriptions of the temporal bone from light microscopic preparations and gave the first detailed report on ossification centers.

DOROTHY WOLFF, U.S.A. (1895–1980)
Otosclerosis: hypothesis of its origin and progress. Arch Otolaryngol, *52:853*, 1950.
With RJ Bellucci and AA Eggston. *Surgical and Microscopic Anatomy of the Temporal Bone*. New York, Hafner Publishing Co, 1971.

Wolff was a meticulous anatomist who will be remembered for her teaching of ear anatomy and for the excellent books on microscopic anatomy of the ear that she co-authored.

JOHN RALSTON LINDSAY, U.S.A. (1898–1981)
Suppuration in the petrous pyramid. Ann Otol Rhinol Laryngol, *47:3*, 1938.
Petrous pyramid of temporal bone: pneumatization and roentgenologic appearance. Arch Otolaryngol, *31:231*, 1940.
Labyrinthine dropsy and Ménière's disease. Arch Otolaryngol, *35:853*, 1942.
Postural vertigo and positional nystagmus. Ann Otol Rhinol Laryngol, *60:1134*, 1951.

Lindsay developed a systematic study of the pathologic conditions of the temporal bone. His surgical approach to suppuration of the petrous apex was based on painstaking studies of pneumatization. He felt that one should first attempt to find a tract from the mastoid to the petrous apex; if that course failed, he suggested an approach to the apex from the middle ear. His first case report of idiopathic endolymphatic hydrops, which appeared only a few years after the initial discovery by Yamakawa and by Hallpike and Cairns, launched three decades of investigation into the pathology and pathophysiology of Ménière's disease. He ascribed the overaccumulation of endolymph found in Ménière's disease to a failure of the endolymphatic sac to perform its resorptive function. His expertise in neuro-otology is exemplified by his classic paper on positional vertigo and nystagmus. In this paper, he detailed the classifications, diagnostic examination, pathogenesis, and treatment of this entity.

GEORG VON BÉKÉSY, HUNGARY, SWEDEN AND U.S.A. (1899–1972)
Zur Physik des Mittelohres und über das Hören bei fehlerhaftem Trommelfell. Akust Ztschr, 1:13, 1936.
Über die Messung der Schwingungsamplitude der Gehörknöchelchen mittels einer kapazitiven Sonde. Akust Ztschr, 6:1, 1941.
Über die mechanische Frequenzanalyse in der Schnecke verschiedener Tiere Akust Ztschr, 9:3, 1944.

Békésy (Nobel laureate, 1961) contributed to our present understanding of the process of sound conduction by the middle and inner ears. His visualization of sound-induced displacements of the basilar membrane made possible by strobomicroscopy led to his formulation of the traveling wave theory of hearing. He hypothesized that the movements of the stapes footplate established traveling waves in the basilar membrane; the maximal amplitude for the waves of low-pitched tones was located in the apex of the cochlea while higher pitched tones were associated with waves whose peak amplitudes occurred more basally. He noted that, in the diseased middle ear, the round window could act as a significant route of sound access to the cochlea as well as effectively cancel the effect of sound entering via the oval window. He described the resting endocochlear potential.

HEINRICH F.G. KOBRAK, U.S.A. (1905–1957)
Zur Physiologie der Binnenmuskeln des Ohres. Beitr Anat Physiol Path Therap Ohres, 28:138, 1930.
The physiology of sound conduction. Ann Otol Rhinol Laryngol, 47:166, 1938.
The Middle Ear. Chicago, University of Chicago Press, 1959.

Through his cinematographic studies of the movements of the ossicular system, Kobrak contributed to our understanding of the vibrating characteristics of the ossicles. He also elucidated the functions of the intratympanic muscles.

Index

Numerals in **boldface** indicate illustrations; numerals followed by **s** indicate stereoscopic view; numerals followed by T indicate table

Bone, enchondral (endochondral) *(cont.)*
　intrachondral. *See* Bone, globuli interossei
　membranous. *See* Embryology, of membra-
　　nous bone
　perichondrial, 263, **268**, 270
　periosteal, 130, 263, 270
Bony bar to head of malleus, 62, 63
Bony labyrinth of inner ear, 129–135, **130**,
　131
　microfissures of, 132–135, **133**
Bony spur(s), epitympanic, 59, **60–62**
Border cell(s) of cochlea, 139
Bursa(e) in stapediovestibular articulation, 76,
　76

Canal(s), accessory, to cochlear aqueduct, 156
　carotid, **26**
　external auditory. *See* External auditory
　　canal
　fallopian (for facial nerve), 164. *See also*
　　Dehiscence(s) of fallopian canal; Em-
　　bryology of facial canal
　internal auditory. *See* Internal auditory canal
　of Cotugno (for inferior cochlear vein), **154**,
　　156
　of Huguier (for chorda tympani nerve), 59
　petromastoid, 5, 121, 125, 128
　Rosenthal's, **131**, 137
　semicircular, 16, 17, **131**, 132, **222s**
　　blue-lining of, **213s**, **214s**, **216s**
　　lateral, 5, 6, **212s**, **214s**
　　posterior, 6, 10, **213s**
　　superior, 5, **216s**
　singular, for posterior ampullary nerve, 9, 93
Canaliculi, paravestibular, **147**, 151–152, **151**,
　152
Canaliculi perforantes (of Schuknecht), 153
Capsular channels (aqueducts). *See* Embryol-
　ogy, of capsular channels
Carotid artery, internal. *See* Artery(ies), ca-
　rotid, internal
Carotid canal, **26**
Cartilage, Meckel's, 243, **244**, 260, **260**
　of auricle (pinna), 36
　of eustachian tube, **96–97**, **97–103**
　Reichert's, 243, **244**, 260, **260**
Cecum, cupular, 137
　vestibular, **30s**, **129**
Central mastoid tract, **112**, **113**, **115**, **116**, **117**,
　118
Cerumen, 42
Channel(s), capsular. *See* Embryology, of cap-
　sular channels
Cholesteatoma, **228s**, **231s**
　congenital, of petrous apex, **232s**
Chordal eminence, 87, 95
Chordal ridge, 88
Cistern, perilymphatic, of vestibule, 8, **19**
Claudius' cells of cochlea, **137**, 140
Cochlea, **30s**, **33s**, 130–131, **131**, **132**
　hook portion of, **31s**, **34s**
　vascular supply of, 202–205, **203**, **206**
Cochlear aqueduct, 153–156, **154–156**, 264
Cochlear duct, 132, 137–140, **137**, **153**
Cochlear nerve. *See* Nerve(s), cochlear
Cochleariform process, 83, **83**, **220s**, **222s**
Common crus (crus commune), 6, 7
Corpora amylacea, 155
Corpuscles, middle ear, 107–109, **107**, **108**
Corti, organ of, 139–140
Cortilymph, 139
Cotugno, canal of, **154**, 156
Crest, semilunar, of round window, **92**
　transverse (falciform), of fundus of internal
　　auditory canal, **23**, 157, **157**

utricular, inferior, 18, **33s**
　vertical, of fundus of internal auditory canal,
　　29s, 157, **157**
　vestibular, 129
Cribriform (cribrose) area(s), 130, **141**, 157
Crista ampullaris, of lateral canal, 6, **29s**, **32s**
　of posterior canal, **31s**, **34s**, 92, 94, 155, **156**
　of semicircular ducts, 144
　of superior canal, **29s**
Crista neglecta, 144–145, **145**
Crista stapedis, 68
Crus (crura), **50**, 68, **68**
Cupping of internal auditory canal, 158, **159**
Cupula(e) of semicircular ducts, **94**, 144
Cupular cecum of cochlear duct, 137

Darwinian (auricular) tubercle, 35, 37, 266
Dehiscence(s) of fallopian canal, 166, 168–
　169, **169–172**
Deiters' cells of cochlea, **137**, 140
Digastric ridge, 118, **211s**
Dissection of temporal bone, surgical, 209,
　209s–223s
Duct(s), cochlear. *See* Cochlear duct
　endolymphatic. *See* Endolymphatic duct
　periotic, 153–156
　saccular, 136, **141**, 142
　semicircular, 143–145, **143**, **144**
　utricular, 136, **141**, 142
Ductus reuniens, **33s**, 136

Eighth cranial nerve and ganglion. *See* Embry-
　ology, of eighth cranial nerve and gan-
　glion
Elliptical recess of vestibule, 129, **131**
Embryology, 240–288
　development to 4 weeks, 240–245
　development to 8 weeks, 245–255
　development to 16 weeks, 255–261
　development 16 + weeks, 261–269
　of annular ligament, 268, **268**
　of arteries, 243–244, 253–254, 261
　　auditory (labyrinthine), internal, 253–
　　　254, **254**
　　stapedial, 253–254, **253**
　of capsular channels, 248, 258, 264–265
　of cochlear aqueduct, 264
　of cochlear duct, 246, 255–256, 261–263
　of eighth cranial nerve and ganglion, 241,
　　247–248
　of enchondral (endochondral) bone, **262**,
　　263–264, 270
　of endolymphatic duct, 247, 263
　of eustachian tube, 106–107, 251, 266
　of external auditory canal, tympanic mem-
　　brane, and tympanic ring, 250–251,
　　259, 266
　of facial canal, 249, 265
　of facial nerve, 242, 248–249, 258–259,
　　265
　of fissula ante fenestram, 258
　of fossula post fenestram, 258
　of lamina stapedialis, 243, 252–253
　of malleus and incus, 243, 251–252, **260**,
　　267–268
　of Meckel's cartilage, 243, **244**, 260, **260**
　of membranous bone, 270
　of membranous labyrinth, 240–241, 245–
　　246, 255
　of ossicular muscles, 261, 269
　of otic capsule, 241, 248, 257–258, 263–
　　264, 271–273
　of perichondrium, 263, **268**, 270
　of perilymphatic spaces, 248, 258, 264
　of pinna, 242, 249–250, **249**, **250**, 265–266